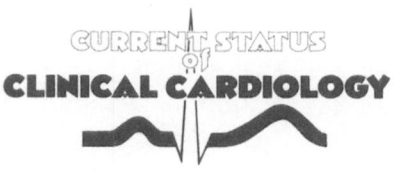

DRUGS
IN THE
MANAGEMENT
OF
HEART DISEASE

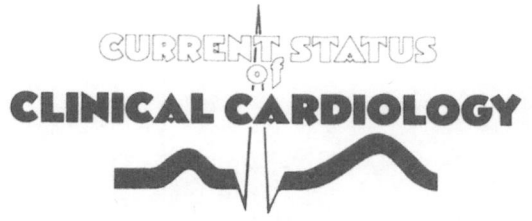

CURRENT STATUS
OF
CLINICAL CARDIOLOGY

Series Editor J.P.Shillingford

DRUGS
IN THE
MANAGEMENT
OF
HEART DISEASE

Edited by A.Breckenridge

Professor of Clinical Pharmacology
University of Liverpool

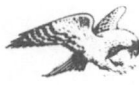 **MTP PRESS LIMITED**
a member of the KLUWER ACADEMIC PUBLISHERS GROUP
LANCASTER / BOSTON / THE HAGUE / DORDRECHT

Published in the UK and Europe by
MTP Press Limited
Falcon House
Lancaster, England

British Library Cataloguing in Publication Data

Drugs in the management of heart disease.—
    (Current status of clinical cardiology)
    1. Heart—Diseases—Chemotherapy
    I. Breckenridge, A.   II. Series
    616.1'2061   RC684.C4

Published in the USA by
MTP Press
A division of Kluwer Boston Inc
190 Old Derby Street
Hingham, MA 02043, USA

Library of Congress Cataloging in Publication Data

Main entry under title:

Drugs in the management of heart disease.
  (Current status of clinical cardiology)
  Includes bibliographies and index.
  1. Heart—Diseases—Chemotherapy. 2. Cardiovascular agents.
  I. Breckenridge, Alasdair.   II. Series.
  (DNLM: 1. Cardiovascular agents—therapeutic use.
  2. Heart diseases—drug therapy. QV 150 D7946)
  RC684.C48D78 1984   616.1'2061   84-25086
  ISBN-13: 978-94-010-8658-5   e-ISBN-13: 978-94-009-4876-1
  DOI: 10.1007/978-94-009-4876-1

Contents

Preface

In any textbook, basic scientific knowledge, and the art of clinical practice should be brought together in a rational manner and this volume on cardiovascular therapy attempts to achieve this aim. It deals with five selected areas – hypertension, angina and coronary artery disease, heart failure and anticoagulant therapy. Clearly not all branches of cardiovascular therapeutics could be included; a separate section on anti-arrhythmic drugs is noticeably absent but it is proposed that this omission will be rectified in other volumes in the series. In general, textbooks on therapeutics tend to be ephemeral; as new discoveries are made and evaluated, medical practice changes. This volume then summarizes current opinion up to mid 1984 and gives, we believe, a reasoned account of present views. The contributors are all clinical pharmacologists with a wealth of clinical experience. The therapeutic advice given is well founded and the underlying scientific basis is clearly explained. The book is aimed at postgraduates, but should the undergraduate care to dip into it, we hope he will be informed and thereby educated.

A. Breckenridge

Series Editor's Note

The last few decades have seen an explosion in our knowledge of cardiovascular disease as a result of research in many disciplines. The tempo of research is ever increasing, so that it is becoming more and more difficult for one person to encompass the whole spectrum of the advances taking place on many fronts.

Even more difficult is to include the advances as they affect clinical practice in one textbook of cardiovascular disease. Fifty years ago all that was known about cardiology could be included in one textbook of moderate size and at that time there was little research so that a textbook remained up to date for several years. Today all this has changed, and books have to be updated at frequent intervals to keep up with the results of research and changing fashions.

The present series has been designed to cover the field of cardiovascular medicine in a series of, initially eight volumes which can be updated at regular intervals and at the same time give a sound basis of practice for doctors looking after patients.

The future volumes will include the following subjects: heart muscle disease; congenital heart disease, invasive and non-invasive diagnosis; ischaemic heart disease; immunology and heart disease; irregularities of the heart beat; and each is edited by a distinguished British author with an international reputation, together with an international panel of contributors.

The series will be mainly designed for the consultant cardiologist as reference books to assist him in his day-to-day practice and keep him up to date in the various fields of cardiovascular medicine at the same time as being of manageable size.

J.P. Shillingford
British Heart Foundation

List of Contributors

Dr Nigel S Baber
International Medical Affairs Department
Pharmaceuticals Division
ICI
Alderley Park
Macclesfield
Cheshire
England

Dr G Davis Johnston
Senior Lecturer
Department of Therapeutics and Pharmacology
Queen's University
Belfast
Northern Ireland

Dr Clive Roberts
Senior Lecturer
Department of Medicine
Bristol Royal Infirmary
Bristol
England

Dr Andrew K Scott
Lecturer in Clinical Pharmacology
University of Aberdeen
Forresterhill
Aberdeen
Scotland

Dr John H Silas
Consultant Physician
Hypertension Unit
Clatterbridge Hospital
Bebington
Wirral
England

1
Drug treatment of hypertension

J.H. SILAS

INTRODUCTION

Hypertension is a very common condition with a prevalence rate which depends on its definition and the age group screened. In patients aged 45 to 64 years, a diastolic blood pressure of 90, 95 and 100 mmHg or more may be found in 40%, 26% and 16% of subjects respectively[1]. Community screening programmes were encouraged by the observation that only half the subjects with high blood pressure had already been identified. However, as 75% of patients considered for treatment have diastolic pressures below 105 mmHg, it is possible that many patients with apparent hypertension may receive life-long drug treatment unnecessarily.

MAKING THE DIAGNOSIS

After initial screening it is essential to confirm that hypertension is sustained. Blood pressure often falls dramatically on repeated examination and at least three further visits are necessary before drug treatment is started. The major trials in mild hypertension have shown that almost a third of patients obtain goal blood pressure (diastolic ≤ 90 mmHg) by periodic observation alone[2,3]. This is independent of the use of placebo tablets or the time between visits.

Avoiding errors

Errors in the measurement of blood pressure often result in inappropriate treatment of spurious hypertension with resultant adverse effects. Guidelines for the measurement of blood pressure have been published[4]. A mercury sphygmomanometer should be used as aneroid sphygmomanometers need frequent calibration. Tight sleeves must be avoided; the arm should be supported so that the cubital fossa is level with the base of the heart. Higher blood pressures are recorded when the arm is dependent or unsupported. The cuff should be deflated at

1

a rate of 2–3 mm per second. The appropriate cuff size must be used, with smaller cuffs in children and larger ones in the obese. The American Heart Association's recommended cuff width/arm circumference ratio is 0.40. The regular cuff which measures 12 × 23 cm is appropriate only for adults with arm circumference of less than 33 cm. For moderately obese subjects (arm circumference 33–41 cm) a large cuff should be used (15 × 33 cm). Use of a standard cuff in obese subjects results in errors proportional to the arm circumference[5]; there is no way of guessing what the blood pressure might have been had the appropriate cuff been used. Rarely a thigh cuff may be required (18 × 36 cm) for arm circumference > 41 cm, but particularly in women this is virtually impossible to use. It has been suggested that a third of normotensive, obese subjects may be wrongly classified as hypertensive.

All major epidemiological and therapeutic surveys in hypertension have based their findings on *sitting* phase 5 diastolic values. Regrettably in most hospital practice supine values are recorded. However, supine blood pressure may be 19/8 mmHg higher than sitting values, suggesting that many patients are receiving inappropriate treatment (Table 1.1)[6].

Table 1.1 Mean blood pressure according to posture[6]

	Normotensive	Untreated hypertensive
Supine	125/64	159/98
Standing (arm horizontal)	102/60	138/90
Sitting (arm horizontal)	108/64	140/90

The number of readings taken at each clinic visit seems less important and suggestions vary from a single reading to the lowest of three and the mean of three. The last averages errors and reduces the number of patients required for clinical trials.

AVOIDING DRUG TREATMENT

Drugs may be avoided if blood pressure can be lowered to acceptable levels by other measures.

Withdrawal of drugs causing hypertension

Some drugs cause a rise in blood pressure and should be withdrawn whenever possible. The main offenders nowadays are non-steroidal anti-inflammatory agents, e.g. indomethacin and steroid drugs. The combined oral contraceptive pill will increase blood pressure slightly in most women[7] even if a 30 μg oestrogen preparation is used. The progesterone component is probably unimportant and in normotensive women the progesterone-only pill does not elevate blood pressure[8].

Weight reduction

Hypertension is the most common risk factor in obesity. It is not an artifact, as the association persists when the appropriate cuff is used. The association may be stronger for women and for diastolic blood pressure. Dietary restriction has been shown to lower blood pressure even without a reduction in salt intake, on average by 2.5-3.0/1.5-2.3 mmHg for each kilogram lost[9]. Most obese patients may not need drugs, but non-compliance rates are high even in committed units. Referral to a dietitian may improve results.

Reducing alcohol intake

Moderate alcohol consumption is associated with a rise in blood pressure[10]. Reducing alcohol consumption may lower blood pressure through weight reduction, but more rapid falls in blood pressure $(-11/7)$ have been observed during abstinence in moderate drinkers (4 pints (2.3 litres) of beer per day)[11]. This work needs to be extended to larger populations. At present it seems reasonable to restrict alcohol consumption to 40 g per day (2 pints of beer or two double whiskies a day) since subjects consuming this quantity do not appear to have higher blood pressures than abstainers.

Reducing salt intake

Although populations consuming very small quantities of salt have a low incidence of hypertension, there is no definite agreement as to the benefits or feasibility of modest salt restriction in the community or of benefits in individual patients except in those with severe renal impairment.

Smoking

Cessation of smoking is justified in its own right, although studies have failed to show a relationship with high blood pressure. In hypertensive patients the risk of cardiovascular death is 3.6 times higher in smokers than in non-smokers, while accelerated hypertension and renovascular hypertension occur only rarely in non-smokers. However, on stopping smoking patients may gain weight and blood pressure may rise slightly; dietary advice is therefore necessary.

THE PRESSURE TO TREAT

There is no doubt of the benefits of treating moderate to severe hypertension (diastolic blood pressure $\geqslant 115$ mmHg) or those in malignant phase. A large proportion of these patients will have cardiovascular complications or symptoms. The place of drug treatment in patients with diastolic pressures above 105 mmHg is also established, although the group studied by the US Veterans Administration was atypical of the general population – comprising only men, 60% of whom had pre-existing cardiovascular disease[12]. The debate about whether to treat mild hypertension is gradually being resolved. The best evidence to date comes from the Australian trial of *uncomplicated* mild hypertension (95–109 mmHg) in men and women aged 18–69 years. The cardiovascular morbidity and mortality was reduced by drug treatment, particularly those with diastolic blood pressure of 100 or more[13,14]. Whether the benefit extends to blood pressures of 95–99 is less certain. What is clear is that we must treat a very large number of people to help a few. Twelve lives were saved and a further 30 complications were prevented as a result of 7000 patient years of treatment. In uncomplicated cases, therefore, treatment is initiated when the diastolic blood pressure is consistently 100 mmHg or more. Contrary to popular practice young patients (<40 years) do not require treatment at lower pressures for they are *less* likely to suffer complications in the succeeding few years.

In contrast, when target organ damage is present (cardiomegaly, ischaemic heart disease, renal impairment, stroke) the risks are much higher, even with diastolic pressures in the 90–99 mmHg range[15] and treatment is therefore advisable. Some of these patients will require treatment for other reasons e.g. β-blockers for ischaemic heart disease, diuretics for heart failure. Diabetes is often ignored as an indication for aggressive treatment. However, epidemiological studies have shown blood pressure to be an important prognostic factor in the development of large and small vessel complications in insulin-dependent and non-insulin-dependent diabetics, even through blood pressures in the 'normal' range[16,17]. Furthermore, there is now evidence to suggest that early treatment of borderline hypertension delays the progression of diabetic nephropathy[18] and I advise treating diabetics with diastolic blood pressures at or above 90 mmHg.

Systolic hypertension

It is unfortunate that trials in hypertension have used diastolic blood pressure as the major criterion for treatment. Systolic blood pressure is probably a better predictor of cardiovascular risk with a 30% increased risk for every 10 mm rise in systolic blood pressure. In hypertension trials diastolic blood pressures of 100 mmHg are usually associated with systolic blood pressures of about 155–160 mmHg. Therefore, pressures of 160 or more may be considered worthy of treatment. When the systolic blood pressure is disproportionately high, i.e. diastolic blood pressure <95 mmHg as occurs in isolated systolic hypertension, the calculation of mean arterial pressure (diastolic$+\frac{1}{3}$ pulse pressure) is a useful guide. For example a blood pressure of 170/90 is equivalent to 152/100 (mean pressure 117 mmHg). I therefore recommend treatment for calculated mean arterial pressures of above 115 mmHg.

Hypertension in the elderly

There is no hard evidence upon which to base the treatment of hypertension in the elderly. The Australian Mild Hypertension Trial included patients up to the age of 69, and I therefore take elderly to mean 70 or over. At this age treatment is only considered if the patient is free from serious non-cardiovascular disorders which may in their own right affect the quality of life or longevity. Physiological age is more important than chronological age. Symptomatic cardiovascular disease warrants treatment in its own right – for example for heart failure, angina and transient cerebral ischaemic attacks. In asymptomatic 70–75-year-olds who are fit, I use drug treatment if mean arterial pressure is 125 mmHg or more. This will include many with isolated systolic hypertension ($\geqslant 200$ mmHg). Their risks are greatly increased and sudden stroke may cause years of disability. The European Working Party on mild hypertension in the elderly has demonstrated that carefully titrated drug treatment is well tolerated, the principles of drug treatment being similar to those in younger subjects.

PRINCIPLES OF DRUG TREATMENT

Drug treatment is a burden for the patient who should understand the reasons for lifelong treatment and the need to continue with non-pharmacological measures. Because a third of patients may be non-compliant, it is important to simplify drug treatment, recommending as few different preparations as possible, preferably on a once-daily basis. It is rarely necessary to exceed the known ceiling dose of a drug and the price of doing so is usually an increase in side-effects. One should be aware that for any given patient the maximum tolerated dose may be lower than the suggested ceiling dose and it is therefore wise to start off with a small dose and increase it gradually, no more often than every 2 weeks. The majority of patients, even with mild hypertension, require more than one drug to control their blood pressure, and in this situation combined preparations are particularly useful but only if they are available in the recommended doses. They should *not* be used as first line treatment. Treatment should be geared towards lowering the blood pressure below 150/90 mmHg (or mean arterial pressure $\leqslant 110$). In the elderly a figure of 160/100 (or mean arterial pressure $\leqslant 120$) may be acceptable. Patients should be free from side-effects and the quality of life should be unchanged or improved. Assessment of blood pressure response should be made in the outpatient clinic and patients rarely need be admitted for treatment, except in the management of emergencies such as accelerated hypertension or heart failure. The stepped care approach to treatment entails starting with a β-blocker or diuretic, then the combination if necessary. A third drug may be added if control is inadequate.

β-ADRENORECEPTOR ANTAGONISTS

From a chance observation these drugs have become first line agents in the treatment of hypertension. Ten different β-blockers are available in the United Kingdom. All attenuate exercise-induced increases in heart rate and lower blood pressure to a similar extent at the appropriate dose. They differ mainly in their ancillary pharmacological properties and in their physiochemistry which influences their fate and some clinical effects. Only the most commonly used agents are considered (Table 1.2).

Table 1.2 Characteristics of commonly used β-blockers

Drug	β_1-Selective	Partial agonist activity	Lipid solubility	Ceiling dose* mg/day
Propranolol	No	No	Yes +	160
Oxprenolol	No	Yes	Yes	160–240
Pindolol	No	Yes + +	Yes	20–30
Metoprolol	Yes	No	Yes	200
Nadolol	No	No	No	80
Atenolol	Yes	No	No	100

*In hypertension

Pharmacokinetics

Differences in lipid solubility correlate well with the kinetic properties of these drugs. The more lipid soluble agents are better absorbed but because they are extensively metabolized they have lower oral bioavailability and short half-lives of elimination (2–5 hours). The metabolism of some β-blockers exhibit polymorphism and wide interpatient variability in plasma drug concentration may be seen. In contrast, water soluble agents are eliminated by the kidney and they have half-lives of 7–20 h. In non-uraemic subjects less interpatient variability in plasma concentration is seen. Lipid soluble agents are more likely to penetrate the central nervous system and this may influence side-effects.

Mechanism of action

This is poorly understood but the principal prerequisite is β_1-blocking activity. The following observations are important:

(1) *Reduction in cardiac output.* There is a fall in cardiac output during acute and chronic dosing but this correlates poorly with

reduction in resting blood pressure both between individuals receiving the same compound and between different compounds. For example, the reduction in cardiac output is less marked with drugs which possess partial agonist activity, yet blood pressure control is similar.

(2) *Effect on total peripheral resistance.* Those who respond to β-blockade may show no change or only a slight reduction in total peripheral resistance long term. In this respect β-blockers differ from other antihypertensive agents.

(3) *Inhibition of the renin angiotensin system.* All β-blockers reduce exercise-stimulated plasma renin activity – an effect which must therefore be mediated via β_1-adrenoreceptors[19]. The majority of studies in selected patients have shown a correlation between blood pressure response and either pretreatment plasma renin activity or a change in plasma renin activity. It is suspected that inhibition of the renin angiotensin system results in a decrease in direct and indirect pressor effects of angiotensin II. Stimulation of angiotensin II presynaptic receptors on the postganglionic neuron enhance the release of noradrenaline. In addition longer term effects through aldosterone may explain why β-blockers do not cause fluid retention and false tolerance unlike most antihypertensive agents, except diuretics and converting enzyme inhibitors.

(4) *Decreased sympathetic outflow.* In contrast to some animal studies there is no evidence in man to support the view that β-blockers reduce sympathetic outflow by a centrally mediated effect. However, stimulation of presynaptic β-adrenoreceptors on the postganglionic neuron augment release of noradrenaline and β-blockers may reduce exercise mediated catecholamine release at this site. Basal plasma catecholamine concentrations, however, are not altered.

(5) *Alteration in baroreflex arc.* A resetting of baroreceptors has been suggested. However, β-blockers do not influence the sensitivity of the baroreceptor reflex arc. Subsequent changes in the reflex may be secondary to long term reduction in blood pressure *per se*.

Dose interval and daily dose

The duration of β-blocking effect is much greater than the half-life as pharmacological activity declines in a linear fashion while the fall in plasma concentration is an exponential one. The antihypertensive effect persists beyond the β-blocking effect and some authorities suggest that even β-blockers with short half-lives (2–4 h) may be prescribed once daily in hypertension. However, this practice may be associated with greater variability in blood pressure control with frank loss of control at some times in the day[20]. These compounds should be prescribed twice daily in hypertension while agents with longer half-lives (>7 h) are best administered once daily.

The ceiling dose of these drugs is much lower than formerly suggested. Increasing the dose beyond that indicated (Table 1.2) should be considered only if non-compliance is excluded and if inadequate β-blockade is demonstrated. In general it is best to start with half the ceiling dose and if necessary to double the dose. The maximum effect may be seen within a fortnight.

Slow release formulations

Several slow release formulations of shorter acting β-blockers are available. Only long acting propranolol 160 mg once daily[21] can be recommended on the strength of its sustained β-blocking and antihypertensive effects. The slow release film-coated formulations of both oxprenolol (160 mg) and metoprolol (200 mg) are ineffective in both respects. The antihypertensive response to oxprenolol is not improved by doubling the dose of this preparation[22]. Metoprolol durules 200 mg once daily result in 10–11% β-blockade at 24 hours. The effectiveness of this preparation over 24 h in hypertension is disputed.

Efficacy

When used correctly β-blockers lower blood pressure in the majority of patients. The fall in blood pressure when used as a single agent varies between 14/10 and 27/19 mmHg, being greater in patients with higher pretreatment blood pressure. In the Veterans Administration (VA) study of mild to moderate hypertension[23] (diastolic blood pressure 95–114 mmHg) propranolol alone reduced diastolic blood pressure to less than 90 in 62% of white patients and 54% of black patients. Significant additive effects are seen with diuretics, a combination which achieves goal blood pressure in 70–80% of patients with mild hypertension[24]. In this respect, however, the combination is marginally less effective than reserpine 0.1 mg daily plus thiazide, emphasizing that the major advantage of β-blockers is their wide margin of safety.

Adverse effects

Some adverse effects of β-blockers are related specifically to unwanted effects on β-adrenoreceptors. As such they may be prevented by prior patient selection and reduction in dose. In general, therefore, patients with a history of asthma should not receive β-blockers as this is the only life-threatening complication of these agents. Previous heart failure is also a contraindication, except when it has been caused by severe hypertension. A large number of other side-effects occur for reasons

8

Table 1.3   Adverse effects leading to withdrawal in hypertensive patients receiving atenolol (n = 543) or propranolol (n = 390)[25]

Adverse effect	Propranolol	Atenolol
Bronchospasm	13	2
Worsening claudication	9	1
Heart failure	1	2
Cold extremities	3	1
Indigestion	3	3
Vivid dreams/insomnia	2	0
Bradycardia	*	1
Depression	2	0
Impotence	1	0
Fatigue	1	0
Paraesthesia	2	0
Diarrhoea	1	1
Dizziness	0	1
Total (%)	38 (9.7%)	12 (2.2%)

*Not assessed in same way

that are not specifically related to the effects on β-adrenoreceptors. The majority are central nervous system effects and fatigue which may be more frequent with lipid soluble agents. For some reason pindolol is particularly liable to cause sleep disturbances. There is some evidence to support the view that side-effects decrease with increasing hydrophilicity and cardioselectivity. This is illustrated in comparisons of side-effects with atenolol and propranolol in the same blood pressure clinic, although high doses of both agents were used[25] (Table 1.3). In the UK Medical Research Council (MRC) trial of mild hypertension cumulative withdrawals over a 5 year period were only 10% higher in those taking propranolol than in the placebo group[26] (Figure 1.1). Most of these withdrawals were due (in decreasing order of importance) to central nervous system disorders (lethargy, nausea, dizziness), breathlessness, cold extremities and impotence. Whether the use of a selective hydrophilic agent would have been associated with fewer withdrawals is uncertain. In one large survey only cold extremities and fatigue were more common after atenolol than placebo[27].

Bradycardia and heart failure

Most people tolerate bradycardia without symptoms, unless there is associated left ventricular dysfunction. Bradycardia is not an indication for drug withdrawal unless the heart rate falls below 40 or heart block supervenes, but occasionally symptomatic ventricular escape beats or dizziness may necessitate a change in treatment. In such patients a switch to an agent with partial agonist activity will result in a return to a near-normal heart rate. Patients who develop heart failure on β-blockers may do so with small doses[28] and regardless of the presence of partial agonist activity.

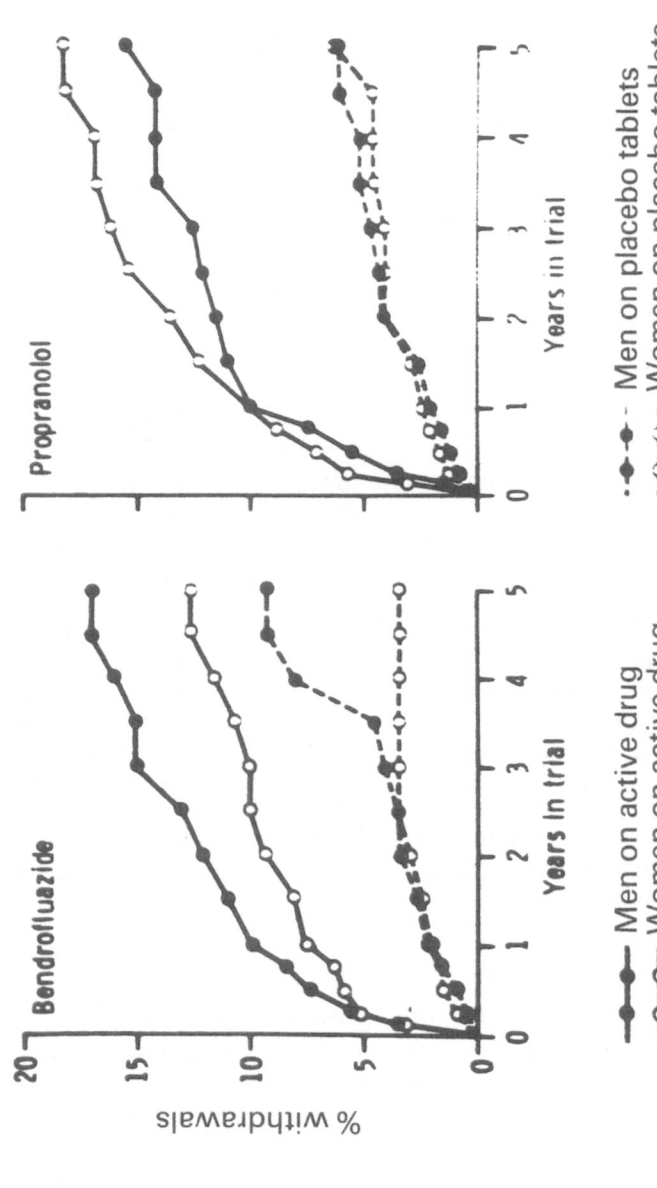

Figure 1.1 Cumulative percentage withdrawals from randomized treatment owing to suspected adverse reactions to primary drug – MRC trial in mild hypertension[26]. (Reproduced with permission from the *Lancet*)

Asthma

On no account should non-selective agents be used in asthmatics. Cardioselective agents protect against this complication but the beneficial effects may be partially lost at higher doses. At the recommended doses used in hypertension atenolol is marginally safer than metoprolol and both are superior to acebutolol. In contrast to non-selective agents, airways obstruction caused by cardioselective agents may be reversed by inhaled β_2 stimulants. Partial agonist activity does not protect against asthma.

Fatigue

It is important to separate the feeling of lethargy from muscle fatigue on exercise. The former is probably a central effect while the effect on skeletal muscle is presumed to be secondary to β_2-receptor blockade on skeletal muscle sites. Muscle fatigue is common after acute dosing with β-blockers, but far less common with chronic dosing, so that many studies have failed to demonstrate the phenomenon on formal submaximal treadmill exercise tests. However, the perception of fatigue is increased in marathon runners who take non-selective β-blockers, with some benefit on substitution of a cardioselective agent.

Cold extremities

Cold extremities are frequently reported in hypertensive patients, particularly women. In the MRC study, after 2 years' treatment 16% of women on placebo or thiazide reported this symptom, compared to 29% on propranolol[26]. Men were less commonly affected. Cardioselective agents and those with partial agonist activity may protect against this symptom and there is some evidence that the reduction in skin blood flow is less.

Claudication

Claudication is said to worsen in patients taking β-blockers. However, when angina is treated with these agents this could well unmask underlying peripheral vascular disease. Formal studies have failed to show an increase in symptoms with drug treatment. However, β-blockers do cause a decrease in muscle blood flow during exercise – but the effect is also seen with other antihypertensive agents such as methyldopa. β-Blockers are not firmly contraindicated in patients with intermittent claudication but they should be used with caution and withdrawn in patients complaining of worsening symptoms or skin changes.

Diabetes

Most authorities claim that in treated diabetics β-blockers mask the symptoms of hypoglycaemia. It is hard to discount anecdotal reports of unconsciousness due to hypoglycaemia, but formal studies in insulin-dependent diabetics have failed to confirm them[29]. Psychological phenomena and sweating are the main symptoms of hypoglycaemia and these are not impaired by β-blockers. Tachycardia is attenuated, however, and following propranolol alone frank bradycardia associated with severe hypertension may accompany hypoglycaemia. Both non-selective and selective agents have been used safely in diabetic clinics without an increase in symptoms or loss of diabetic control[29]. Nevertheless, studies indicate that the delay in spontaneous recovery from insulin-induced hypoglycaemia is less marked with selective agents[30]. Most insulin-dependent diabetics treat hypoglycaemia with oral glucose and therefore the implications of these observations are not as clear as they first seem. Clearly cardioselective β-blockers are not contraindicated in insulin-dependent diabetes and may be used with considerable benefit. However, patients should be warned to look out for a change in symptoms of hypoglycaemia.

Plasma lipids

Standard antihypertensive doses of propranolol, oxprenolol, atenolol and metoprolol lead to an increase in plasma very low density lipoprotein (LDL) and triglyceride and a decrease in high density lipoprotein (HDL). There is a concomitant reduction in HDL/LDL ratio[31]. The changes may be more marked with non-selective agents but the implications of these findings are unclear.

DIURETICS

Diuretics are the most widely used antihypertensive agents. Generally the longer acting thiazide related compounds are preferred because in uncomplicated hypertension they are superior to loop diuretics such as frusemide[32]. Drugs such as xipamide have an intermediate duration of action but they have no advantage over the conventional compounds with regard to efficacy or side-effects. Thiazides are less effective in renal impairment (creatinine greater than $250\,\mu$mol/l) when loop diuretics should be used. More potent diuretics are also important in the treatment of resistant hypertension, as will be discussed later in this chapter.

Potassium sparing compounds are commonly used in combination with thiazides to prevent hypokalaemia. However, spironolactone and amiloride are effective in their own right, but they should be avoided in patients with renal impairment and must never be prescribed with potassium supplements. The antihypertensive effect of thiazide diuretics and spironolactone lasts for at least 24 hours. The dose-response curve is relatively flat, therefore there is little to be gained by exceeding the recommended daily doses since the symptomatic and biochemical side-effects are dose related. The probable ceiling doses are bendrofluazide 5 mg, hydrochlorothiazide 25 mg, cyclopenthiazide 0.5 mg, chlorthalidone 25 mg, spironolactone 100 mg.

Mechanism of action

Diuretics lower blood pressure by promoting sodium and water loss. Suggestions that they exert a direct vasodilatory effect independent of their diuretic action have been discounted, partly because thiazides are less effective in renal failure and a hypotensive effect is seen with diuretics unrelated to thiazides. The initial effects of diuretics are to reduce plasma volume, extracellular fluid (ECF) volume, body weight and cardiac output while increasing urinary sodium excretion. Blood pressure falls after the first dose. Within 6–8 weeks, however, cardiac output returns to normal but even at 6 months a slight reduction in plasma volume, ECF and body weight remain. These changes are modest, with a fall in plasma volume of 300 ml and that of ECF and body weight of 1.4 kg. The long term antihypertensive effect is associated with a fall in total peripheral resistance. This may reflect decreased arteriolar responsiveness to pressor agents as a result of a reduction of intracellular sodium in arterial smooth muscle. The hypotensive effects of diuretics may be offset by salt loading. The magnitude of the response correlates inversely with both pretreatment plasma renin activity and the 'compensatory' rise in aldosterone following treatment.

Efficacy

Thiazide diuretics are highly effective first line agents in the treatment of mild to moderate hypertension. The VA study reported a mean reduction in blood pressure of 18/12 mmHg and over half the patients attained a goal diastolic blood pressure of less than 90 mmHg[23]. The response is greater in black subjects and those with more severe hypertension and possibly the elderly. In addition diuretics potentiate the effects of other antihypertensive agents and therefore should be continued if target blood pressure is not attained.

Adverse effects

Until recently it was assumed that thiazide diuretics rarely caused symptoms; two major studies have dispelled this view, but both used large doses – up to 10 mg bendrofluazide in the MRC Study[26] and 200 mg chlorothiazide in the VA Study[33]. In these studies drug withdrawal was more likely in men than in women. This was mainly because of reversible erectile impotence during the first year of treatment and gout. Dry mouth, paraesthesiae and gastrointestinal symptoms were more common in women, but they nevertheless tolerate diuretics better than propranolol (Figure 1.1). The major concern over the use of thiazides lies in their potentially deleterious biochemical effects. It has also been suggested that they predispose to cardiac arrhythmias and sudden death.

In contrast to thiazide diuretics the biochemical changes associated with the use of spironolactone (100 mg) are unimportant in patients with normal renal function and normal potassium intake. There is a slight rise in serum urea and potassium. Nausea may necessitate dividing the dose. Men commonly complain of gynaecomastia and impotence, in which case the dose may need to be reduced below 100 mg daily. Women may experience menstrual irregularities.

Hypokalaemia

Thiazides increase renal clearance of potassium with little if any fall in total body potassium. Serum potassium falls by 0.5 to 0.6 mmol/l in hypertensive patients[26]. In one survey[34] this resulted in hypokalaemia (<3.5 mmol/l) in 43% of patients receiving bendrofluazide without potassium supplements. The incidence is dose related, being 55% in those receiving 10 mg daily and 33% in those receiving 5 mg daily. However, only 6% have more serious hypokalaemia (<3.0 mmol/l). Symptoms due to hypokalaemia are rare, but there is growing concern that the likelihood of cardiac arrhythmias is increased. There is no agreement as to when to treat hypokalaemia with potassium supplements or potassium sparing agents, but routine supplementation is not indicated. Their use in those with serum potassium below 3.3 mmol/l would limit additional treatment to 15% of patients or possibly less if used in combination with β-blockers. The following equivalent daily doses of potassium supplements and potassium sparing agents elevate serum potassium by 0.3–0.4 mmol/l: potassium chloride 32 mmol, amiloride 10 mg, spironolactone 25 mg, triamterene 50 mg[35].

Cardiac arrhythmias

Concern that diuretic-induced hypokalaemia may cause serious arrhythmias arose initially from observations in digoxin-treated patients. However, mild chronic hypokalaemia (3.0–3.5 mmol/l) is generally well tolerated. Recently the MRC reported its findings in hypertensive patients[36]. In unselected patients receiving 5 or 10 mg of bendrofluazide there was no increase in ventricular ectopic activity when compared to placebo. When the larger dose was used for greater than 2 years, however, there was a trend to more frequent ventricular ectopic activity, though the actual numbers of ventricular extrasystoles were small and there was a poor correlation with serum potassium. Nevertheless the prevalence of the more serious forms (multifocal beats, couplets, R on T beats and bigeminy) were more common with bendrofluazide 10 mg than placebo and they were more likely to occur in association with hypokalaemia.

The major complication of treated hypertension is myocardial infarction. Ventricular fibrillation in the peri-infarction period is often associated with hypokalaemia but the relationship may not be causal. Severe 'stress' from any cause leads to a rise in plasma adrenaline which stimulates skeletal muscle β_2-adrenoreceptors resulting in potassium influx and hypokalaemia. In the experimental 'stress' situation, prior thiazide treatment causes more profound hypokalaemia but does not influence the magnitude of the fall in serum potassium nor the prolongation of the QT interval on E.C.G.[37]. The link between potassium and clinically important arrhythmias remains unproven but diuretics are not necessarily exonerated. It is possible that diuretic treated patients are more likely to develop ventricular fibrillation irrespective of serum potassium.

Glucose intolerance

Hypertension and diabetes are both important risk factors for cardiovascular disease. Therefore it is unfortunate that thiazide diuretics impair glucose tolerance[38]. In younger patients this may take more than 5 years to develop but it is possibly seen sooner in the elderly, in obese patients and in those with pre-diabetic glucose tolerance tests. In most cases glucose tolerance improves within 7 months of thiazide withdrawal and frank diabetes requiring treatment is uncommon particularly in women.

The mechanism of glucose intolerance is unclear. It is assumed to be a direct pancreatic effect but the data are conflicting. There is a correlation with hypokalaemia but this may be indirect or related to dose. It is interesting that one study showed no rise in glucose over 6 years when smaller diuretic doses and potassium supplements were used[39]. How important is this clinically? Frank diabetes occurs only in borderline diabetics and rarely is the control of established diabetes worsened. In the majority of patients we do not know whether the small increase in blood glucose is of importance. I avoid thiazides in borderline diabetics or those receiving oral hypoglycaemic agents; in these patients potassium sparing diuretics or β-blockers are preferable. However, if these agents are poorly tolerated, small doses of thiazides may be used with caution.

Hyperuricaemia

Hyperuricaemia is common in untreated hypertension and its prevalence may double following treatment with thiazides. However, gout is a problem mainly confined to men, with an attack rate of 12 per thousand patient years[26]. Less than half the cases develop in the first year. Men with a family history of the condition should have their serum urate monitored and a non-thiazide should be substituted if symptoms occur or if the serum urate exceeds 0.6 mmol/l. Propranolol may also increase serum urate.

Hyperlipidaemia

Thiazide diuretics cause a slight rise in serum cholesterol and a greater rise in fasting triglycerides. The ratio of total cholesterol to HDL cholesterol is not radically altered.

Other biochemical changes

A slight rise in serum calcium is seen with thiazides but not with loop or potassium sparing diuretics. Occasionally hyponatraemia may occur and this may be an important cause of confusion in elderly patients.

THE CHOICE BETWEEN β-BLOCKERS AND DIURETICS

When compared for efficacy and tolerability there is little to choose between β-blockers and diuretics. The former may be preferred in younger patients, in men, those with ischaemic heart disease and in non-insulin-dependent diabetes. Diuretics have advantages in the elderly, in females, those with peripheral vascular symptoms, fluid retention or asthma. Many clinicians use β-blockers as first line agents in the hope of primary prevention of myocardial infarction. Some have argued that the failure to reduce mortality from myocardial infarction in treated hypertension is due to adverse effects of diuretics which have hitherto been used as the first step. The adverse effects on plasma lipids are common to both classes of drugs and the importance of the other biochemical effects must await the result of the MRC trial in mild to moderate hypertension. It may be argued, however, that some adverse effects of diuretics were due to a high dose of bendrofluazide. Two studies[40,41] have been widely quoted by those who are strongly against the use of diuretics in mild hypertension. The multiple risk factor intervention trial[40] (MR FIT) was not specifically a hypertension trial. In fact, the mean baseline blood pressure was 136/91. Men who were considered to be at high risk from coronary artery disease were randomized to receive either usual care (UC) from their practitioner or were assigned to special intervention (SI), including counselling on diet and smoking as well as stepped care for hypertension. Even the mildest hypertensives with diastolic blood pressures between 90 and 94 mmHg received diuretics. At the end of the 6 year follow-up there was *no difference* in mortality between the two groups. On analysis of

Table 1.4 Mortality among previously untreated hypertensives in the MR FIT Study[40]

Baseline blood pressure (mmHg)	Coronary Heart Disease SI	Coronary Heart Disease UC	Total SI	Total UC
90–94	17	12	47	31
95–99	19	19	43	39
≥ 100	16	22	25	45

None of the differences were significant

blood pressure the final diastolic blood pressure was 80 mmHg with SI and 84 mmHg with UC. In hypertensive patients coronary heart disease and total mortality were similar in both groups being 80 versus 79 and 174 versus 169 for SI and UC respectively. A subgroup of these hypertensive patients who had not received hypotensive treatment prior to the trial were further subdivided for initial blood pressure and the data compared (Table 1.4). It is argued that in the mildest hypertensives diuretics may be responsible for the apparent excess death from coronary heart disease in the SI group. It is hard to explain the greater

Table 1.5 Mortality rate/100 000 days and total infarcts or sudden death in relation to severity of hypertension and regimen[41]

Diastolic blood pressure (mmHg)	Treatment	Mortality rate	Fatal infarcts
< 95	None	7.91	3
95–110	None	9.25	2
	Diet	8.00	2
	Thiazide	19.23*	10
	β-Blocker	7.66	4
≥ 110	Thiazide	6.03	2
	β-Blocker	9.97	2

*Statistically significant

excess *total* mortality on this basis or why patients with significant hypertension (diastolic blood pressure ≥ 100 mgHg) should be protected from these effects. After data splitting the final numbers were very small and statistically insignificant. The second study[41] was a comparison of different antihypertensive regimes in elderly hypertensive men. The results were stratified in relation to severity of hypertension (Table 1.5). There was a significant excess death, including deaths from myocardial infarction, in mild hypertensives treated with thiazide. Amazingly this was not seen in more severe hypertensives where the mortality rate was *lower* than in untreated and β-blocker-treated patients with mild and moderate hypertension. Collectively the results from the two papers are ambiguous and may well be spurious.

CONVENTIONAL THIRD DRUGS IN HYPERTENSION

Approximately 20–30% of hypertensive patients will not achieve adequate blood pressure control despite the use of optimal doses of a β-blocker plus a diuretic. A third drug is then added. Numerous agents are available but many have rightly been abandoned because of a high incidence of adverse effects. For this reason clonidine, indoramin, and the postganglionic blocking agents will not be discussed. Low dose reserpine (maximum 0.2 mg daily), which is probably as effective as β-blockers[24] has long since fallen from favour in the UK and I have little experience with it. The conventional third drugs are α-methyl-dopa and four vasodilators which have direct effects on arteriolar smooth muscle (hydralazine, minoxidil) or which block α-adrenorecep-tors (prazosin, labetalol). These agents have recently been compared in patients without severe renal impairment (creatinine < 300 μmol/l) who were uncontrolled on a β-blocker plus diuretic[42]. Because it has β-blocking effects, labetalol was substituted for the other β-blocker used. The results suggest that hydralazine and prazosin are the best tolerated (Table 1.6). Minoxidil, in those who could tolerate this drug, was more effective than the other agents which lowered blood pressure to a similar extent (Figure 1.2).

Table 1.6 Withdrawal rate and complaints in the 'Third Drug' Study[42]

	Placebo	Hydralazine	Prazosin	Methyldopa	Minoxidil	Labetalol
Withdrawals %	4	20	21	33	57	78
Complaints/ patient	0.4	1.8	2.8	4.1	2.6	3.9

Hydralazine

This is one of the oldest antihypertensive agents, having been intro-duced in 1953.

Mechanism of action and pharmacological effects

Hydralazine lowers blood pressure by a direct relaxant effect on arter-iolar smooth muscle with little if any effect on capacitance vessels; postural effects are not seen. Even with chronic administration there is a reflex tachycardia due probably to increase in sympathetic nervous activity and withdrawal of vagal tone. Hydralazine itself is twice as effective in the presence of a β-blocker[43], which also prevents the increase in heart rate.

Pharmacokinetics

Hydralazine is completely and rapidly absorbed. It is then subject to first pass N-acetylation which is the major determinant of its bioavail-

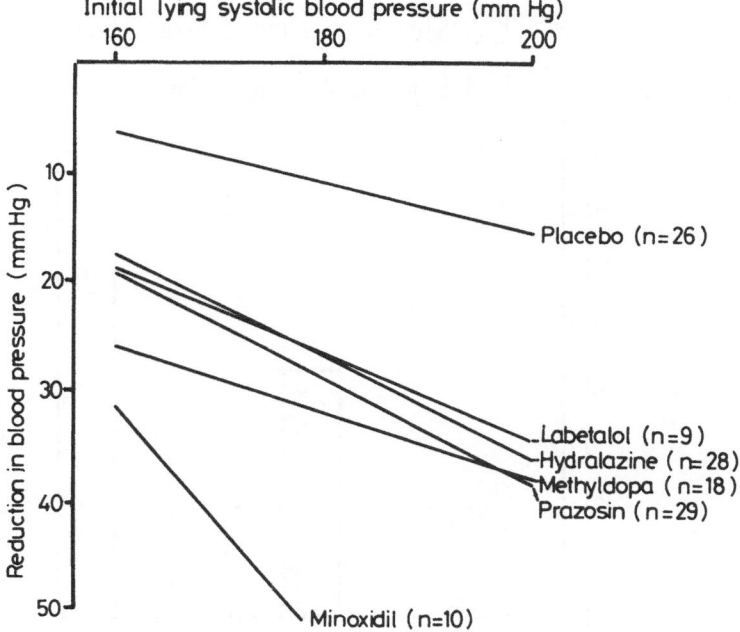

Figure 1.2 Regression lines relating reduction in blood pressure to initial lying systolic pressure for each drug group – Third Drug Study[42]. (Reproduced with permission from the *British Medical Journal*)

ability. The pathway exhibits polymorphism similar to that seen with sulphadimidine; 60% of subjects in the UK are slow acetylators and 40% are rapid acetylators. With multiple dosing the bioavailability in rapid acetylators is 6.6% compared to 39.3% in slow acetylators, and peak plasma hydralazine concentrations are correspondingly higher in the latter group. Plasma hydralazine half-life on multiple dosing is short[44], 20 minutes in rapid acetylators and 40 minutes in slow acetylators, but the differences are less marked after intravenous administration, presumably because of considerable non-enzymatic metabolism to hydrazones in plasma.

Acetylation phenotype and response

The hypotensive effect of hydralazine correlates well with its oral bioavailability and therefore slow acetylators respond better and require smaller doses of hydralazine[45] (Figure 1.3). When hydralazine is added to a β-blocker plus diuretic the dose should be increased gradually from 50 mg to a maximum of 200 mg daily. When used in this way most slow acetylators achieve target blood pressure, but the majority of rapid acetylators do not. Hydralazine should be administered twice

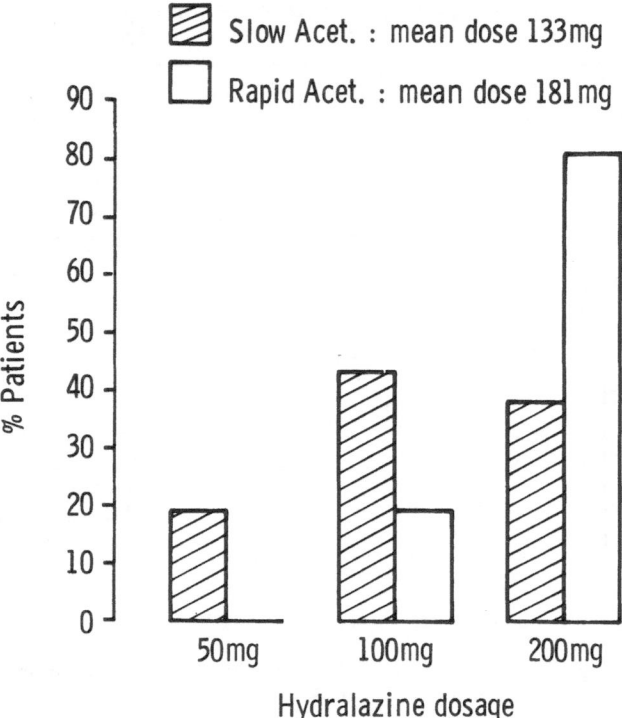

Figure 1.3 Final dose of hydralazine required in relation to phenotype[45]. (Despite the higher dose only 27% of rapid acetylators were controlled.) (Reproduced with permission from the *European Journal of Clinical Pharmacology*)

daily in rapid acetylators but it is effective in slow acetylators when given once daily[46].

Adverse effects

Although hydralazine is the best-tolerated third drug, the withdrawal rate because of side-effects (20%) is higher than that seen with the first line agents. When used without a β-blocker and in doses higher than 200 mg daily, the incidence of adverse effects is doubled. Headache remains the most common complaint when used with a sympathetic blocker. The non-immune side-effects are not related to acetylator phenotype[45].

Lupus syndrome

Hydralazine fell into disrepute in Britain largely because long term use was commonly associated with a syndrome that mimicked systemic lupus erythematosus. In Perry's series of 44 patients[47] who developed

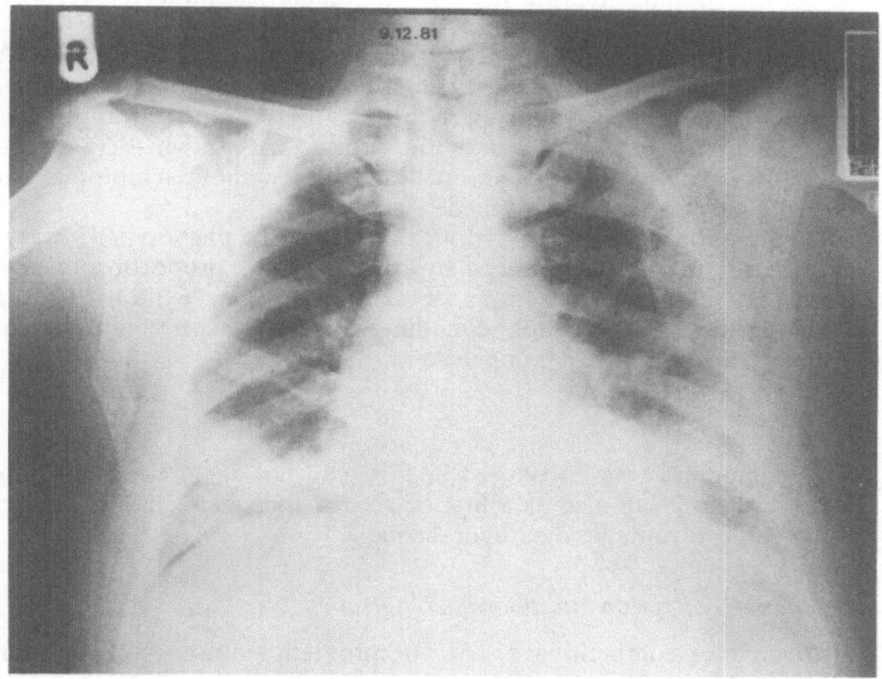

Figure 1.4 Chest x-ray showing hydralazine-induced pneumonitis. (Reproduced with the permission of Dr L.E. Ramsay)

this condition, all but one had been taking a dose in excess of 200 mg daily. The concept that a dose of up to 200 mg is safe has been shattered; the prevalence with these low doses is about 4%. The syndrome is rare when the daily dose falls below 100 mg. Those affected are almost invariably slow acetylators who have been taking the drug for at least 6 months but usually for a year or more. The sex ratio is four to one in favour of females and, unlike spontaneous lupus erythematosus (LE), toxicity is associated with the HLA-DRW4 antigen (73% of cases). It has been suggested that women who are slow acetylators have a 12% chance of developing the syndrome after 1 year on 200 mg daily, but if they are DRW4 all develop the syndrome[48]. Negroes are rarely affected. The syndrome itself may present as an acute or chronic illness mimicking rheumatoid arthritis, spontaneous LE or systemic malignancy, with musculoskeletal symptoms, profound weight loss, anaemia, thrombophlebitis, pneumonitis (Figure 1.4) with or without haemoptysis. Hepatosplenomegaly is not uncommon. In addition to these features documented by Perry, cutaneous vasculitis and rarely renal involvement has been described. In contrast to spontaneous lupus, the central nervous system is spared. Symptoms resolve within weeks of stopping hydralazine and the diagnosis should be reconsidered if it does not or if corticosteroids are necessary.

Antinuclear antibodies are always present in high titre but anti-DNA antibodies and hypocomplementaemia are rare. There is a polyclonal increase in immunoglobulins, particularly IgM. Antinuclear antibodies may persist for many years after the drug is withdrawn. Between 30 and 50% develop a positive antinuclear factor without symptoms, but the drug need not be discontinued.

Ideally patients receiving hydralazine should be phenotyped. Acetylator status may be determined by measuring the proportion of acetylated metabolite in a sample of plasma or urine 6 hours after a 10 mg/kg oral dose of sulphadimadine. Plasma is a better guide than urine, particularly in renal impairment.

Prazosin

This compound was introduced in 1970 and has been useful not only as a third drug but also as a first or second line agent. In this respect it has some advantages over hydralazine.

Mechanism of action and pharmacological effects

Prazosin is a competitive α_1-adrenoceptor antagonist which acts on both resistance and capacitance vessels. Its effect is highly selective for postsynaptic sites, unlike the older α-blockers which also antagonized presynaptic α_2-adrenoreceptors. Acute dosing causes postural hypotension and reflex tachycardia, but these are less evident with chronic treatment.

Pharmacokinetics

Prazosin is probably well absorbed but its bioavailability varies, averaging about 60% as a result of extensive first pass hepatic metabolism predominantly via o-dealkylation[49]. The metabolites are excreted in bile and only 6% of the parent compound appears unchanged in urine. Peak plasma prazosin concentrations occur at about 2 hours and the plasma elimination half-life is about 2.5-3 h. Prazosin is highly bound to plasma proteins, but this is diminished in uraemia when half-life is prolonged by 50%. This may account for the suggestion that the drug is more effective in renal failure. Generally however, plasma prazosin concentrations correlate poorly with the chronic antihypertensive effects.

Adverse effects

Prazosin is less well tolerated than hydralazine but probably only marginally so[42]. Unlike hydralazine it is devoid of long-term complications, making it more convenient for follow-up. The side-effects which occur more frequently than with hydralazine are postural dizziness without hypotension, drowsiness and lethargy. Sexual dysfunction, nightmares, dry mouth and urinary incontinence may occur. In elderly patients spontaneous postural dizziness and urinary incontinence are so common that the addition of prazosin may well confuse the picture and should be avoided.

First dose phenomenon

In general α-blockers need to be introduced gradually if they are to be tolerated. The first dose phenomenon describes the adverse cardiovascular effects resulting from too large a starting dose and may be seen occasionally with large dose increments. The clinical effects of initial doses as low as 1–2 mg are well documented. There is a marked postural fall in blood pressure with an associated reflex tachycardia. Despite a rise in plasma catecholamines, a proportion of patients experience not merely dizziness but syncope. These patients develop sudden bradycardia presumed to be vagally mediated[50]. The magnitude of the fall and its duration (2–6 h) depend on the dose, plasma prazosin concentration and concomitant therapy. For example, the effects are enhanced by diuretics because of plasma volume depletion and by β-blockers because they attenuate the compensatory reflex tachycardia. It is believed that some of the postural effects are due particularly to blockade of receptors on capacitance vessels, a view supported by the absence of such symptoms in patients with heart failure and therefore high venous pressure.

Efficacy and clinical use

When used as a third drug the hypotensive effect is comparable to that seen with hydralazine and methyldopa. As a first line agent its effects are comparable to β-blockers and diuretics. Because of the first dose effect the drug must be introduced gradually starting with 0.5 mg twice daily. A starter pack is available. Many surveys show that most patients achieve control with daily doses of less than 10 mg but the ceiling is 20 mg. Like many other agents with a short plasma half-life it is effective when given twice daily.

α-Methyldopa

In the last 10 years the use of α-methyldopa has declined in hospital clinics, but the drug is still popular with general practitioners. It does not have to be used in conjunction with a β-blocker or diuretic but because the frequency of side-effects is higher than with either of these agents it is best used when the first line agents have failed.

Pharmacokinetics

α-Methyldopa is an amino acid. By analogy with L-Dopa its absorption is likely to be an active process (in contrast to most drugs) and may therefore be impaired if taken with food. The proportion of the dose absorbed varies from 26 to 74% between patients, but the oral bio-availability averages only 25% because of first pass sulphate conjugation[51,52]. Peak plasma concentrations of α-methyldopa occur at 3–6 hours. After absorption and first pass metabolism methyldopa is largely eliminated, unchanged in urine. Equal proportions of parent drug and metabolites, mainly sulphate conjugates, appear in urine. The elimination half-life of methyldopa in plasma is about 2 h. The compound is widely distributed, entering peripheral adrenergic neurons and the central nervous system (c.n.s.) where a small proportion is metabolized first by dopa decarboxylase to α-methyldopamine, then to α-methylnoradrenaline. Like endogenous catecholamines these are cleared by methyl transferase enzymes thereby increasing the urinary recovery of 'metanephrines'. Unlike noradrenaline, α-methylnoradrenaline is not a substrate for monamine oxidase and the urinary recovery of VMA is unchanged.

Mechanism of action and pharmacodynamics

The activity resides in the (−)-isomer, but, unlike the other drugs discussed, α-methyldopa must be metabolized to α-methylnoradrenaline in the c.n.s. to achieve its hypotensive effect[51]. Dopa decarboxylase inhibitors prevent the physiological effects of α-methyldopa only if they cross the blood brain barrier. α-Methylnoradrenaline is believed to stimulate α$_2$-adrenoceptors which inhibit sympathetic outflow from the vasomotor centre. Its mode of action therefore is similar to that of clonidine.

The maximum fall in blood pressure after oral dosing takes 4–6 h to come on, but then wanes slowly and lasts over 24 h. However, twice daily dosing is best. Peripheral resistance falls with little alteration in heart rate or cardiac output. Postural hypotension is usually mild but reports vary and the fall in standing blood pressure in excess of supine may be between 2/4 and 16/10 mmHg.

Efficacy

Methyldopa is a highly effective antihypertensive agent and blood pressure reduction is comparable to that seen with β-blockers, whether used as a single agent or in combination with a diuretic. As a third drug its effects are equivalent to those of hydralazine or prazosin. The maximum dose usually recommended is 2 g a day but the ceiling dose is probably much lower. As 1.5 g is not superior to 750 mg per day[53] I advise against increasing the dose above a gram when the frequency of side-effects can be expected to increase. In most patients the slight postural fall in blood pressure is not a problem.

Adverse effects

Methyldopa commonly causes side-effects and a third of patients may be unable to tolerate it when the ceiling dose is 2 g per day. In addition, it is now accepted from questionnaires that many adverse effects are unreported or unrecognized. However, it is not clear to what extent the tolerability of methyldopa would be improved if the dose were limited to a gram a day. The drug should always be introduced gradually, starting with 125 mg b.d. The principal reasons for drug withdrawal are drowsiness, lethargy, nausea, dry mouth and nasal stuffiness. Erectile impotence in men is common. Use of the drug is associated with a rise in serum prolactin concentration which may also explain why galactorrhoea can complicate treatment. Although there are numerous anecdotal reports of depression, formal studies have failed to confirm this.

A number of more serious side-effects have been reported; 20% of patients treated for 6 months or more develop a Coombs positive direct antiglobulin test. The incidence is dose related being 36% with doses above 2 g and 11% in those receiving less than half this dose. Haemolytic anaemia, however, is rare (0.1–0.2% of patients) and usually arises within 18 months of initiation of treatment[54]. Drug withdrawal is essential if haemolysis occurs and occasionally corticosteroids may be required. The antibody persists for several months after drug withdrawal. The mechanism of the anaemia is obscure but neither the drug nor its metabolites act as haptens. Genetic factors are important, as most patients with antibodies are HLA-B7. It has been proposed that methyldopa reacts with lymphocytes resulting in inhibition of T cell function with loss of control over B cell antibody production[55]. A number of other uncommon, but serious side-effects have been described – hepatitis, rashes, pancreatitis, malabsorption and blood dyscrasias.

Minoxidil

Minoxidil is a potent vasodilator which has been used largely in resistant hypertension or in severe renal disease. As a result there are few comparative studies in hypertension. Its use has also been limited by fluid retention despite thiazide treatment and by hirsutes, making it unacceptable to most women.

Mechanism of action and pharmacodynamics

The mechanism of action and pharmacodynamics of minoxidil are similar to but more profound than hydralazine. Peripheral resistance falls but there is a marked reflex tachycardia which persists on chronic dosing. The drug *must* therefore be given with a β-blocker.

The effects of minoxidil are seen 2-6 hours after dosing, but a fall in blood pressure may persist for up to 2-5 days. The magnitude of these effects is dose related in the therapeutic range of 5-40 mg daily. However, the profound fall in blood pressure with higher doses necessitates twice-daily administration when the dose exceeds 15 mg. With smaller doses once-daily treatment is feasible.

Pharmacokinetics

Minoxidil is rapidly and fully absorbed from the gastro-intestinal tract. Peak plasma concentrations occur at about an hour. The drug is not significantly bound to plasma proteins and seems to be concentrated in arteriolar smooth muscle but not in skeletal or cardiac muscle.

Elimination is by metabolism to a glucuronide conjugate and other water soluble metabolites which are then excreted by the kidneys. The half-life of elimination is about 4 hours[56], much shorter than the biological effects. The kinetics are not influenced by dose or duration of treatment. However, in severe renal failure the absorption rate may be delayed, the metabolites accumulate and appear in the faeces. In patients undergoing haemodialysis the plasma minoxidil concentration falls by a third following dialysis but this is probably not important clinically because of the prolonged effect on arteriolar sites.

Efficacy

Minoxidil is undoubtedly an extremely potent hypotensive agent. Assessment of its efficacy during chronic dosing has, however, been complicated by the need to introduce large doses of loop diuretics to counteract fluid retention, evidenced by weight gain or oedema. As we shall see, frusemide itself will enhance the effects of triple therapy. Comparative studies have failed to allow for the fact that minoxidil-treated patients were receiving additional frusemide, often in high doses of 300-400 mg daily. Nevertheless, minoxidil (maximum dose 40 mg) was at least as effective as high dose hydralazine (maximum 400 mg daily) when both groups of patients received a β-blocker and high dose frusemide[57]. In the Third Drug Study minoxidil lowered blood pressure in men more than the other agents. However, the drug was only tolerated in those with mild hypertension (systolic 160-180 mmHg) because larger doses of 20 mg or more were associated with oedema.

Adverse effects

The most frequent side-effects are hirsuties, fluid retention and occasionally gynaecomastia. Hirsuties occurs in most patients treated for more than 4 weeks. Hair growth involves areas of the face not normally covered by hair even in men. For this reason women should only rarely receive the drug and then hair may be removed with calcium thioglycolate depilatory.

Fluid retention

Even in the absence of moderate renal impairment the majority of minoxidil-treated patients require frusemide to control fluid retention. The likelihood of severe fluid retention, oedema, left ventricular failure or pericardial effusion are all greater in patients with moderate or severe renal impairment and a higher dose of diuretics is required to control the symptoms. Nevertheless, fluid retention occurs without deterioration in renal function. Although plasma renin activity increases, aldosterone is unchanged during chronic treatment. Minoxidil, and to a lesser extent other vasodilators, are believed to enhance proximal tubular salt and water reabsorption probably through redistribution of renal blood flow from outer cortex to the juxtaglomerular cortex.

Cardiac effects

T wave changes on E.C.G. may be seen in the majority of patients during the first 2 weeks of treatment and in most cases revert spontaneously to normal. The changes are not related to ischaemia. An increase in pulmonary artery pressure has been described in patients receiving minoxidil, but only when used without a β-blocker. Myocardial necrosis described in dogs and rats does not occur in man.

Labetalol

Labetalol may be used as a first line agent, but many would prefer to substitute it where a conventional β-blocker is inadequate.

Mechanism of action and pharmacodynamics

Labetalol is a non-selective β-blocker which also antagonizes α_1-adrenoceptors. The relative potency for β:α sites is 4:1. As a result its α-blocking effects are less evident at doses below 400 mg daily. Its mechanism of action and pharmacodynamics reflects combined adrenoceptor blockade. After acute dosing peak effects occur at 2 h. There is a rapid fall in blood pressure due to a reduction in peripheral resistance, only slight reduction in basal heart rate, and no fall in cardiac output at rest. Postural effects on blood pressure are only troublesome with modest initial doses or with larger doses administered chronically (> 800 mg daily). The duration of the effect is less than 24 h and the drug must be administered twice daily.

Pharmacokinetics

Like other lipid soluble β-blockers, labetalol is completely absorbed and undergoes extensive first pass metabolism. Oral bioavailability is about 33% in healthy subjects. The elimination half-life in plasma is 3 h and less than 5% of the unchanged drug appears in urine.

Efficacy

The hypotensive effects of modest doses of labetalol are equivalent to those of other β-blockers but doses above 800 mg may be superior. The dose may be increased to a maximum of 3200 mg daily when labetalol plus a thiazide diuretic may be equivalent in effect to conventional three drug combinations.

Adverse effects

Labetalol is less well tolerated than most β-blockers. It is probable, however, that to some extent this may be due to injudicious use. Like all α-blockers small starting doses must be administered (50–100 mg b.d.) even when it is substituted for a β-blocker. The dose may be increased after a few days. Side-effects on chronic dosing are also dose related, therefore the withdrawal rate may be as low as 4%[58] with doses below 400 mg a day and 25%[59] with double this dose. In the Third Drug Study[42] the withdrawal rate and long term complaints were higher than in either of these trials, possibly because of a high initial dose. Only a quarter of those withdrawing did so in the first 2 weeks and complaints were not specifically related to receptor blockade. The main problems with this compound are nausea, tiredness, aching limbs and tingling skin. Labetalol is not immune from conventional β-blocker side-effects such as asthma or heart failure although there are suggestions that these may be less common. In conclusion, although labetalol may be used as a first line agent, in most patients there is little to recommend it over a conventional β-blocker. As a substitute for a third drug in dual therapy failures it seems attractive because it may simplify the regimen. However, as other β-blockers are available in fixed dose combination with diuretics, this facility may be more apparent than real.

NEWER ANTIHYPERTENSIVE AGENTS

Angiotensin converting enzyme inhibitors

These are exciting new compounds developed to lower blood pressure by inhibiting the renin angiotensin system. Renin released from the kidney catalyses the formation of angiotensin I which is converted by 'converting enzymes' into angiotensin II. Inhibition of angiotensin converting enzyme (ACE) leads to a fall in angiotensin II and concurrently to a rise in plasma renin and angiotensin I reflecting the loss of a negative feedback loop. Two orally active ACE inhibitors, captopril and enalapril, have undergone clinical trials.

Mechanism of action and pharmacodynamics

The fall in blood pressure is due to a reduction in peripheral resistance; there is no change in heart rate, cardiac output or postural hypotension. The effect on blood pressure is closely correlated with inhibition of converting enzyme, both during acute and chronic dosing, but complete inhibition is unnecessary[60] (Figure 1.5).

Its duration is longer than inhibition of the enzyme in plasma would predict, possibly because of an effect on renin in resistance vessels. The precise mode of action is unclear since a wide range of responses may be seen both in renin dependent (renal or renovascular) and low renin hypertension. Angiotensin II and the kallerkrein–kinin system are important.

(1) *Fall in plasma angiotensin II.* This is probably the most important mechanism through reduction of direct pressor activity. However, the reduction in plasma angiotensin II levels correlates better with the immediate hypotensive effect than with the long term fall in blood pressure. Furthermore, hypotensive effects have been noted despite pretreatment with salarasin, a competitive inhibitor of angiotensin II. Plasma aldosterone concentration is influenced by angiotensin II and therefore falls during treatment. This may explain the further gradual reduction in blood pressure over a 2–3 week period, the rise in serum potassium and the lack of fluid retention. The decrease in angiotensin II may lead to reduction in sympathetic outflow by centrally mediated effects on baroreceptor function.

(2) *Increase in blood or tissue kinins.* ACE, also known as kininase II, is one of the enzymes responsible for the inactivation of kinins, such as bradykinin, which possess vasodilator properties. Failure to inactivate kinins may explain some of the hypotensive effect, particularly in low renin hypertension. Circulating venous bradykinin concentrations however may not be altered but urinary kinins increase with ACE inhibition, and there are suggestions that tissue kinin levels increase too. Bradykinin may be responsible for the documented rise in prostaglandin concentrations which could also lead to vasodilatation.

Pharmacokinetics

Captopril is very rapidly absorbed. Peak plasma concentrations are seen between 0.5 and 1.5 h after dosing. Food reduces the absorption

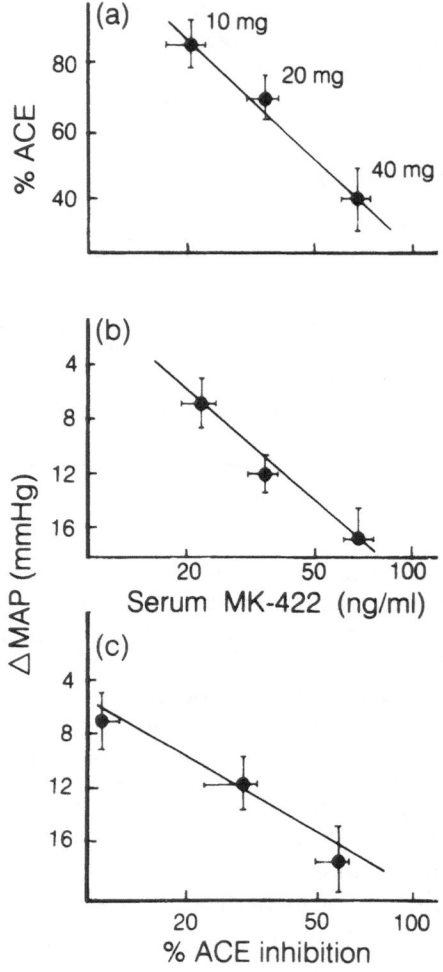

Figure 1.5 (a) Percentage ACE activity plotted against serum MK-422, (b) fall in mean arterial blood pressure (Δ MAP) plotted against serum MK-422 and (c) plotted against percentage ACE inhibition after chronic administration of enalapril to patients with hypertension. Each point is the mean ± s.e.m. of several determinations in patients on 10, 20 and 40 mg enalapril daily. (Reproduced with permission from the *Journal of Hypertension*)

slightly: plasma protein binding is low. The elimination is via metabolism to inactive metabolites and by renal tubular secretion in equal proportions. The half-life in patients with normal renal function is about 2 h, but this would be prolonged in renal failure or with administration of probenecid. The measurement of captopril in plasma is technically difficult and correlation between plasma concentration and effect is not reliable. The onset of effect may be as short as 15 minutes, maximal at 2 h and then wanes over the next 8 h.

Enalapril (MK 421) is an ester which is well absorbed and undergoes hydrolysis in the liver to its active metabolite enalaprilic acid (MK 422), which is then excreted by the kidney. The bioavailability is not influenced by food. The peak plasma concentrations of enalapril occur 1 h after administration while enalaprilic acid concentrations peak at 4 h. The elimination half-life of the acid is 35 h. The hypotensive effect reflects the gradual appearance of the active agent in plasma and acute hypotension is not seen. The maximum fall in blood pressure occurs between 4 and 12 h and lasts for at least 24 h. Plasma enalaprilic acid concentrations correlate well with ACE inhibition and with hypotensive response (Figure 1.5).

Efficacy

Almost by design captopril was introduced as an agent for severe or resistant hypertension and was commonly administered to patients with renal or renovascular disease. In the UK it is primarily licensed for severe hypertension when other therapy has failed (ABPI Data Sheet Compendium, 1984–1985). Initial studies were therefore uncontrolled but suggested that resistant hypertension in patients with renal disease could be managed solely with the combination of captopril and a diuretic. Several controlled studies have shown that captopril lowers blood pressure in essential hypertension. The effects are probably greater when added to a diuretic. It has been suggested that patients uncontrolled on captopril plus a diuretic derive little additional benefit from the addition of a β-blocker, but this is strongly disputed.

The advice on dosage and administration of captopril in the 1984–1985 data sheet is hopelessly out of date. Although it was initially used on a thrice daily basis there is evidence that it is effective when given twice daily. Furthermore small doses may be as effective as larger ones and the dose of 150 mg per day should not be exceeded. The ceiling dose may be 75 mg or less[61], and the starting dose is probably 12.5 mg b.d. Patients with renal impairment should receive smaller doses.

Enalapril may be available in 1985. Like captopril it is effective in renovascular, renal and essential hypertension. Large multicentre trials have shown that when used as monotherapy in essential hypertension enalapril has similar antihypertensive effect to propranolol 240 mg daily or to atenolol 100 mg daily[62]. Once daily dosing is satisfactory. The dose used has been 10–40 mg daily.

Adverse effects

Serious penicillamine-like adverse effects with captopril have been attributed to the presence of a sulphydryl group. The majority of reports have occurred in patients receiving high doses (> 150 mg daily) despite renal disease and sometimes in association with collagen vas-

Table 1.7 Serious adverse effects with captopril in relation to dose and renal impairment[63]

	Neutropenia	Proteinuria	Rash	Ageusia
No renal impairment + Dose ≤ 150 mg	0.02%	0.2%	1.4%	0.5%
Renal impairment + Dose > 150 mg	7.2%*	3.5%	5.1%	2.9%

*Mainly patients with collagen vascular disease

cular disease requiring immunosuppressive agents. It is not always easy to separate out the primary pathology from drug effects or drug–disease interactions. An up-to-date review summarizes the present position[63] (Table 1.7). Clearly neutropenia is a rare occurrence except in predisposed individuals. Proteinuria greater than 1 g per 24 h may lead to nephrotic syndrome in 25% of cases. Although initial reports suggested immune complex glomerulonephritis following captopril treatment the consensus view is that many of these patients had pre-existing disease. The pathogenesis of captopril-induced rash is poorly understood. It is not an allergic reaction; it is dose related and may not recur with rechallenge. Enalapril which is free of SH groups rarely causes such reactions and may be substituted for captopril with resolution of rash, taste disturbance and proteinuria. Nevertheless, to date its use has been carefully controlled. Long term confirmation of its safety is necessary.

First dose effects

Following the first dose of captopril, there may be a severe reduction in supine or standing blood pressure which lasts for up to 3 h. The phenomenon is not described with enalapril and must be related in part to its rapid absorption and ACE inhibition. The reaction is more common in hypertension secondary to renal or renovascular disease, in patients with high pretreatment plasma renin and angiotensin II[64]. Diuretics increase the risk in those with secondary hypertension but captopril dose is not important possibly because maximum inhibition of ACE occurs with lower doses although the duration of this effect is then short lived. Initial dosing need be supervised only in high risk patients.

Reversible renal impairment

This may occur in patients with renal artery stenosis following treatment with captopril and enalapril. Indeed, a rise in serum creatinine may identify patients with renovascular disease particularly those with a solitary functioning kidney or with bilateral stenoses. Only 50% of patients with these conditions suffer renal impairment but the magnitude of blood pressure reduction and dose are unimportant[65]. Renal artery stenosis is associated with a decreased blood pressure in the afferent arteriole which stimulates angiotensin II production. Its pressor effects are most marked in the efferent arteriole leading to a rise in filtration pressure. Angiotensin converting enzyme inhibition, however, prevents these homeostatic mechanisms. Isotope renography may be used to monitor the effects of captopril and loss of function is an indication for drug withdrawal[66] (Figure 1.6).

Tolerability

Despite the problems related to the use of ACE inhibitors, the majority of patients report an improvement in well-being, particularly if the drug has satisfactorily been substituted for several other agents. Unproductive cough has been reported with both captopril and enalapril. When used prudently in essential hypertension captopril and enalapril are as well tolerated as existing first line agents[61,62] but the place of ACE inhibitors has yet to be determined. In view of their cost, they should not replace β-blockers or diuretics as first line agents. They may be used in diuretic failures when β-blockers are contraindicated, in patients with resistant hypertension or cautiously in patients with renal or renovascular hypertension.

Calcium antagonists

Nifedipine and verapamil are important antianginal agents and will be described in detail in Chapter 2 of this book. Although their use in hypertension is widely promoted there are few published data to support their case, except where other agents have failed or if there is coexistent angina. Nifedipine is useful in Raynaud's disease and it may be rational where cold extremities are a problem.

Mechanism of action and pharmacodynamics

Calcium antagonists interfere with calcium fluxes upon which smooth muscle contraction depends. This leads to vasodilatation in resistance vessels, a decrease in peripheral resistance and a fall in blood pressure. Much has been made of the fact that these effects are prominent in hypertensive patients but less evident in normotensive subjects. However, the effect of most antihypertensive agents is correlated with pretreatment blood pressure. The suggestion that these compounds correct a specific abnormality in hypertension[67,68] is disputed and perhaps irrelevant to their clinical use.

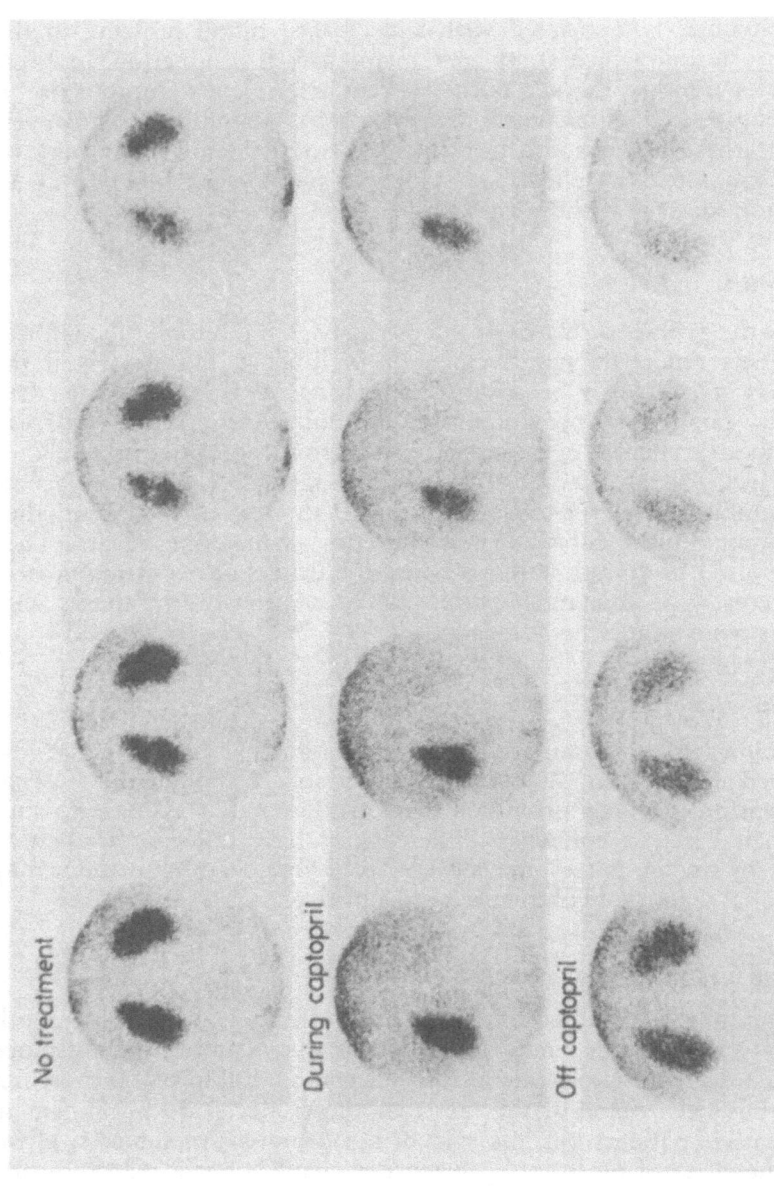

Figure 1.6 Sequential ⁹⁹ᵐTc-DTPA kidney scans (at 2, 5, 10, 15 min) in patient with unilateral renal artery stenosis before, after 4 weeks of captopril and 1 week after stopping captopril. (Reproduced with permission from the *British Medical Journal*)

Nifedipine

After acute oral administration of nifedipine capsules the hypotensive effect is seen within half an hour and may last only 6–8 hours. Thrice-daily dosing is essential even with chronic treatment. The initial reflex tachycardia disappears with repeated administration, despite a fall in blood pressure. This has been attributed to resetting of baroreceptors. Nifedipine Slow Release tablets are probably more suitable for patients with hypertension. They are more slowly absorbed and probably effective when administered twice daily[69].

Verapamil

Acute oral administration of verapamil is associated with relatively short-lived effects on blood pressure. During chronic treatment however the hypotensive effect persists for at least 12 h[70], probably because the half-life of both verapamil and norverapamil is prolonged. There may be a slight fall in heart rate but cardiac output does not change except in incipient heart failure.

Efficacy

Nifedipine is probably the more effective antihypertensive agent, but properly controlled trials are lacking. To date the data suggest that when added to a β-blocker and diuretic the effect is similar to that seen with other third drugs, but some postural effect may be observed[71]. Unlike some vasodilators response is not dependent on concomitant use of a β-blocker. The recommended dose range is 10–30 mg capsules thrice daily or 20–60 mg tablets twice daily.

Verapamil should not be used with a β-blocker as both may depress the myocardium and the atrio-ventricular node. Few controlled trials are published. When compared with optimal doses of β-blocker, verapamil 120 mg t.d.s. or 160–240 mg b.d. lowered blood pressure to a similar extent[70].

Adverse effects

Side-effects are common with nifedipine treatment and 14–31% of patients may withdraw. It is not certain whether the tolerability is improved by using the slow release tablets or by co-administration of the β-blocker and diuretic[72]. The principal problems are facial flushing, palpitations, headache and ankle oedema. Nifedipine may precipitate angina and lower serum potassium.

Verapamil should be avoided if the left ventricular function is compromised as it may precipitate heart failure. Heart block is another contraindication since the PR interval increases slightly and occasionally A.V. dissociation may be precipitated. The most common side-effect is constipation which occurs in a third of patients. In previously asymptomatic hypertensives this may be unacceptable, although trialists report a low withdrawal rate. Flushing, palpitations and oedema are less common than with nifedipine. There have been several reports of hepatitis occurring shortly after introduction of verapamil.

RESISTANT HYPERTENSION

As many as 20% of patients may be uncontrolled despite triple therapy as recommended above. Where interactions and non-compliance have been excluded as a cause, further investigation and additional treatment will be necessary.

Interactions

The principal offender is the use of non-steroidal anti-inflammatory agents. Most commonly they are inappropriately prescribed when paracetamol will suffice. Other compounds which may elevate blood pressure should be withdrawn if possible. The intake of alcohol should be reviewed. In patients with renal impairment excessive salt intake should be avoided.

Compliance

Non-compliance is the most common cause of apparent resistance to treatment. Tablet counting is probably the best way of making the diagnosis in a routine clinic but this necessitates issuing all the tablets from one pharmacy so that the excess tablets returned may be estimated. Patients who take more than 85% of their medication are considered compliant. Non-comprehension, polypharmacy, frequent drug dosing and adverse effects are all important causes of poor compliance and must be avoided. Regular counselling or supervision is important for this group, who therefore require more time. Patients suspected of non-compliance should *not* be admitted for observation. Blood pressure falls dramatically in over 50% of untreated hypertensives or fully compliant resistant hypertensives when they are admitted, only to rise again on discharge. The mechanism may be a reduction in sympathetic outflow with a decrease in venous tone and cardiac output[73].

Further investigations

When apparent resistance is excluded, further investigation is indicated as there is an increased chance of finding a specific cause.

Conn's syndrome

Primary hyperaldosteroidism should be reconsidered if hypokalaemia has been present in the past. Many drugs alter serum potassium and withdrawal of all drugs for a month may be necessary before full investigation can be carried out. Patients with bilateral adrenal hyperplasia may have borderline low or normal serum potassium even when sampled correctly, i.e. fasting, without a tourniquet and spun immediately. The diagnosis is based on high urinary and plasma aldosterone and an inappropriate plasma renin activity (low or normal). Tumours are best localized by CT scanning and should be removed. Bilateral hyperplasia should be treated with spironolactone 100–400 mg daily.

Renovascular or renal disease

Few patients require extensive renal investigations at presentation. Resistance is an indication for intravenous pyelography (i.v.p.) and dynamic renography. Previous accelerated hypertension, smoking, peripheral vascular disease and advancing years increasing the likelihood of atheromatous renal artery stenois. Ten per cent of cases may be missed with non-invasive techniques and renal arteriography may be necessary. Significant stenosis is best treated by angioplasty which carries low morbidity with a 66% chance of improvement and a 20% chance of a cure[74]. Reconstructive surgery is rarely advised as it carries a 5% mortality. A unilateral small kidney on i.v.p. may be due to renal artery stenosis or occlusion or congenital or acquired renal disease. Resection is only indicated if it is non-functioning and this may be determined by dynamic scans. In my experience the majority of such patients are unsuitable for surgery because of poor physical condition. Surgical treatment is never indicated for unilateral pyelonephritis as results are poor and some renal function usually remains.

Drug treatment

There are few drug trials in this field. Adding a fourth agent may be effective. The choice should be rational, avoiding two compounds with identical mechanisms of action. Prazosin may be added to hydralazine and methyldopa to either vasodilator. In rapid acetylators of hydralazine it is often best to assume that resistance is secondary to kinetic factors and to substitute another conventional third drug. Substitution of minoxidil in severe hypertension must be accompanied by additional diuretic and this may not be particularly attractive. Captopril can be substituted for other third drugs but despite glowing reports in essential hypertension, I have found that this manœuvre leads to control in less than 50% of cases. However, in some instances – particularly in patients with renal hypertension – dramatic responses do occur and may permit the withdrawal of all other agents except diuretics.

Additional diuretic treatment

Despite the use of thiazide diuretics all third drugs lead to fluid retention which may antagonize their hypotensive action. This phenomenon of 'false tolerance' occurs with an increase in body weight of approximately 1 kg and may be opposed by increasing the diuretic regime[73]. Ramsay[75-77] has studied a number of diuretic regimens as an alterna-

Table 1.8   Fall in blood pressure with different diuretic regimens in patients uncontrolled on conventional triple drug therapy[75-77]

Regimen*	Fall in blood pressure (mmHg)		Change in body weight (kg)
	Supine	*Standing*	
Bendrofluazide 10 mg	14/4	4/4	+0.4
Frusemide 80 mg	18/7	15/8	−0.5
Bendrofluazide 5 mg and Spironolactone 100 mg	28/12	30/17	−0.9
Bendrofluazide 5 mg and Frusemide 80 mg	52/23	67/21	−1.5

* Substituted for bendrofluazide 5 mg

tive to conventional fourth drugs (Table 1.8). A significant response is associated with a reduction in body weight reflecting fluid loss. *Increasing bendrofluazide* dose carries little added benefit. *Substituting frusemide* (80 mg daily) for a thiazide has a significant effect and few side-effects except urinary frequency for a few hours in the day. However, less than 40% will be controlled by this manœuvre, possibly because of the short duration of action. Whether twice daily dosing would be better is uncertain but probably less convenient. *Adding spironolactone* 100 mg to a thiazide diuretic is very helpful when tolerated. Gynaecomastia in men is the main difficulty. Postural hypotension is not a problem despite a fall in body weight. This regimen must be restricted to patients with serum creatinine less than 200 μmol/l. Larger doses may be used but they are less well tolerated. *Adding frusemide* 40-80 mg daily has profound effects on blood pressure. However complaints are common, mainly postural hypotension, serious hypokalaemia (<3.0 mmol/l in 40%), occasional symptomatic hyponatraemia and a significant rise in serum urea, creatinine and urate. Potent diuretics should be used when renal impairment is present, although severe dehydration could pose a serious problem. As with all these regimens, close biochemical monitoring is essential. *The rational choice* of diuretic in resistant hypertension may be to add spironolactone when possible and then, if necessary, substitute frusemide 40 mg for a thiazide, increasing the dose to 80-120 mg once daily. This should lower blood pressure with less hypokalaemia and hyperuricaemia although some of the problems will remain. Eighty per cent of resistant patients may be controlled in this way, i.e. with a total of four drugs. Increasing the diuretic dose is preferred in females, in whom fluid retention is more common. Male patients may be better off with a conventional antihypertensive agent.

URGENT MANAGEMENT OF HYPERTENSION

Nowadays rapid reduction of blood pressure is seldom indicated except under the following circumstances.

(1) Accelerated hypertension suggested by fundoscopy findings of haemorrhages, exudates or papilloedema. Care should be taken not to confuse retinal vein occlusion with malignant hypertension. The former, which produces unilateral haemorrhages often limited to a single quadrant (branch vein occlusion), may be associated with hypertension but its occurrence is not related to blood pressure control.

(2) Hypertension associated with acute left ventricular failure invariably requires specific antihypertensive treatment in addition to parenteral diuretics.

(3) Hypertension associated with myocardial infarction. In the light of benefits from β-blockers in acute myocardial infarction these agents should be used to deal with hypertension in the immediate postinfarction period.

(4) Hypertensive encephalopathy is associated with headache, confusion, drowsiness, neurological signs and papilloedema. The condition should not be confused with hypertension following a stroke where grade III or IV retinopathy is absent and where abrupt reduction in blood pressure may worsen the condition. In patients with acute hypertension, hypertensive encephalopathy may occur at levels of diastolic pressure as low as 110 mmHg. Typically patients have either eclampsia or acute renal failure.

(5) Eclampsia. This may occur abruptly with warning symptoms for only 24 h or so and invariably necessitates delivery in addition to blood pressure control.

(6) Aortic dissection.

Oral therapy

In patients with chronic hypertension dramatic reduction of blood pressure may lead to stroke, myocardial infarction or blindness. Cerebral autoregulation is set at a higher level[78] and dramatic blood pressure reduction to normal levels leads to cerebral ischaemia without hypotension. Unless the patient is *in extremis*, bed rest and oral therapy are all that are required. The aim should be to reduce diastolic pressure no lower than to 100 mmHg over 24 h. Standard therapy such as β-blockers or labetalol will usually suffice in the first instance. Other standard drugs may be added over the next few weeks. Oral nifedipine 10–20 mg has been recommended as a first line agent in accelerated hypotension. Unless the patient is *in extremis*, bed rest and oral therapy are all that are required. The aim should be to reduce diastolic pressure no lower than to 100 mmHg over 24 h. Standard therapy such vascular disease suggest caution. Patients with accelerated hypertension should be investigated for a primary cause; in some series renovascular hypertension has been found in as many as 40% of men but this observation has been disputed.

Parenteral drugs

Parenteral treatment is indicated to deal with acute left ventricular failure, encephalopathy, eclampsia and aortic dissection. In acute hypertensive crises the aim should be to bring blood pressure down to normal.

Labetalol

This is probably the easiest agent to use and probably the drug of choice in labour. It may be administered as bolus doses of 25 mg or by constant infusion starting at 25 mg per hour and increasing the dose as required. The full effect is seen within 5 minutes of a bolus. It may be used cautiously in left ventricular failure caused by severe hypertension since reduction in blood pressure will usually improve left ventricular function.

Diazoxide

This is an arteriolar vasodilator. The standard 300 mg rapid bolus is no longer recommended as precipitous falls in blood pressure may occur with disastrous consequences. A 50 mg bolus may be effective and if it is not, the dose should be increased to 100–150 mg. Peak effects occur within 5 minutes and may last for several hours[80]. Repeated bolus doses lead to fluid retention and serious hyperglycaemia and treatment beyond 24 h is not advised. If continued parenteral treatment is required an alternative agent is recommended. If used in pregnancy it should be remembered that occasionally it may inhibit labour.

Nitroprusside

This dilates both arterioles and venules, invariably lowering blood pressure with only a slight increase in heart rate[81]. The effect of an intravenous infusion is immediate but equally short lived. Its great advantage is that dose titration enables precise control of blood pressure provided that intra-arterial monitoring is performed. Therefore, although nitroprusside is the ideal agent in severe hypertension with acute left ventricular failure, it is often easier and quicker to try the effects of labetalol or diazoxide first. Nitroprusside should be used in aortic dissection. It works even in hypertensive crises due to pheochromocytoma. Its use in eclampsia is more controversial as it may reduce uterine blood flow, but this may be a secondary consideration when other vasodilators fail. Nitroprusside solution must be prepared immediately before use; 50 mg in a 500 ml 5% dextrose solution. Infusion bottles should be protected from the light with aluminium foil. The dose may be regulated with a microdrop regulator. Two drops per minute (12.5 µg per minute in 0.2 ml) is a suitable starting dose which may be adjusted every 2–3 minutes. Only if nitroprusside is used for several days is it necessary to measure thiocyanate plasma concentrations. This metabolite is excreted by the kidney and accumulates in renal failure.

Other agents

Hydralazine is a popular drug in emergency situations probably because it can be given both i.v. and i.m. There is little to justify its use over the agents mentioned above and its effect takes 20 min to come on and reaches a maximum at 30–40 min. Therefore clinicians are often tempted to administer additional treatment in the interim and this may lead to serious hypotension. Furthermore, the incidence of side-effects is high, with flushing, tachycardia and headache. In pregnancy there is no particular reason to favour its use over labetalol.

Methyldopa should not be used parenterally since its onset of action is slow (4–6 hours). When used intravenously it is given as its ester methyldopate which must be metabolized to methyldopa before it can be effective.

Phentolamine as a 2–5 mg bolus or via i.v. infusion of 1 mg per minute should be reserved for patients with suspected pheochromocytoma. Significant response is not diagnostic of this condition.

HYPERTENSION IN PREGNANCY

Hypertensive disease remains the most common cause of maternal deaths in England and Wales, nearly half from cerebral haemorrhage[82]. The majority of these patients have at least one avoidable factor. In addition hypertension particularly when associated with proteinuria of greater than 0.5 g per 24 h increases the incidence of perinatal deaths and complications such as respiratory distress syndrome[83]. Superficially there seems a strong case for treating all cases of pregnancy-associated hypertension, whether mild (140/90), moderate (diastolic $\geqslant 100$) or severe($\geqslant 170/110$). However, except in the last group, complications are so closely related to the *development* of proteinuria that the value of routine treatment is disputed.

Pre-existing hypertension

When uncomplicated by pre-eclampsia, that is a further rise in blood pressure and proteinuria, the complication rate is lower than in normotensive women. However, the chances of developing pre-eclampsia is increased fivefold and may occur in as many as 25% of women with raised blood pressure at booking[83].

Mild to moderate pre-eclampsia

A rise in blood pressure after 20 weeks, unassociated with proteinuria, is not associated with an increase in perinatal mortality. However, blood pressure must be closely watched because of the risk of maternal death. The use of drug treatment therefore is controversial. Many obstetricians admit patients for bed rest although there is no evidence of efficacy. An alternative approach is to treat the blood pressure and continue close outpatient observation of blood pressure, proteinuria, and warning symptoms of eclampsia, such as headache, vomiting and visual problems. In the best trial to date[84] this approach was used to compare atenolol against placebo. Active treatment was associated with significantly better blood pressure control, it prevented proteinuria and it reduced the number of hospital admissions. The perinatal morbidity rate, principally respiratory distress syndrome, was also lower but mortality was unaffected. However, patients in the placebo group were withdrawn from the study when severe changes supervened. Other studies have shown a reduction in midtrimester abortions with methyldopa, reduction of growth retardation with oxprenolol and a decrease in neonatal deaths with metoprolol.

Severe pre-eclampsia

Admission and drug treatment are clearly indicated and parenteral treatment may be necessary. Termination of the pregnancy is usually performed.

Drugs used

All the drugs recommended below seem free from teratogenic effects and do not increase the risk to the fetus. Methyldopa, several β-blockers, labetalol and hydralazine have been well studied. The ceiling dose is probably double that I have recommended for non-pregnant patients, because of an increase in both hepatic and renal drug clearance. Anecdotal reports of adverse fetal effects caused by β-blockers cannot be substantiated and the only complication may be isolated neonatal bradycardia which is unlikely to be significant. Although β-blockers cross the placenta they do *not* mask the signs of fetal distress, as fetal heart rate is predominantly under parasympathetic control[85]. Diuretics are less commonly used in pregnancy as they are less effective and the rise in serum urate may be misleading. The drugs used appear in breast milk, but they have no significant effect on the fetus. Following delivery, if blood pressure is normal, those drugs started after the midterm should be withdrawn. The need for continued treatment must be reviewed over the next 3–4 months. Twenty-five per cent of patients with pregnancy-associated hypertension develop hypertension within 12 years[86].

CONCLUSIONS

The treatment of hypertension has been reviewed. Particular emphasis has been placed upon how drugs may be avoided in patients with spurious hypertension or where non-pharmacological measures may be an alternative. Only the important antihypertensive agents are discussed. The choice of drug is based largely on tolerability since most compounds are equally effective. β-blockers and low dose thiazides remain the cornerstone of treatment. The best choice third drugs are hydralazine and prazosin. Newer compounds such as the ACE inhibitors and calcium antagonists are welcome since existing agents cause a withdrawal rate of at least 20%; however, their place in routine practice is not established. Even in the most difficult cases it is unnecessary to use more than four compounds to control blood pressure.

References

1. Hawthorne, V.M., Greaves, D.A. and Beevers, D.G. (1974) Blood pressure in a Scottish town. *Br. Med. J.*, 3, 600–603
2. Management Committee of the Australian Therapeutic Trial in Mild Hypertension. (1982). Untreated mild hypertension. *Lancet*, 1, 185–91
3. Medical Research Council Working Party on Mild to Moderate Hypertension. (1977). Randomised controlled trial of treatment for mild hypertension; design and pilot trial. *Br. Med. J.*, 1, 1437–40
4. Memorandum from the WHO/ISH Meeting. (1983). Guidelines for the treatment of mild hypertension. *Lancet*, 1, 457–8
5. Maxwell, M.H., Waks, A.U., Schroth, P.C., Karam, M. and Dornfield, L.P. (1982). Error in blood pressure measurement due to incorrect cuff size in obese patients. *Lancet*, 2, 33–6
6. Webster, J., Newnham, D. and Petrie, J.C. (1983). Influence of arm position on the measurement of blood pressure by sphygmomanometer. *J. Hypertension*, 1, 319
7. Weir, R.J., Briggs, E., Mack, A., Naismith, L., Taylor, L. and Wilson, E. (1974). Blood pressure in women taking oral contraceptives. *Br. Med. J.*, 1, 533–5

8. Weir, R.J., Wilson, E.S.B., Cruikshank, J. and McMaster, M., (1983). Effects on blood pressure of low dose oestrogen and progesterone only oral contraceptives. *J. Hypertension*, 1 (Suppl. 2), 100–101

9. Reisen, E., Abel, R., Mordan, M., Silverbergh, D.S., Eliahou, H.E. and Modan, B. (1978). Effect of weight loss without salt restriction on the reduction of blood pressure in overweight hypertensive patients. *N. Engl. J. Med.*, 298, 1–6

10. Clatsky, A.L., Freedman, G.D., Siegelaub, A.B. and Gerrard, M.J. (1977). Alcohol consumption and blood pressure. Kieser Permanente Multiphasic Health Examination Data. *N. Engl. J. Med.*, 196, 1194–1200

11. Potter, J.F. and Beavers, D.G. (1984). Pressor effect of alcohol in hypertension. *Lancet*, 1, 119–22

12. Veteran's Administration Co-operative Study Group on Anti-hypertensive Agents. (1970). Effects of treatment on morbidity in hypertension. II. Results in patients with diastolic blood pressure averaging 90 through 114 mm Hg. *J. Am. Med. Assoc.*, 213, 1143–52

13. Report by the Management Committee. (1979). Initial results of the Australian therapeutic trial in mild hypertension. *Clin. Sci.*, 57, (Suppl. 5), 449–52

14. Report by the Management Committee. (1980). The Australian therapeutic trial in mild hypertension. *Lancet*, 1, 1261–7

15. Veteran's Administration Co-operative Study Group on Anti-hypertensive Agents. (1972). Effects of treatment on morbidity in hypertension III. Influence of age, diastolic blood pressure and prior cardiovascular disease; further analysis of side effects. *Circulation*, 45, 991–1004

16. Fuller, J.H., Shipley, M.J., Rose, G., Jarrett, R.J. and Keen, H. (1983). Mortality from coronary heart disease and stroke in relation to degree of glycaemia; The Whitehall Study. *Br. Med. J.*, 287, 867–70

17. Knowler, W.C., Bennett, P.H. and Ballintine, E.J. (1980). Increased incidence of retinopathy in diabetics with elevated blood glucose. *N. Engl. J. Med.*, 302, 645–50

18. Parving, H.K., Andersen, A.R., Smidt, U.M. and Svendsen, P.A. (1983). Early aggressive anti-hypertensive treatment reduces rate of decline in kidney function in diabetic nephropathy. *Lancet*, 1, 1175–9

19. Buhler, F.R. (1981). Anti-hypertensive actions of beta-blockers. In Laragh, J.H., Buhler, F.R. and Seldon, D.W. (eds) *The Frontiers in Hypertension Research*, pp. 423–5. (New York: Springer)

20. Floras, J.S., Jones, J.V., Hassan, M.O. and Sleight, P. (1983). Ambulatory blood pressure during once daily randomised, double-blind administration of atenolol, metoprolol, pindolol and slow release propranolol. *Drugs*, 25, (Suppl. 2) 19–25

21. Petrie, J.C., Jeffers, T.A., Robb, O.J., Scott, A.K. and Webster, J. (1980). Atenolol, slow release oxprenolol and long-acting propranolol in hypertension. *Br. Med. J.*, 280, 1573–5

22. Wilcox, R.G. and Hampton, J.R. (1981). Comparative study of atenolol, metoprolol, metoprolol durules and slow release oxprenolol in essential hypertension. *Br. Heart J.*, 46, 498–502

23. Veteran's Administration Co-operative Study Group on Anti-hypertensive Agents. (1982). Comparison of propranolol and hydrochlorothiazide for the initial treatment of hypertension I. *J. Am. Med. Assoc.*, 248, 1996–2003

24. Veteran's Administration Co-operative Study Group on Anti-Hypertensive Agents. (1977). Propranolol in the treatment of essential hypertension. *J. Am. Med. Assoc.*, 237, 2303–10

25. Zacharias, F.J., Cowen, K.J., Cuthbertson, P.J.R., Johnson, T.W.B., Prestt, J., Thompson, J., Vickers, J., Simpson, W.T. and Touson, R. (1977). Atenolol in hypertension: a study of long-term therapy. *Postgrad. Med. J.*, 53, (Suppl. 3), 102–110

26. Report of M.R.C. working party on mild to moderate hypertension. (1981). Adverse reactions to bendrofluazide and propranolol for the treatment of mild hypertension. *Lancet*, 2, 539–43

27. Cruikshank, J.M. (1983). How safe are beta-blockers. *Drugs*, **25**, (Suppl. 2) 331–40.
28. Greenblatt, D.J. and Koch-Weser, J. (1974). Adverse reactions to beta-adrenergic receptor blocking drugs. A report from the Boston Collaborative surveillance programme. *Drugs*, **7**, 118–29
29. Barnett, A.H., Leslie, D. and Watkins, P.J. (1980). Can insulin treated diabetics be given beta-blocking drugs? *Br. Med. J.* **1**, 976–8
30. Lager, I., Blohme, G. and Smith, U. (1979). Effective cardio-selective and non-selective beta-blockade on the hypoglycaemic response in insulin dependent diabetes. *Lancet*, **1**, 458–62
31. Day, J.L., Metcalfe, J. and Simpson, C.W. (1982). Adenergic mechanisms in control of plasma lipid concentration. *Br. Med. J.*, **284**, 1145–8
32. Anderson, J., Godfrey, B.E., Hill, D.M., Munro-Faure, A.D. and Sheldon, J. (1971). A comparison of the effects of hydrochlorothiazide and of frusemide in the treatment of hypertensive patients. *Q. J. Med.*, **40**, 541–60
33. VA Co-operative Study Group on Anti-hypertensive Agents. (1982). Comparison of propranolol and hydrochlorothiazide for the initial treatment of hypertension II. Results of longterm study. *J. Am. Med. Assoc.*, **248**, 2004–11
34. Ramsay, L.E., Boyle, P. and Ramsey, M.H. (1977). Factors influencing serum potassium in treated hypertension. *Q. J. Med.*, **46**, 401–10
35. Ramsay, L.E., Hettiarchi, J., Frazer, R. and Morton, J.J. (1980). Amiloride, spironolactone and potassium chloride in thiazide treated hypertensive patients. *Clin. Pharmacol. Ther.*, **27**, 533–43
36. M.R.C. Working Party on mild to moderate hypertension. (1983). Ventricular extrasystoles during thiazide treatment. Substudy of M.R.C. mild hypertension trial. *Br. Med. J.*, **287**, 1249–53
37. Struthers, A.D., Whitesmith, R. and Reid, J.C. (1983). Prior thiazide diuretic treatment increases adrenaline-induced hypokalaemia. *Lancet*, **1**, 1358–61
38. Murphy, M.B., Lewis, P.J., Koehner, E., Schumer, B. and Dollery, C.T. (1982). Glucose intolerance in hypertensive patients treated with diuretics. A 14 year follow up. *Lancet*, **2**, 1293–5
39. Bergman, G. and Andersson O. (1981). Betablocker with diuretics in hypertension. A six year follow up of blood pressure and metabolic side effects. *Lancet*, **1**, 744–7
40. Multiple risk factor intervention trial research group. (1982). Multiple risk factor intervention trial; Risk factor changes and mortality results. *J. Am. Med. Assoc.*, **248**, 1465–77
41. Morgan, F.O., Adam, W.R., Hodgson, M. and Gibbar, R.S. (1980). Failure of therapy to improve prognosis in elderly males with hypertension. *Med. J. Austr.*, **2**, 27–31
42. McAreavey, D., Ramsay, L.E., Latham, L. *et al.* (1984). 'Third Drug' Trial; A comparative study of antihypertensive agents added to treatment when blood pressure remains uncontrolled by a betablocker plus thiazide diuretic. *Br. Med. J.*, **288**, 106–11
43. Zacest, R., Gilmore, E. and Koch-Weser, J. (1972). Treatment of essential hypertension with combined vasodilation and beta-adrenergic blockade. *N. Engl. J. Med.*, **286**, 617–22
44. Shepherd, A.M.M., Ludden, T.M., McMay, J.L. and Lynn, M.S. (1980). Hydralazine kinetics after single and repeated oral doses. *Clin. Pharmacol. Ther.*, **28**, 804–11
45. Ramsay, L.E., Silas, J.H., Ollerenshaw, J.D., Tucker, G.T., Phillips, F.C. and Freestone, S. (1984). Should the acetylator phenotype be determined when prescribing hydralazine for hypertension? *Eur. J. Clin. Pharmacol.*, **26**, 39–42
46. Silas, J.H., Freestone, S. and Ramsey, L.E. (1982). Hydralazine once daily in hypertension. *Br. Med. J.*, **284**, 1602–4
47. Perry, H.M. (1973). Late toxicity to hydralazine resembling system lupus erythematosus or rheumatoid arthritis. *J. Am. Med. Assoc.*, **54**, 58–72

48. Bachelor, J.R., Walsh, K., Tenoko, R.M. *et al.* (1980). Hydralazine induced systemic lupus erythematosus; influences of HLA DR and sex on susceptibility. *Lancet*, **1**, 1107–9

49. Jaillon, P. (1980). Clinical pharmacokinetics of prazosin. *Clin. Pharmacokinetics*, **5**, 365–76

50. Rubin, P.C. and Blaschke, J.F. (1980). Studies on the clinical pharmacology of prazosin I. Cardiovascular, catecholamine and endocrine changes following a single dose. *Br. J. Clin. Pharmacol.*, **10**, 23–32

51. Sjoerdsma, A., Vendslau, A. and Engleman, K. (1963). Studies on the metabolism and mechanism of action of methyldopa. *Circulation*, **28**, 492–502

52. Kwan, K.C., Faltz, E.L., Breault, G.O., Baer, J.E. and Tataro, J.A. (1976). Pharmacokinetics of methyldopa in Man. *J. Pharmacol. Exp. Ther.*, **198**, 264–77

53. Webster, J., Jeffers, T.A., Galloway, D.B., Petrie, J.C. and Barker, M.P. (1977). Atenolol, methyldopa and chlorthalidone in moderate hypertension. *Br. Med. J.*, **1**, 76–8

54. Carstairs, K.C., Worrlledge, S.M., Dollery, C.T. and Breckenridge, A. (1966). Methyldopa and haemolytic anaemia. *Lancet*, **1**, 201

55. Kirkland, H.H., Mohler, D.N. and Horowitz, D.A. (1980). Methyldopa inhibition of suppressor lymphocyte function. A proposed cause of an auto-immune haemolytic anaemia. *N. Engl. J. Med.*, **302**, 825–32.

56. Campese, D.M. (1981). Minoxidil: a review of its pharmacological properties and therapeutic use. *Drugs*, **22**, 257–78

57. Johnson, B.F., Black, H.R., Beckner, R., Vyner, B. and Angeletti, F. (1983). A comparison of minoxidil and hydralazine in non-azotaemic hypertensives. *J. Hypertension*, **1**, 103–7

58. Takeda, T., Kaneko, Y., Omae, T., Yoshinga, K., Masuyama, Y., Nukada, T. and Shigiya, R. (1982). The use of labetalol in Japan: results of multicentre clinical trials. *Br. J. Clin. Pharmacol.*, **13**, (Suppl. 1), 49S–58S

59. Waal-Manning, H.J. and Simpson, F.O. (1982). Review of long-term treatment with labetalol. *Br. J. Clin. Pharmacol.*, **13**, (Suppl. 1) 65S–74S

60. Johnson, C.I., Jackson, B., McGrath, B., Matthews, G. and Arnolda, L. (1983). Relationship of antihypertensive effect of enalapril to serum MK 422 levels and angiotensin converting enzyme inhibition. *J. Hypertension*, **1** (Suppl. 1), 71–5

61. VA Co-operative study group on antihypertensive agents. (1982). Captopril: evaluation of low doses twice daily doses and the addition of diuretic for the treatment of mild to moderate hypertension. *Clin. Sci.*, **63**, 433S–445S

62. Arr, S.M., Burgess, J., Cooper, W.D. *et al.* (1984). A comparative study of enalapril and atenolol in moderate to severe hypertension. *Br. J. Clin. Pharmacol.*, **18**, 31P

63. Dollery, C.T. (1983) Safety and efficacy of enalapril: summing up the evidence. *J. Hypertension (Suppl. 1)*, **1**, 155–7

64. Hodsman, G.P., Isles, C.G., Murray, G.D., Usherwood, T.P., Webb, D.J. and Robertson, J.I.S. (1983). Factors related to the first dose hypotensive effect of captopril prediction and treatment. *Br. Med. J.*, **286**, 832–4

65. Hrick, D.E., Browning, P.J., Kopelman, R., Goorna, W.E., Madias, N.E. and Dazu, D.J. (1983). Captopril induced functional renal insufficiency in patients with bilateral renal artery stenosis or renal artery stenosis in a solitary kidney. *N. Engl. J. Med.*, **308**, 373–6

66. Wenting, G.J., Tan-Tjiong, H.L., Derkx, F.H.M. *et al.* (1984). Split renal function after captopril with unilateral renal artery stenosis. *Br. Med. J.*, **288**, 886–90

67. Robinson, B.F., Dobbs, R.J. and Bayley, S. (1982). Response of forearm resistance vessels to verapamil and sodium nitroprusside in normotensive and hypertensive men: Evidence for a functional abnormality of vascular smooth muscle in primary hypertension. *Clin. Sci.*, **63**, 33–42

68. Heagerty, A.M., Bing, R.F., Thurston, H. and Swales, J.D. (1983). Calcium antagonists in hypertension: Relation to abnormal sodium transport. *Br. Med. J.*, **287**, 1405–7

69. Hornung, R.S., Gould, B.A., Jones, R.I., Sonecha, T. and Raftery, E.B. (1983). Nifedipine tablets for hypertension. A study using continuous ambulatory intra-arterial monitoring. *Postgrad. Med. J.* 59, (Suppl. 2) 95-7
70. Hornung, R.S. (1983). Calcium antagonists in hypertension. In Jackson, W. (ed.) *Calcium Antagonists Today and Tomorrow*, pp. 49-53. (Medicine Publishing Foundation)
71. Murphy, M.B., Scriven, A.J. and Dollery C.T. (1983). Role of nifedipine in treatment of hypertension. *Br. Med. J.*, 287, 257-9
72. Yagil, Y., Leibel, B., Kobrin, I., Stressman, J. and Ishay, D.B. (1983). A combination of propranolol and nifedipine in the treatment of hypertension: Acute and longterm effects. *Postgrad. Med. J.*, 59, (Suppl. 2) 114-18
73. Dunstan, H.P., Tarazi, R.C., Bravo, E.L. (1976). False tolerance to antihypertensive drugs. In Sambhi, M.P. (ed.) *Systemic Effects of Antihypertensive Agents*, pp. 51-73. (New York: Stratton)
74. Geyskes, G.G., Puylaert, C.B.A., Dei, H.Y. and Dorhout Mees, E.J. (1983). Follow up study of 70 patients with renal artery stenosis treated by percutaneous transluminal dilation. *Br. Med. J.*, 287, 333-6
75. Ramsay, L.E., Silas, J.H. and Freestone, S. (1980). Diuretic treatment of resistant hypertension. *Br. Med. J.*, 281, 1101-3
76. Freestone, S., Ramsay, L.E. and Silas, J.H. (1982). A controlled trial of frusemide versus high dose thiazide in resistant hypertension. *Br. J. Clin. Pharmacol.*, 14, 137P-138P
77. Freestone, S., Ramsay, L.E. and Silas, J.H. (1982). Hypertensive effect of spironolactone when added to bendrofluazide in resistant hypertension. *Br. J. Clin. Pharmacol.*, 151, 622P-623P
78. Strandgaard, S. (1976). Autoregulation and cerebral blood flow in hypertensive patients. *Circulation.* 53, 720-7
79. Bertel, O., Connen, D., Radu, E.W., Miller, J., Lang, C. and Duback, U.C. (1983). Nifedipine in hypertensive emergencies. *Br. Med. J.*, 286, 19-20
80. Koch-Weser, J. (1976). Diazoxide. *N. Engl. J. Med.*, 294, 1271-4
81. Palmer, R.F. and Lasseter, K.C. (1975). Sodium nitroprusside. *N. Engl. J. Med.*, 294, 294-7
82. Report on confidential enquiries into maternal deaths in England and Wales (1979) (Department of Health & Social Security 1973-75), pp. 21-9. (London: HMSO)
83. Chamberlain, G. (1981). Raised blood pressure in pregnancy. The foetus in hypertension. *Br. J. Hosp. Med.*, 26, 127-133
84. Rubin, P.C., Butters, L., Clark, D.M. *et al.* (1983). Placebo-controlled trial of atenolol treatment of pregnancy associated hypertension. *Lancet*, 1, 431-4
85. Rubin, P.C. (1981). Betablockers in pregnancy. *N. Engl. J. Med.*, 305, 1323-6
86. Svensson, A., Andersch, B. and Hansson, L. (1983). Prediction of later hypertension following a hypertensive pregnancy. *J. Hypertension*, 1 (Suppl. 2), 94-6

2
Drug treatment of angina pectoris

G.D. JOHNSTON

INTRODUCTION

Although this chapter is concerned mainly with the use of drugs in the symptomatic treatment of angina pectoris, it is important to examine other forms of therapy at the onset, in particular coronary artery surgery, in order to select the appropriate therapy for the individual patient.

The decision to embark on medical or surgical treatment depends on many factors such as the patient's age, his occupation, the degree of disability, site and severity of the lesions, myocardial function, psychological make-up and the presence of associated conditions such as diabetes mellitus, hypertension and renal and pulmonary disease. Even if surgery is considered to be the treatment of choice, drug therapy may be required afterwards. Stable angina associated with single or double vessel coronary disease is probably best treated medically. Unstable angina, significant left main coronary stenosis and high grade triple vessel coronary disease are indications for surgical intervention. In making the decision, however, myocardial function, the presence of other medical conditions and patient preference must be taken into consideration[1].

In addition, before embarking on medical treatment for angina, certain other aspects of therapy should be considered. Epidemiological evidence indicates that the incidence of ischaemic heart disease is increased in smokers as is the risk of developing a myocardial infarction[2]. This, combined with the tendency of smoking to increase heart rate, systolic blood pressure and hypoxia[3], makes it essential for the patients with angina to stop smoking. A reduction in dietary saturated fat intake is probably beneficial as is an increase in the proportion of polyunsaturated fats although the evidence is by no means conclusive[4]. The use of cholesterol lowering drugs is more contentious. Recent studies with clofibrate suggest that this drug, although appearing to reduce the incidence of non-fatal ischaemic heart disease, does not

49

prevent coronary deaths, and the risk of dying from other causes appears to be increased[5]. The place for cholesterol lowering drugs now seems to be limited to the high risk individuals with familial hypercholesterolaemia[5]. A reduction in weight is clearly beneficial but unsuccessful in the majority of patients in the long term. An increase in exercise has become a very popular intervention. Although evidence is at present lacking that such patients live longer if they exercise, beneficial effects have been described in selected cases[6].

RATIONALE FOR THE USE OF DRUGS IN ANGINA PECTORIS

Pathophysiology of angina pectoris

Angina pectoris occurs when there is an imbalance between myocardial oxygen supply and demand. Myocardial oxygen supply is principally dependent on coronary blood flow while demand depends on a variety of factors including heart rate and arterial blood pressure[7].

Control of coronary blood flow

There are three main determinants of coronary blood flow – aortic diastolic pressure (perfusion pressure), the duration of diastole and coronary vascular resistance. During exercise and conditions associated with increased sympathetic activity, increased heart rate and duration of diastole are the limiting factors. The main determinant of coronary blood flow, however, is vascular resistance which is controlled by the small coronary arteries and arterioles where vessel diameter can be varied considerably. Changes in diameter result from contraction of vascular smooth muscle (autoregulation) or extravascular myocardial compression due to ventricular contraction. During ventricular systole, compression causes a marked decrease in vascular resistance which effectively prevents coronary blood flow during this part of the cardiac cycle. These compressive forces are not uniform across the ventricular wall and are greatest in the subendocardium and least in the subepicardium[8]. Tone of the resistance vessels is modified by neurogenic, humoral and myogenic factors, but principally by local myocardial metabolism[9].

Advanced coronary artery atherosclerosis interferes with the regulation of coronary blood flow by adding fixed resistance in series with the resistance vessels. If stenosis is severe or metabolic demands increase, metabolic needs cannot be maintained and myocardial ischaemia results. Because of systolic compression, the subendocardium is more sensitive to coronary artery narrowing and is most vulnerable to myocardial ischaemia.

An equally serious obstruction to flow can arise as a result of intense vasospasm in the coronary artery in the absence of atheroma. Such a mechanism underlies the variant of angina described by Prinzmetal[10], which characteristically affects younger people and comes on at rest and not after exertion.

Factors influencing myocardial oxygen demand

Unlike skeletal muscle, human cardiac muscle cannot maintain any measure of oxygen debt during stress and pay this back later. Heart muscle also maintains greater cellular activity at rest than skeletal muscle, extracting 75% of the available oxygen under basal conditions[1]. Both factors clearly render the heart more vulnerable when coronary blood flow is reduced.

Myocardial oxygen requirements increase when there is an increase in heart rate, contractility (as with exercise or emotion), arterial pressure (hypertension) or ventricular volume (heart failure)[11,12]. Other factors which may play a part include basal metabolic rate, activation of contraction and fibre shortening which can become major determinants of myocardial oxygen in certain pathological conditions[12] (Figure 2.1).

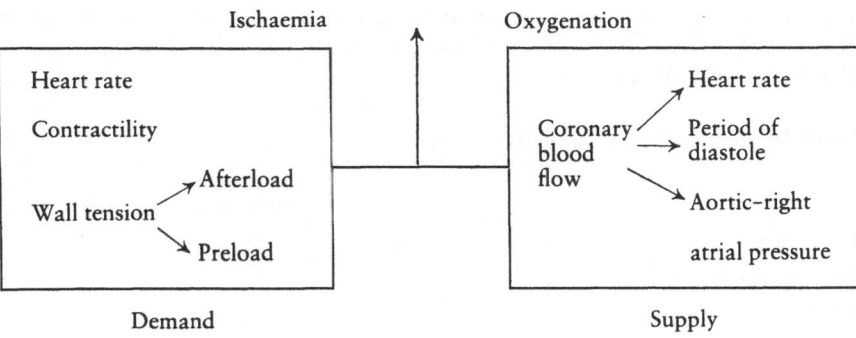

Figure 2.1 The oxygen supply/demand balance

The purpose of therapy in angina pectoris is twofold: firstly to relieve the symptoms and secondly to arrest or delay progression of the underlying disease. Until recently the emphasis in the treatment of myocardial ischaemia was symptomatic and this chapter is mainly devoted to this area of therapy. The possibility of improving survival in ischaemic heart disease is fast moving from a theoretical concept to a practical reality and has led to the idea of cardioprotection.

Cardioprotection – the possible role of anginal drugs

Evidence is growing to show that some antianginal drugs may protect the myocardium from irreversible damage during a period of ischaemia. For example there is experimental evidence to show that β-adrenoceptor blocking agents reduce the high catecholamine levels associated with ischaemia and so reduce the risk of arrhythmia and thrombus formation[13,14]. Similarly it has been demonstrated in animals that calcium antagonists reduce the extent of myocardial damage occurring after ischaemia and reperfusion by limiting the entry of calcium into ischaemic cells[15]. As yet no satisfactory clinical study of a calcium antagonist has been completed but the majority of the evidence now points to a significant protective effect of certain β-adrenoceptor blocking drugs in patients during the period following a myocardial infarction[16-19]. One might speculate that a similar protective effect might occur in patients with angina who have not had a myocardial infarction. As yet no convincing data on primary prevention are available.

Symptomatic relief – the role of antianginal drugs

It is clear from the discussion on the pathophysiology of angina pectoris that to produce symptomatic improvement, a drug must increase the blood supply to the myocardium and/or reduce demand. The main effects of the commonly used antianginal drugs are summarized in **Table 2.1**. The effects of combined therapy with all three groups of drugs are also illustrated.

Table 2.1 Main effects of antianginal drugs

	Nitrates	β-Blockers	Calcium antagonists	Combination
Heart rate	↑ *	↓	* ↑→	↓
Blood pressure	↓	↓	↓	↓
Wall tension	↓	↑	↓	↓
Contractility	↑ *	↓	↓	↓
Coronary flow	↑	↑	↑	↑

Actions of each class of drug alone or in combination
*Reflex changes mediated by the sympathetic nervous system

Nitrates

The nitrates have been the mainstay of treatment of angina pectoris since the use of amyl nitrate was described by Brunton in 1867[20]. Twelve years later Murrel described the use of nitroglycerin for this condition[21].

Chemistry and mode of action

The nitrates used in the treatment of angina pectoris are simple nitric acid esters of polyalcohols (Figure 2.2).

All therapeutically active agents in this group release nitrate ions (NO_2) in vascular smooth muscle which then react with specific receptors containing sulphhydryl ($-SH$) groups. Little is known about the steps linking receptor binding of the nitrate ion to vascular smooth muscle but experimental evidence suggests that cGMP[22] and vasodilatory prostaglandins (PGE_2 and PGI_2)[23,24] are involved.

The basic pharmacological effect of the nitrates is the widespread and non-specific relaxation of smooth muscle. The most striking cardiovascular responses are in the peripheral circulation where marked dilatation of the capacitance vessels results in a gravity dependent reduction in venous pressure and decreases in the left ventricular volume[25-27]. In addition there is dilatation of the large conductance arteries and to a lesser degree, the small arterioles. The overall effect is a modest decrease in systemic vascular resistance[25-27]. This and the decrease in venous pressure usually result in a slight overall decrease in

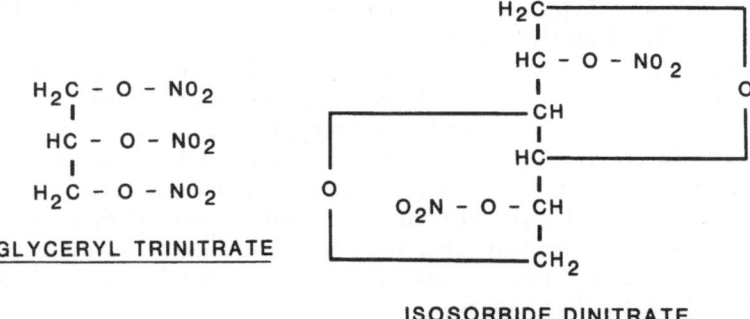

Figure 2.2 Structure of nitrates used in treatment of angina pectoris

arterial blood pressure. Decreases in ventricular volume and systolic blood pressure combine to decrease ventricular wall tension, a major determinant of myocardial oxygen requirements. Although nitrates induce a reflex increase in heart rate and myocardial contractility which tend to increase myocardial oxygen demand, this is overshadowed by the reduction in ventricular wall tension previously described.

Nitrates also appear to alter the haemodynamic responses to exercise[28,29]. End-diastolic and peak systolic pressures are reduced as is the response of the ischaemic myocardium to adrenergic stimulation.

Although not a major mode of action, coronary dilatation occurs in certain clinical situations. In angina pectoris with fixed stenosis, nitrates probably do not increase total coronary blood flow although causing coronary artery dilatation. However, improved regional blood flow to ischaemic areas may be important in some patients, although there is controversy as to the beneficial effects of nitrates on collateral coronary and subendocardial vessels where blood supply tends to be poorest[30–35]. Coronary artery dilatation probably accounts for most of the therapeutic benefit seen in patients with coronary artery spasm[36].

Choice of nitrate (administration and dose)

Glyceryl trinitrate has been the mainstay of treatment for angina pectoris for over a century. The haemodynamic effects of glyceryl trinitrate last only for about 30 minutes, however, so that various attempts have been made recently to prolong the duration of effect of the nitrates and so make them suitable for prophylactic use. Therefore – in addition to sublingual preparations – oral, chewable, transdermal, transmucosal and intravenous forms are now available.

Sublingual glyceryl trinitrate

Sublingual nitroglycerin should be administered initially at the smallest possible dose (300 μg) and this increased to a maximum of 1200 μg if required. The drug should be taken as early as possible after the onset of angina, or preferably used prophylactically before activities which might cause angina such as walking uphill, emotional upset and sexual intercourse. If chest pain persists, glyceryl trinitrate can be repeated at 5-minute intervals until pain relief is achieved. Clearly if relief is not obtained, medical advice should be sought. It is important to explain carefully the use of glyceryl trinitrate to the patient. Patients often do not take glyceryl trinitrate promptly because they believe that it may be an addicting analgesic or take too large an initial dose, with resulting headache and hypotension.

Oral nitrates

There is some debate concerning the oral administration of long acting nitrates such as isosorbide dinitrate[37,38]. When nitrates are orally administered they undergo extensive first pass metabolism suggesting that the oral route is likely to be ineffective[39]. However, clinical studies seem to show definite beneficial haemodynamic effects up to 4–6 hours with oral nitrates[40–42] and there is evidence that isosorbide mononitrate has a reduced biotransformation during first pass through the liver[43].

When long acting oral nitrates are used in adequate doses (for example isosorbide dinitrate doses of up to 240 mg/day) and are carefully titrated to produce maximum effect with minimum adverse effects in the individual patient, they can be of considerable value in the symptomatic treatment of angina pectoris. Orally acting nitrates can also provide effective relief of coronary arterial spasm in both induced and spontaneous forms although they do not appear to be as effective as calcium antagonist drugs in this situation.

Buccal nitrate

This is a form of glyceryl trinitrate in which the chemical is impregnated into an inert polymer matrix allowing diffusion from the tablet across the buccal mucosa. The tablet surface rapidly develops a gel-like coating which forms a surrounding seal and allows the tablets to adhere to the mucosal surface of the mouth. Absorption occurs provided the pill remains in an intact form. Chewing the tablet negates the desired effect and can cause a large amount of the drug to be absorbed unless immediately swallowed. Buccal nitrate formulation has an onset of action comparable to that of sublingual glyceryl trinitrate but achieves its maximum effect about 30 min later. Activity is sustained for up to 6 h, the tablet remaining pharmacologically active provided it remains in the mouth. Studies to date indicate that this formulation is well tolerated in most patients and provides prompt and sustained relief of symptoms in angina[44].

Transdermal nitrates

The use of cutaneous nitroglycerin was described as early as 1955[45] but this route of administration did not become popular until 1974, when a sustained therapeutic effect was demonstrated[46]. The two most common preparations are glyceryl trinitrate ointment which lasts about 4–6 h and slow release preparations which allow continuous absorption over a 24 h period.

For the standard ointment, the delay in onset is about 30 min and the time course is similar to oral isosorbide dinitrate. The absorption is dependent on site and blood flow[47] and large doses are often required to produce adequate therapeutic effect (up to 30 g). Because of the cumbersome nature of the treatment, skin irritation and variable absorption, there is little to recommend this form of therapy at the present time.

Various slow release preparations have recently been marketed. Each uses a nitroglycerin reservoir which allows gradual absorption over a 24 h period. Despite the recent popularity of these methods of nitrate administration, convincing data on their efficacy and duration of effect are not yet available. Adequate doses of oral nitrates are probably equally effective and less expensive.

Intravenous nitrates

Intravenous nitrates are useful in managing unstable or variant angina pectoris unresponsive to other medical therapy[48,49]. The doses required for pain relief vary widely[50] and there appears to be little correlation between the infusion rate, plasma concentration and haemodynamic effects[51]. Intravenous glyceryl trinitrate has a short elimination half-life and is extensively metabolized to less active metabolites, all of which are excreted within the urine within 24 h[52]. Episodes of angina have been reported to decrease by 70–90% and some patients may require less narcotic analgesia[53,54].

The dosage of intravenous glyceryl trinitrate is usually started at 5 μg/min and adjusted until maximum pain relief is achieved[55]. Dose adjustment is difficult because the drug is absorbed to the polyvinyl chloride infusion sets. The haemodynamic responses are therefore different during the first 4 hours when the plastic is becoming saturated with the drug[56].

Intravenous glyceryl trinitrate is generally well tolerated with careful monitoring. Hypotension occurs in approximately 20% of patients but can be controlled by reducing the infusion rate or stopping the drug. Headaches are reported in only 2% of patients and are usually mild. Sinus bradycardia (4%) and tachycardia (1%), probably related to autonomic effects, have been reported[54,55].

Pharmacokinetics

The use of organic nitrates is strongly influenced by the presence of a high capacity hepatic organic nitrate reductase which inactivates the drug[57]. The bioavailability of most orally administered organic nitrates is very low (typically less than 10%). If therapeutic levels of the drug are required rapidly, the sublingual route is preferred. Both glyceryl trinitrate and isosorbide dinitrate are absorbed efficiently by this route and achieve therapeutic plasma levels within a few minutes. If sufficient doses of oral, buccal, and possibly dermal, nitrate preparations are used, adequate plasma concentrations can be achieved despite extensive first pass hepatic metabolism. Intravenous glyceryl trinitrate is rapidly effective and extensively metabolized but there is little correlation between plasma concentration of the drug and clinical effect[58].

Unchanged nitrates have half-lives of only 2–8 min. The principal metabolites have longer elimination half lives (1–3 h) but are less potent vasodilators. Excretion mainly as the glucuronide occurs via the kidney.

Adverse effects

The major acute toxic effects of the organic nitrates are direct extensions of therapeutic vasodilatation: orthostatic hypotension, tachycardia and throbbing headache which are more severe when combined with other vasodilators, including alcohol. Occasionally, excessive tachycardia occurs in response to hypotension and angina may be worsened. Glaucoma, once thought to be a contraindication, is not made worse by the use of these drugs but nitrates are still contraindicated in the presence of raised intracranial pressure. Long term therapy with long acting nitrates, even in large doses, is not associated with clinically important tolerance[59,60]. Nitrate ions react with haemoglobin (containing ferrous iron) to produce methaemoglobin (containing ferric iron). The amount of methaemoglobin formed is small and unimportant clinically even if large doses of organic nitrate are used. There is no evidence of physical dependence to therapeutic doses of organic nitrates.

Interactions with nitrates

Phenobarbitone enhances the metabolism of glyceryl trinitrate[60] but this effect is probably clinically unimportant[61]. Ethanol on the other hand acts as an enzyme inhibitor and appears to increase the drug's vasodilator activity[60]. The hypotensive effects of tricyclic antidepressants are increased when the drugs are used with nitrates[60] and preliminary data suggest that indomethacin inhibits the peripheral vasodilatory effects of the nitrates, probably by reducing prostaglandin E synthesis[62].

β-Adrenoceptor blocking drugs

Mechanism of action in angina pectoris

Agents used to treat angina pectoris work either by increasing myocardial oxygen supply and/or by reducing myocardial oxygen consumption. β-Adrenoceptor blocking drugs antagonize the effects of catecholamines at the β-adrenoceptor receptors by occupying the receptors and competitively reducing catecholamine receptor occupancy. This results in prominent cardiac effects which are predictable from the known effects of catecholamines. β-Blocking drugs therefore reduce heart rate, particularly exercise heart rate, myocardial contractility and systemic blood pressure. The net effect is to reduce myocardial oxygen consumption, although in some clinical situations decreased myocardial contractility can lead to enlargement of the heart and increased oxygen consumption[63].

Canine experiments with propranolol suggest that propranolol improves blood flow in ischaemic myocardial segments[64]. However, this has not been confirmed in man[65].

Undesirable effects of β-adrenoceptor blocking drugs include an increase in end-diastolic volume which accompanies the bradycardia and increase in ejection time. The increases in myocardial oxygen requirements associated with these changes can largely be balanced by the concomitant use of nitrates.

Choice of β-blocker

A variety of β-adrenoceptor blocking compounds are available for use in angina pectoris. Several studies have confirmed that most presently available β-blocking drugs are equally effective in the treatment of angina pectoris provided the doses of drug are equipotent[66]. Two properties which could influence one's choice of β-adrenoceptor blocking drug include intrinsic sympathomimetic activity (ISA) and β_1 selectivity. It is doubtful whether ISA confers any real advantages in the treatment of angina pectoris[67] but agents with this property probably have less effects on the peripheral circulation. ISA may also protect against congestive heart failure, depression of atrioventricular conduction and bradycardia[68–70] associated with β-blockade. These potentially useful properties are counterbalanced by the consideration that partial agonist activity may be undesirable in angina occurring at rest or at low exercise levels[71].

Although cardioselectivity theoretically offers some advantages by not blocking the coronary β_2-receptors which oppose the vasoconstrictor effects of α-stimulation, no clinical superiority has been demonstrated.

Selection of patients

Since there is growing evidence that β-adrenoceptor blocking agents improve survival after a myocardial infarction[72] and may be of value in primary prevention, there would seem to be a case for treating even mild cases of angina with β-adrenoceptor blocking drugs. Some characteristics of the patients with angina will influence the choice of preparation. Patients with bradycardia at rest may benefit from a drug with intrinsic sympathomimetic activity while a β-blocker without this property would be preferable in a patient with angina at rest. Patients with asthma or insulin-dependent diabetes are less likely to develop problems with cardioselective agents, although it is probably better to prescribe a calcium antagonist or nitrate in these circumstances. Drugs with ISA and cardioselectivity are probably preferable in patients with peripheral vascular disease[68] but again, if possible, β-blocking drugs are best avoided in this situation.

Dose adjustment

The plasma concentration–effect relationships of the β-adrenoceptor antagonists in angina are complex. Calculations of maximum β-blockade based on competitive antagonism to isoprenaline or reduction of an exercise tachycardia do not always relate easily to the clinical situation. Plasma concentration measurement is rarely helpful in dose adjustment. It has been suggested that maximum blockade with propranolol occurs at plasma concentrations around 100 ng/ml although levels as high as 500 ng/ml have been recorded in some patients[73,74]. There is no evidence that plasma concentration measurement is of any value for dose selection with any of the other β-adrenoceptor blocking drugs.

It has also been suggested that a resting heart rate of 50–60 beats/

minute represents adequate β-blockade. This is often a poor guide in many patients because resting heart rate is largely determined by vagal activity and varies widely between individuals. Lower heart rates are often acceptable provided the patient is asymptomatic. Clearly the resting heart rate cannot be used as a measure of β-blockade with drugs which have intrinsic sympathomimetic activity. Exercise heart rate is a better measure of drug effect but does not lend itself to routine assessment of patients with angina pectoris[75].

Pharmacokinetics

Most drugs in this class are well absorbed after oral administration, with peak concentrations about 1-3 hours after ingestion. Sustained release preparations are available. Oral bioavailability is variable largely due to variations in 'first pass' metabolism (Table 2.2).

Table 2.2

	Elimination half-life (hours)	Bioavailability (%)
Propranolol	3-6	30
Metoprolol	3-4	50
Atenolol	6-9	40
Nadolol	14-24	30
Timolol	4-5	50
Pindolol	3-4	100

The drugs are rapidly distributed and have large volumes of distribution. Most are rapidly eliminated (Table 2.2). Propranolol and metoprolol are extensively metabolized in the liver with little unchanged drug appearing in the urine. Pindolol and atenolol are less completely metabolized. Nadolol is excreted unchanged in the urine and has a longer elimination half-life. The elimination of drugs with extensive first pass metabolism is prolonged in the presence of liver disease, reduced liver blood flow or hepatic enzyme inhibition. The elimination half-life of nadolol is prolonged in renal failure. It is worth remembering that the clinical effects of these drugs are often prolonged beyond the time predicted from the half-life data[67].

Adverse effects

A variety of minor adverse effects occur with propranolol. Central nervous system effects include sedation, sleep disturbance and depression. Rash, fever and other allergic manifestations are rare.

The major adverse effects of β-receptor antagonist drugs relate to the predictable pharmacological results of β-blockade. Drugs with β_2-receptor blocking activity tend to make obstructive airways disease worse and mild asthma may become severe after β_2-blockade. While

β_1-selective drugs may have less effect on airways than the non-selective group, they must be used very cautiously, if at all, in patients with reversible airways obstruction.

β-Receptor blockade depresses myocardial contractility and excitability. In patients with abnormal myocardial function, cardiac output can depend on increased sympathetic activity. Removal of this activity can result in cardiac decompensation and even small doses (e.g. 10 mg propranolol) can provoke severe cardiac failure in susceptible individuals. Great caution must be exercised in using this group of drugs in patients following an acute myocardial infarction or with compensated congestive heart failure. Five per cent of patients on propranolol have symptoms closely resembling those of Raynaud's phenomenon, or complain that their claudication is worse[76]. This is in part due to unopposed α-stimulation but reduced cardiac output also contributes, especially in patients with ischaemic heart disease.

Catecholamines increase glycogenolysis and cause increases in blood glucose levels. In addition lipolysis is enhanced and free fatty acids are released from adipose tissue. β-Blocking drugs (especially non-selective) antagonize these metabolic effects and reduce insulin secretion. Hypoglycaemic reactions have been reported during β-blocking therapy both in diabetics using insulin and healthy volunteers receiving sulphonylureas. Of greater clinical importance is their effect on antagonizing adrenergic responses to hypoglycaemia. This prolongs the duration of the attack and makes the diagnosis of insulin- or drug-induced hypoglycaemia more difficult. The true incidence of this condition is unknown and many patients receiving insulin with β-adrenoceptor blocking drugs do not suffer from adverse effects. However it would be advisable to avoid these drugs in insulin-dependent diabetics, especially those who are liable to develop hypoglycaemia if alternatives are available. β_1-Selective adrenoceptor blocking agents are considered to be safer in this situation.

Other adverse effects of β-adrenoceptor blocking agents include nausea, constipation and diarrhoea; these effects are mostly mild and rarely necessitate drug withdrawal[76]. Renal function sometimes deteriorates during treatment with β-blocking drugs, probably due to impaired renal blood flow.

Sudden withdrawal of β-blockade

Present evidence suggests that patients with ischaemic heart disease may be at increased risk of developing sudden deterioration in their clinical condition following withdrawal of their β-adrenoceptor blocking agent[77,78]. The mechanism of this effect is uncertain but might involve 'up regulation' in the number of β-receptors. Patients should be warned of the possible dangers of stopping the drugs suddenly and, in those in whom withdrawal is indicated, gradual tapering rather than abrupt cessation should be employed.

Use in variant and unstable angina

Although there is growing evidence that coronary bypass surgery should be undertaken early in the management of unstable angina[79], medical therapy also has a part to play[80].

The use of large doses of β-blockers in this condition remains controversial. Episodes of unstable angina are frequently due to coronary artery spasm which can be made worse by this group of drugs, probably as a result of unopposed α-agonist activity in the coronary arteries[81,82]. Since the drugs are useful in patients with fixed stenosis, it is important to identify this group when therapy with β-adrenoceptor blocking drugs is embarked upon. Some patients with variant angina may benefit, however, from treatment with β-blocking drugs, but as a general rule it is preferable to prescribe a calcium antagonist and/or a nitrate.

Calcium antagonists

Chemistry and mode of action

Verapamil, the first clinically useful member of the group, was the result of attempts to synthesize more active analogues of papaverine, a vasodilator alkaloid found in the opium poppy. Since then several substances of widely varying structure have been shown to have the same fundamental pharmacological action (Figure 2.3).

The calcium antagonists act by inhibiting post-excitation influx of calcium into myocardial cells and the cells of vascular smooth muscle. This interferes with the action of calcium dependent ATPase which is required for the energy needs of myocardial contractility and smooth muscle contraction. The overall effect is a reduction in myocardial contractility and dilatation of vascular smooth muscle. The agents selectively block calcium channels and leave the sodium channels relatively unaffected. Therefore myocardial contractility (dependent on calcium ions) is reduced while myocardial depolarization (dependent on sodium ions) is largely unaffected. In patients with angina pectoris the overall effect is to reduce myocardial oxygen demands and reflex tachycardia does not appear to be a problem. The vasodilating properties are not confined to systemic arteries, but also affect the coronary arteries so that under certain clinical conditions oxygen supply to the myocardium can be increased. It is probably this property which makes them the drugs of first choice in the treatment of angina where arterial spasm plays a major role[83]. Occasionally calcium antagonists aggravate angina pectoris[84,85], possibly by vasodilatation of the coronary circulation and a redistribution of blood away from ischaemic areas.

Although these drugs have a common mode of action, they differ significantly with respect to myocardial contractility, systemic vascular

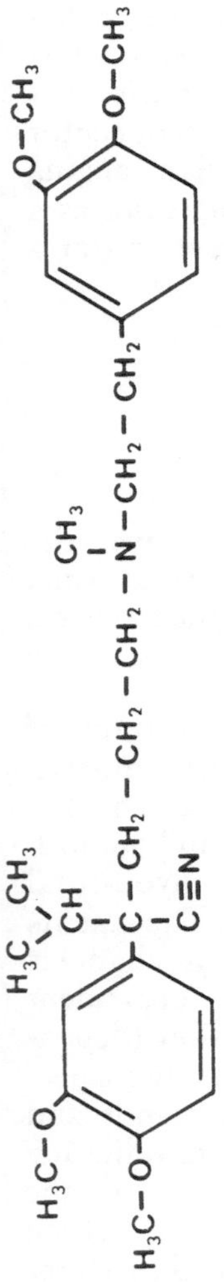

VERAPAMIL

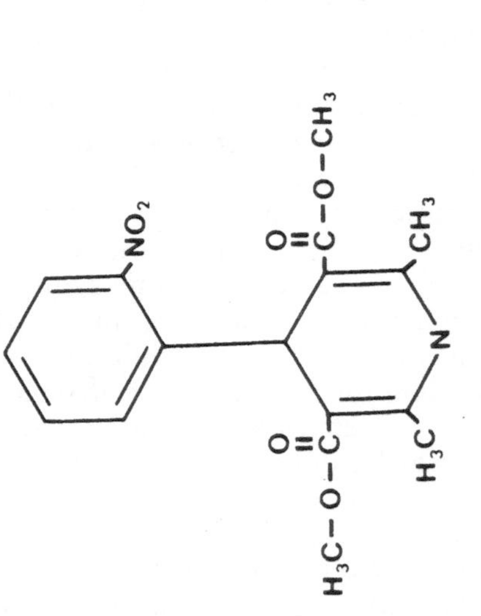

NIFEDIPINE

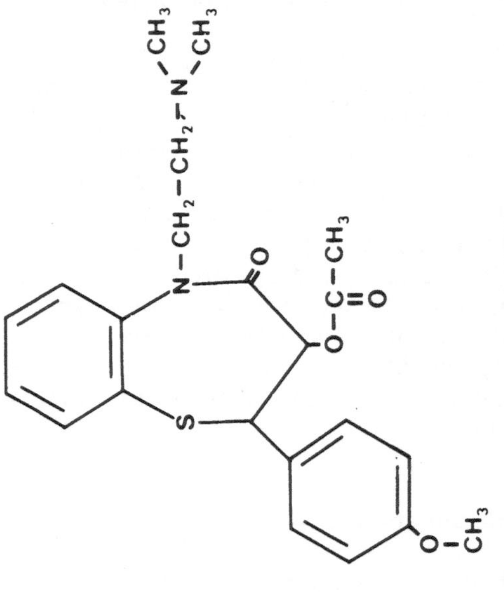

DILTIAZEM

Figure 2.3 Structures of verapamil, nifedipine and diltiazem

resistance, coronary vasodilatation, veno motor tone and antiarrhythmic activity. Perhexiline, in addition to its calcium antagonist activity, has also some type I antiarrhythmic activity, is a weak diuretic and reduces exercise heart rate. Lidoflazine also attenuates the heart rate responses to exercise (Table 2.3).

Table 2.3

	Negative inotropic activity	Delayed AV conduction	Smooth muscle relaxation
Nifedipine	+	−	+ + +
Verapamil	+ +	+ +	+ +
Diltiazem	−	+ +	+ +
Lidoflazine	−	+	+
Perhexiline	−	+	+
Prenylamine	+	+	+ +

Choice of calcium antagonist

Although the calcium antagonists share a common mode of action, their chemical structures are very different and they have different cardiovascular and pharmacokinetic effects. Nifedipine produces a very rapid and marked decrease in blood pressure with an increase in heart rate due to secondary sympathetic stimulation[86]. These effects start within a few minutes of ingestion, peak at 30 minutes and persist for 3–4 hours. By contrast, the vasodilating effect of diltiazem occurs 15 min after oral ingestion, reaches a maximum at 3 h and lasts for 6–8 h. Unlike nifedipine, diltiazem slows heart rate and appears to have no effect on myocardial contractility. Verapamil produces a drop in blood pressure starting 15–30 min after oral ingestion with a peak activity at 1–2 h[87]. Verapamil has the greatest depressant effect of the group on the sinoatriol (SA) and atrioventricular (AV) nodes, and possesses some negative inotropic effects especially in patients with congestive heart failure.

Perhexiline has a variety of actions, some unrelated to its calcium antagonist activity. It reduces an exercise tachycardia similar to β-blockers[88], has quinidine-like properties and is a mild diuretic[89]. The drug appears to have no negative inotropic activity or adverse effects on airways resistance[15,90]. Lidoflazine has similar properties with impaired heart rate responses to exercise and no effects on myocardial contractility or conduction[15].

When maximal vasodilatation is the main aim of therapy, nifedipine or verapamil are at present the most appropriate choices. In the presence of congestive heart failure, nifedipine should be used because reduction of increased afterload in heart failure tends to improve cardiac output[87]. Verapamil is probably best avoided in this situation because of its negative inotropic properties. Diltiazem would appear to be as useful a drug as verapamil or nifedipine in angina pectoris, since it reduces myocardial oxygen demands by reducing heart rate and systolic blood pressure. Verapamil and diltiazem decrease atrio-ventricular nodal conduction and are effective in the management of supraventricular re-entry tachycardia and in decreasing ventricular responses in atrial fibrillation or flutter.

Stable angina

Calcium entry blockers are effective in the long term management of chronic stable angina. A number of studies have demonstrated an increase in exercise duration and a significant delay in the onset of angina pain. The clinical effectiveness of verapamil in this condition has been demonstrated in several studies[91-93] and comparisons with β-adrenoceptor blocking agents have been favourable[94-96]. The improvement achieved with verapamil is maintained on long term therapy[97] and when combined with propranolol may produce further benefit[98], although adverse effects on conduction and inotropic function are more likely to occur. Nifedipine, in a large open study, showed a 70% improvement in the frequency of anginal attacks[99], a value which has been confirmed by single and double blind studies in stable angina pectoris[100-102]. Nifedipine has also been shown to improve exercise tolerance and decrease the blood pressure/heart rate product at a given workload by decreasing blood pressure[101,102]. Exercise tolerance can be further improved by the addition of a β-blocking drug, due to either a further decrease in systolic blood pressure or an associated improvement in coronary blood flow[103,104].

Long term administration of diltiazem in a double blind study showed a protective effect in patients with angina pectoris and minimal adverse effects[105,106]. Diltiazem and verapamil appear similar in their clinical efficacy[107].

Unstable angina

Evidence is now accumulating that calcium antagonists are particularly useful in the management of unstable angina[108-110]. Gerstenblith and colleagues[111] assessed the efficacy of adding nifedipine to conventional treatment of unstable angina and demonstrated its effectiveness especially in those with ST segment elevation during chest pain. Controlled studies in small numbers of patients have confirmed the efficacy of nifedipine in unstable angina[112,113] while others have demonstrated improvement in coronary artery spasm documented by angiography[114].

Similar findings have been obtained with verapamil. In a large series by Severi and colleagues[115], the frequency and severity of angina was reduced in all but 14 of 120 patients following discharge from hospital. These findings were confirmed by Kinura and Kishida[116], and the drug has been shown to be effective in reducing the severity of ergonovine-induced coronary artery spasm[117].

Evidence exists as to the effectiveness of diltiazem in variant angina[117] and in coronary artery spasm induced by ergonovine[117] and alkalosis[118].

As with stable angina there is no evidence that these drugs differ in their effectiveness in variant angina[117].

Although both perhexiline[119,120] and lidoflazine[15] have been demonstrated as being effective in angina pectoris, both are limited by the considerable delay between starting therapy and achieving a therapeutic response. The use of perhexiline is further limited by frequent and severe adverse effects[15].

Dosage and adjustment of therapy

Due to extensive 'first pass' metabolism, the oral bioavailability of verapamil is low (10-20%)[121]. The effective oral doses required to produce a clinical effect in angina pectoris (up to 480 mg daily) are therefore much higher than the doses required intravenously. Plasma concentrations of the drug vary widely between patients and there is no easy relationship between plasma concentration and effect. Measurements of plasma concentration may be helpful in some patients who fail to respond to verapamil because of very low levels (<100 ng/ml) but clinical monitoring remains the only way of assessing therapy.

Nifedipine is usually given orally in 10 mg doses three times a day to initiate therapy, and the dose increased depending on the clinical response. As with verapamil, plasma concentration measurement is of limited value in managing patients with angina pectoris. Sublingual nifedipine 20 mg has also been shown to be clinically and haemodynamically effective, producing a response within 30 minutes of drug administration[122]. Oral doses of diltiazem vary from 120 to 240 mg/ day but clinical experience is insufficient for definite recommendations[123].

Pharmacokinetics

Verapamil undergoes extensive biotransformation with the N-demethylated form as the only active metabolite. Oral absorption is rapid and almost complete but bioavailability is low (Table 2.4) because of extensive first pass hepatic extraction. A relationship between plasma concentrations and effect has been described for the antiarrhythmic activity[124,125] but data in angina pectoris are lacking.

On the other hand, nifedipine although rapidly and almost completely absorbed after oral administration has a first pass metabolism of about 65% and has no active metabolites[126]. A relationship between plasma nifedipine and vascular resistance in hypertensive patients has been described[127] and although plasma concentration effect relations have not been described in angina, a dose dependent relationship has been alluded to in variant angina[128,129]. Perhexiline is rapidly absorbed

Table 2.4

Drug	Absorption	Onset of action	Plasma half-life	Disposition
Verapamil	>90% after oral administration	<1½ min i.v. <30 min orally	3–7 h	90% protein bound in plasma 85% first pass metabolism 70% renal elimination
Nifedipine	>90% after oral administration	<1 min i.v. <3 min sublingual <20 min orally	4 h	90% protein bound in plasma 80% urinary excretion (drug + metabolites)
Diltiazem	>90% after oral administration	<3 min i.v. <3 min orally	4 h	Low protein binding 80–90% metabolism

and extensively metabolized in the liver with an elimination half-life of 2–5 days. Slow hydroxylators (9%) are particularly likely to suffer adverse effects. The dose should be reduced in patients with liver and/or renal disease[15,130]. Lidoflazine also undergoes extensive hepatic metabolism and has an elimination half-life of 1–2 days. There appears to be no relationship between plasma concentrations at steady state and clinical effect in angina, and full clinical effect may not be seen for several months[15]. Little pharmacokinetic information is available on other calcium antagonists and plasma level effect relationships have not yet been described.

Adverse effects and drug interactions

Verapamil is well tolerated during chronic therapy. Symptoms such as dizziness, headache, constipation and nausea can occur but usually disappear with continued therapy. The drug is well tolerated in patients with obstructive airways disease and no disturbances of the immune system have been described[131]. During chronic administration verapamil appears to decrease the renal clearance of digoxin by 50%, resulting in a dose dependent increase in plasma digoxin levels[132].

Most common adverse effects of nifedipine include dizziness, flushing headache and palpitations – features associated with vasodilatation. Nausea and vomiting are relatively common but no abnormalities of renal, haematological or immune systems have been reported[133]. No clinically significant interactions with other drugs have as yet been reported, including the β-adrenoceptor blocking agents, nitrates, diuretics and oral anticoagulants[133]. Nifedipine has also been reported to increase plasma digoxin levels but the clinical significance has not as yet been established.

Diltiazem produces symptoms related to its vasodilator activity but reported clinical experience is inadequate to establish conclusions regarding long term toxicity or drug interactions. The use of perhexiline is severely limited because of severe dose-related adverse effects – impaired liver function, peripheral neuropathy, hypoglycaemia, weight loss, headache and nausea. Other neurological adverse effects include tremor, incoordination, myopathy, papilloedema, and cerebellar and extrapyramidal syndromes[15].

Drugs with α-adrenoceptor blocking properties

Coronary artery vasospasm is mediated via the sympathetic α-receptors[134-136] and therefore some clinicians have used α-adrenoceptor blocking agents, both non-selective[137-139] and selective[140], in the treatment of this condition. Alternatively a drug which has both α- and β-adrenoceptor blocking properties can also be used[141]. In a series of open studies with relatively small numbers of patients, labetalol was shown to be at least as effective as other forms of antianginal therapy, particularly in patients with hypertension, and adverse effects on left ventricular function and peripheral blood flow were less than with other β-blockers[142-145]. The overall incidence of adverse effects appeared to be greater due to the additional α-blocking activity – postural hypotension, reduced libido, failure of erection, scalp tingling and difficulty with micturition[146]. Phentolamine has also to be shown to be of value in the treatment of angina pectoris[139]. When given orally the drug improved exercise tolerance and reduced the frequency of chest pain in twelve patients with stable angina pectoris and intravenous administration reduced the ST segment and wedge pressure in another small group of patients. Clinical information is inadequate at present to recommend non-specific α-adrenoceptor blocking drugs – phentolamine[137] or phenoxybenzamine[138] for the routine management of angina patients.

Non-selective α-blocking drugs may also have deleterious cardiac effects because of their ability to block the presynaptic α-receptors. The increase in the release of noradrenaline results in positive inotropic and chronotropic effects with increased myocardial oxygen consumption. Prazosin, on the other hand, blocks the post synaptic α_1-receptors with almost no α_2 effects[147]. There are theoretical advantages therefore for using this agent in angina pectoris. In a group of six patients with variant angina recovering from acute myocardial infarction, the addition of prazosin 8–30 mg/day to a therapeutic regime of isosorbide dinitrate and nifedipine resulted in improvement in five patients and unacceptable hypotension in one[140]. Further studies are clearly required before the role of prazosin in Prinzmetal's and possibly other forms of angina pectoris is established.

Alinidine

Alinidine is a derivative of clonidine which reduces heart rate, blood pressure and myocardial oxygen consumption. These effects do not appear to be mediated by β-adrenergic blockade. The haemodynamic effects should be beneficial in the treatment of angina pectoris. A preliminary study[148] suggested that this may be the case, but larger studies are required before the full potential can be realized, in particular whether the drug is a useful alternative to β-adrenoceptor blocking agents.

Combination therapy

Until recently, the standard treatment of chronic stable angina pectoris was a combination of nitrates and β-adrenoceptor blocking drugs. There is growing evidence that greater control can be achieved if calcium antagonists are added to this regimen[149,150]. Subramanian *et al.*[98] showed that the combination of propranolol and verapamil was more efficacious than either alone, at least in terms of exercise tolerance, and similar results have been obtained with propranolol and nifedipine in patients with angina pectoris[149].

In patients with severe symptoms, all three agents may be used to advantage as each has different properties that collectively can lead to a balance between myocardial oxygen demand and delivery. Thus, the nitrates provide for reduction in preload, the β-blockers for a reduction in heart rate and myocardial oxygen demand, while calcium antagonists diminish arteriolar resistance, systolic blood pressure and afterload.

Present opinion would suggest that patients whose angina is not responding adequately to calcium channel or β-adrenoceptor blockers alone merit consideration of combined therapy. Nifedipine seems to be the calcium antagonist of choice in this situation since it is less likely to cause electrophysiological adverse effects when combined with β-blockers than verapamil or diltiazem. For the majority of patients who require such a combination it is effective and safe especially in patients with associated hypertension, and in some clinical situations it may be possible to reduce the dose of the β-adrenoceptor blocking drug[150].

Selection of drug therapy

The sequence in which these drugs should be introduced is not completely clear. In variant angina, the calcium channel blocking drugs appear to be the agents of first choice. If full doses of these drugs are inadequate, nitrates should be added. In some clinical situations it may be more appropriate to start with a nitrate. In chronic stable angina, β-blockers would usually be the treatment of first choice because of the documented effect upon survival following myocardial infarction. The calcium channel blockers are probably best prescribed next and finally nitrates if adequate response is not achieved. Careful monitoring of the clinical response, preferably with sequential treadmill testing, is helpful in assessing the drug response and the need for further pharmacological or surgical intervention.

GENERAL MANAGEMENT OF THE PATIENT WITH ANGINA PECTORIS

The treatment of angina pectoris is aimed at providing symptomatic relief and prolonging life. The most important prognostic factors are the degree of left ventricular dysfunction, the extent of coronary atherosclerosis and the severity of myocardial ischaemia. Clearly these factors are interrelated. In patients with chronic stable angina, the degree of left ventricular dysfunction and the severity of the obstructive coronary artery disease should be determined in most patients before a therapeutic plan is offered. Echocardiography can give some information regarding left ventricular function while useful data on the severity and extent of coronary atherosclerosis can be obtained by treadmill exercise testing with or without thallium 201 myocardial scintigraphy. In the high risk patient, coronary arteriography should be performed. If significant left main coronary artery disease or severe proximal triple vessel disease is detected, coronary artery bypass surgery is indicated[151,152]. In selected patients relief of coronary obstruction can be achieved by coronary angioplasty.

In the absence of high risk coronary artery lesions or in patients in whom surgery would be particularly hazardous, the pharmacological approach is preferred. Diseases which predispose to angina should be treated – hypertension, anaemia, thyrotoxicosis, obesity, heart failure and chronic anxiety states. The patient should be asked to stop smoking and avoid overeating and although regular exercise should be encouraged it is probably best to avoid exercise after meals. Antianginal agents provide symptomatic treatment for patients but there is no convincing evidence that they have any beneficial effect on the underlying disease process.

Nitrates are the drugs of choice for the immediate relief of angina. For the long term management of patients with chronic stable angina, a combination of nitrates and β-adrenoceptor blocking drugs provide substantial benefit in most patients. Calcium influx-blocking drugs can produce further improvement and should be considered if nitrates and β-blocking therapy fail to produce a satisfactory response. If the symptoms of angina pectoris persist despite full drug therapy, surgical revascularization or angioplasty should be considered.

In unstable angina, immediate therapy with full doses of nitrates and β-blocking drugs provide relief in approximately 50% of patients and the addition of calcium entry-blocking agents will prevent recurrence of rest angina in an even larger proportion of patients. In patients who remain symptomatic, early coronary arteriography should be undertaken with a view to surgical revascularization or angioplasty. Even in patients who get adequate relief from medical therapy, elective coronary arteriography is desirable to determine whether surgical intervention is likely to be beneficial.

Since coronary artery spasm is an important mechanism in variant angina, nitrates and calcium antagonists tend to be used before β-adrenoceptor blocking drugs, although this group of drugs can be useful in patients who have additional obstructive coronary artery disease. Patients who do not respond to medical treatment should undergo coronary arteriography to determine whether significant obstructive coronary artery disease is present. In the absence of fixed coronary artery obstruction, pharmacological treatment should be continued. In the presence of such lesions, surgical revascularization or angioplasty should be considered.

References

1. Frankl, W.S. and Brest, A.N. (1983). What is optimal drug therapy in angina pectoris? *Cardiovasc. Clin.*, **13**, 209-20
2. Gordon, T., Kannel, W.B., McGee, D. and Dawber, T.R. (1974). Death and coronary attacks in men after giving up cigarette smoking: a report from the Framingham Study. *Lancet*, **2**, 1345-8
3. Vokonas, P.S., Cohn, P.F., Klein, M.D., Laver, M.B. and Gorlin, R. (1974). Hemoglobin affinity for oxygen in the anginal syndrome with normal coronary arteriograms. *J. Clin. Invest.*, **54**, 409-15
4. Miettinen, M., Turpeinen, O., Karvonen, M.J., Elosuo, R. and Paavilainen, E. (1972). Effect of cholesterol-lowering diet on mortality from coronary heart-disease and other causes. A twelve-year clinical trial in men and women. *Lancet*, **2**, 835-8
5. Committee of Principal Investigators (1978). A co-operative trial in the primary prevention of ischaemic heart disease using clofibrate. *Br. Med. J.*, **40**, 1069-1118
6. Clausen, J.P. and Trap-Jensen, J. (1976). Heart rate and arterial blood pressure during exercise in patients with angina pectoris. Effects of training and of nitroglycerin. *Circulation*, **53**, 436-42
7. Williams, D.O. (1981). Effects of antianginal agents on the coronary circulation. *Am. Heart J.*, **101**, 473-9
8. Hoffman, J.I.E. and Buckberg, G.D. (1979). Transmural variations in myocardial perfusion. In Yu, P.N. and Goodwin, J.F. (eds) *Progress in Cardiology*. (Philadelphia: Lea & Febiger)
9. Rubio, R. and Berne, R.M. (1975). Regulation of coronary blood flow. *Prog. Cardiovasc. Dis.*, **18**, 105-22
10. Prinzmetal, M., Kennamer, R., Merliss, R., Wada, T. and Bor, N. (1959). Angina pectoris. I. A variant form of angina pectoris: preliminary report. *Am. J. Med.*, **27**, 375-88
11. Sonnenblick, E.H., Ross, J. Jr and Braunwald, E. (1968). Oxygen consumption of the heart: newer concepts of its multifactorial determination. *Am. J. Cardiol.*, **22**, 328-36
12. Sonnenblick, E.H. and Skelton, C.L. (1971). Myocardial energetics: basic principles and clinical implications. *N. Engl. J. Med.*, **285**, 668-75
13. Frishman, W.H., Weksler, B., Christodoulon, P., Smithen, C. and Killup, T. (1974). Reversal of abnormal platelet aggregability and change in exercise tolerance in patients with angina pectoris following oral propranolol. *Circulation*, **50**, 887-96
14. Nayler, W.A. (1981). Protection of the ischaemic heart. *Res. Clin. Forums*, **3**, 59-71
15. MacClean, D. and Feely, J. (1983). Calcium antagonists, nitrates, and new antianginal drugs. *Br. Med. J.*, **286**, 1127-30
16. The Norwegian Multicentre Study Group (1981). Timolol induced reduction in mortality and reinfarction in patients surviving myocardial infarction. *N. Engl. J. Med.*, **304**, 801-7

17. Beta Blocker Heart Attack Study Group (1981). The beta-blocker heart attack trial. *J. Am. Med. Assoc.*, **246**, 2073-4

18. Hansteen, V., Moinichen, E., Lorentsen, E., Anderson, A., Strom, O., Soiland, K., Dyrbekk, D., Refsum, A.-M., Tromsdal, A., Knudsen, K., Eika, C. and Bakken, J. Jr (1982). One year's treatment with propranolol after myocardial infarction: preliminary report of Norwegian Multicentre Trial. *Br. Med. J.*, **184**, 155-60

19. Fox, K.M., Chopra, M.P., Portal, R.W. and Aber, C.P. (1975). Long term beta blockade: possible protection from myocardial infarction. *Br. Med. J.*, **1**, 117-19

20. Brunton, T.L. (1867). On the use of nitrate of amyl in angina pectoris. *Lancet*, **2**, 97-9

21. Murrell, W. (1879). Nitroglycerin as a remedy for angina pectoris. *Lancet*, **1**, 113-15

22. Axelsson, K.L., Wikberg, J.E.S. and Andersson, R.G.G. (1979). Relationship between nitroglycerin, cyclic GMP and relaxation of vascular smooth muscle. *Life Sci.*, **24**, 1779-86

23. Morcillio, F., Reid, P.R., Dubin, N., Chodgoonkar, R. and Pitt, B. (1980). Myocardial prostaglandin E release by nitroglycerin and modification by indomethacin. *Am. J. Cardiol.*, **45**, 53-7

24. Anderson, G.H. Jr, Hueber, P., Sterling, C., Twan, E. and Schroeder, E.T. (1980). Effect of nitroglycerin on prostacyclin production in rat aorta. *Circulation*, **62**, (Suppl. III), 326. No. 1257

25. Cohn, P.F. and Gorlin, R. (1974). Physiologic and clinical actions of nitroglycerin. *Med. Clin. N. Am.*, **58**, 407-15

26. Burggraf, G.W. and Parker, J.O. (1974). Left ventricular volume changes after amyl nitrate and nitroglycerin in man as measured by ultrasound. *Circulation*, **49**, 136-43

27. Mason, D.T. and Braunwald, E. (1965). The effects of nitroglycerin and amyl nitrate on arteriolar and venous tone in the human forearm. *Circulation*, **32**, 755-66

28. Battock, D.J., Alvarez, H. and Chidsey, C.A. (1969). Effects of propranolol and isosorbide dinitrate on exercise performance and adrenergic activity in patients with angina pectoris. *Circulation*, **39**, 157-69

29. Epstein, S.E. and Braunwald, E. (1968). Inhibition of the adrenergic nervous system in the treatment of angina pectoris. *Med. Clin. N. Am.*, **52**, 1031-9

30. Cohen, M.V., Downey, J.M., Sonnenblick, E.H. and Kirk, E.S. (1973). The effects of nitroglycerin on coronary collaterals and myocardial contractility. *J. Clin. Invest.*, **52**, 2836-47

31. Goldstein, R.E., Stinson, E.B., Scherer, J.L. Seningen, R.P., Grehl, T.M. and Epstein, S.E. (1974). Intraoperative coronary collateral function in patients with coronary occlusive disease. Nitroglycerin responsiveness and angiographic correlations. *Circulation*, **49**, 298-308

32. Moir, T.W. (1972). Subendocardial distribution of coronary blood flow and the effect of antianginal drugs. *Circ. Res.*, **30**, 621-7

33. Forman, R., Kirk, E.S., Downey, J.M. and Sonnenblick, E.H. (1973). Nitroglycerin and heterogeneity of myocardial blood flow. *J. Clin. Invest.*, **52**, 905-11

34. Gorlin, R., Brachfeld, N., MacLeod, C. and Bopp, P. (1959). Effect of nitroglycerin on the coronary circulation in patients with coronary artery disease or increased left ventricular work. *Circulation*, **19**, 705-18

35. Horwitz, L.D., Gorlin, R., Taylor, W.J. and Kemp, H.G. (1971). Effects of nitroglycerin on regional myocardial blood flow in coronary artery disease. *J. Clin. Invest.*, **50**, 1578-84

36. Distante, A., Maseri, A., Severi, S., Biagini, A. and Chierchia, S. (1979). Management of vasospastic angina at rest with continuous infusion of isosorbide dinitrate. *Am. J. Cardiol.*, **44**, 533-9

37. Sweatman, T., Strauss, G., Selzer, A. and Cohn, K.E. (1972). The long acting hemodynamic effects of isosorbide dinitrate. *Am. J. Cardiol.*, **29**, 475-80

38. Goldstein, R.E., Rosing, D.R., Redwood, D.R., Beisser, G.D. and Epstein, S.E. (1971). Clinical and circulatory effects of isosorbide dinitrate: comparison with nitroglycerin. *Circulation*, 43, 629–40

39. Needleman, P., Lang, S. and Johnson, E.M. Jr (1972). Organic nitrates: Relationship between biotransformation and rational angina pectoris therapy. *J. Pharmacol. Exp. Ther.*, 181, 489–97

40. Winsor, T., Kaye, H. and Mills, B. (1972). Hemodynamic response of oral long-acting nitrates: Evidence of gastrointestinal absorption. *Chest*, 62, 407–13

41. Franciosa, J.A., Mikulic, E., Cohn, J.N., Jose, E. and Fabie, A. (1974). Hemodynamic effects of orally administered isosorbide dinitrate in patients with congestive heart failure. *Circulation*, 50, 1020–4

42. Williams, D.E., Bommer, W., Merwin, R., Morrison, S., Miller, R.R. and Mason, D.T. (1976). Prolonged effectiveness of oral vasodilator therapy in chronic congestive heart failure with isosorbide dinitrate. *Am. J. Cardiol.*, 37, 182

43. Schanzenbacher, P. (1983). Isosorbide mononitrate or dinitrate in coronary disease? *Dtsch. Med. Wochenschr.*, 108, 807–809

44. Abrams, J. (1982). New nitrate delivery systems: Buccal nitroglycerin. *Am. Heart J.*, 105, 848–54

45. Davis, J.A. and Wiesel, B.H. (1955). The treatment of angina pectoris with nitroglycerin ointment. *Am. J. Med.*, 21, 230–59

46. Reichek, N., Goldstein, R.E., Redwood, D.R. and Epstein, S.E. (1974). Sustained effects of nitroglycerin ointment in patients with angina pectoris. *Circulation*, 50, 348–52

47. Hansen, M.S., Woods, S.L. and Willis, R.E. (1979). Relative effectiveness of nitroglycerin ointment according to the site of the application. *Heart*, 8, 716–20

48. Roubin, G.S., Harris, P.J., Eckhardt, J., Hensley, W. and Kelly, D.T. (1982). Intravenous nitroglycerin in refractory unstable angina pectoris. *Aust. NZ Med.*, 12, 598–602

49. Day, L.J., Thibank, G.E. and Sowton, B. (1977). Acute coronary insufficiency. Review of 46 patients. *Br. Heart J.*, 39, 363–70

50. Mikolich, J.R., Nicoloff, N.B., Robinson, P.H. and Logue, R.B. (1980). Relief of refractory angina with continuous intravenous infusion of nitroglycerin. *Chest*, 77, 375–9

51. Armstrong, P.W., Armstrong, J.A. and Marks, G.S. (1980). Pharmacokinetic-haemodynamic studies of intravenous nitroglycerin in congestive cardiac failure. *Circulation*, 62, 160–6

52. McNiff, E.F., Yacobi, A., Young-Chang, F.M., Golden, L.H., Goldfarb, A. and Fung, H.L. (1981). Nitroglycerin pharmacokinetics after intravenous infusion in normal subjects. *J. Pharm. Sci.*, 70, 1054–8

53. Kaplan, K., Davison, R., Parker, M., Teagarden, R. and Lesch, M. (1981). Efficacy of intravenous nitroglycerin in the treatment of angina at rest unresponsive to standard nitrate therapy. *Circulation*, 64, (Suppl. IV), iv–11

54. Flaherty, J.T. (1982). Intravenous nitroglycerin. *Johns Hopk. Med. J.*, 151, 36–40

55. Kaplan, K., Davison, R., Parker, M., Przybylek, J., Teagarden, J.R. and Lesch, M. (1983). Intravenous nitroglycerin for the treatment of angina at rest unresponsive to standard nitrate therapy. *Am. J. Cardiol.*, 51, 694–8

56. Baaske, D.M., Amanin, A.H., Wagenknecht, D.M., Mooers, M., Carter, J.E., Hoyt, H.J. and Stoll, R.G. (1980). Nitroglycerin compatibility with intravenous fluid filters, containers and administration sets. *Am. J. Hosp. Pharm.*, 37, 201–5

57. Needleman, P. and Johnson, E.M. (1973). Mechanism of tolerance development to organic nitrates. *J. Pharmacol. Exp. Ther.*, 184, 709–15

58. Pitt, W.A., Friedman, R.G., Gross, S.A., Glassman, J., Keating, E.C. and Mazure, J.H. (1982). Effect of intravenous nitroglycerin on haemodynamics of congestive heart failure. *Angiology*, 33, 294–301

59. Elkayam, U. and Aronow, S.W. (1982). Glyceryl trinitrate ointment and isosor-

bide dinitrate: A review of their pharmacological properties and therapeutic use. *Drugs*, **23**, 165-94

60. Di Carlo, F.J. (1975). Nitroglycerin revisited: chemistry, biochemistry, interactions. *Drug Metab. Rev.*, **4** (i), 1-38
61. Dauwe, F., Affaki, G., Waters, D.D., Theroux, P. and Mizgala, H.F. (1979). Intravenous nitroglycerin in refractory unstable angina. *Am. J. Cardiol.*, **43**, 416
62. Van Dusen, J. and Fischl, S.J. (1981). Inhibition of nitroglycerin effect in humans by suppression of prostaglandins. *Am. J. Cardiol.*, **47**, 390
63. Frick, M.H. and Luurila, O. (1976). Double blind titrated dose comparison of metoprolol and propranolol in the treatment of angina pectoris. *Ann. Clin. Res.*, **8**, 385-92
64. Becker, L.C., Fortuin, N.J. and Pitt, B. (1971). Effect of ischaemia and antianginal drugs on the distribution of radioactive microspheres in the canine left ventricle. *Circulation*, **28**, 263-9
65. Frick, M.H., Korhola, O. and Valle, M. (1978). Effect of beta-blockade by metoprolol on global and regional left ventricular myocardial perfusion in coronary heart disease. *Eur. J. Cardiol.*, **7**, 317-25
66. Thadani, U., Davidson, C., Singleton, W. and Taylor, S.H. (1979). Comparison of the immediate effects of five beta adrenoceptor blocking drugs with different ancillary properties in angina pectoris. *N. Engl. J. Med.*, **300**, 750-5
67. Conolly, M.E., Kersting, F. and Dollery, C.T. (1976). The clinical pharmacology of beta adrenoceptor blocking drugs. *Prog. Cardiovasc. Dis.*, **19**, 203-4
68. Kostis, J.B., Frishman, W., Hosler, M.H., Thorsen, N.L., Gonasum, L. and Weinstein, J. (1982). Treatment of angina pectoris with pindolol: the significance of intrinsic sympathomimetic activity of beta blockers. *Am. Heart J.*, **104**, 496-504.
69. Clark, B.J. (1982). Beta-adrenoceptor blocking agents: Are pharmacologic differences relevant? *Am. Heart J.*, **104**, 334-45
70. Louis, W.J., McNeil, J.J., Jarrott, B. and Drummer, O.H. (1983). Beta adrenoceptor blocking drugs: Current status and the significance of partial agonist activity. *Am. J. Cardiol.*, **52**, 104A-107A
71. Kostis, J.B., De Felice, E.A., Frichman, W., Hosler, M.H., Krieger, S.K., Aglitz, N. and Kuo, P.T. (1981). Clinical relevance of intrinsic sympathomimetic activity of beta blockers used in angina. *Angiology*, **32**, 780-7
72. Wilhelmsson, C. and Vedin, A. (1983). Beta blockers in ischaemic heart disease. *Am. J. Cardiol.*, **52**, 108A-112A
73. Pine, M., Favrot, L., Smith, S., McDonald, K. and Chidsey, C.A. (1975). Correlation of plasma propranolol concentration with therapeutic response in patients with angina pectoris. *Circulation*, **52**, 886-93
74. George, C.F., Fenyvesi, T. and Dollery, C.T. (1973). Pharmacological effects of propranolol in relation to plasma levels. In Davies, D.S. and Prichard, B.N. (eds) *Biological Effects of Drugs in Relation to their Plasma Concentration*, p. 123. (London: Macmillan)
75. Jackson, G., Atkinson, L. and Oram, S. (1975). Reassessment of failed beta blocker treatment in angina pectoris by peak-exercise heart rate measurements. *Br. Med. J.*, **3**, 616-18
76. Oates, J.A., Conolly, M.E., Prichard, B.N.C., Shand, D.G. and Schapel, G. (1977). The clinical pharmacology of antihypertensive drugs. In Gross, F. (ed.) *Antihypertensive Agents*. (Berlin: Springer)
77. Alderman, E.L., Coltart, J., Wettach, G.E. and Harrison, D.C. (1974). Coronary artery syndromes after sudden propranolol withdrawal. *Ann. Intern. Med.*, **81**, 625-7
78. Miller, R.R., Olsen, H.G., Amsterdam, E.A. and Mason, D.T. (1975). Propranolol withdrawal rebound phenomenon. *N. Engl. J. Med.*, **293**, 416-18
79. Golding, L.A.R., Loop, F.D., Sheldon, W.C., Taylor, P.C., Groves, L.K. and Cosgrove, D.M. (1978). Emergency revascularisation for unstable angina. *Circulation*, **58**, 1163-6

80. National Co-operative Study Group to compare surgical and medical therapy. Unstable angina pectoris (1978) II. In hospital experience and initial follow up results in patients with one, two and three vessel disease. *Am. J. Cardiol.*, **42**, 839–48

81. Maseri, A., L'Abbate, A., Baroldi, G., Chierchia, S., Marzilli, M., Ballestra, A.M., Severi, S., Parodi, O., Biagini, A., Distante, A. and Pesola, A. (1978). Coronary vasospasm as a possible cause of myocardial infarction. A conclusion derived from the study of pre-infarction angina. *N. Engl. J. Med.*, **299**, 1271–7

82. Yasue, H., Touyama, M., Shimamoto, M., Kato, H., Tanaka, S. and Akiyama, F. (1974). Role of the autonomic nervous system in the pathogenesis of Prinzmetal's variant form of angina. *Circulation*, **50**, 534–9

83. Goldberg, S., Reicheck, N., Wilson, J., Hirshfield, J.W. Jr, Muller, J. and Kastor, J.A. (1979). Nifedipine in the treatment of Prinzmetal's (variant) angina. *Am. J. Cardiol.*, **44**, 804–810

84. Rodger, C. and Stewart, A. (1978). Side effects of nifedipine. *Br. Med. J.*, **1**, 1611–20

85. Jariwalla, A.G. and Anderson, E.G. (1978). Production of ischaemic cardiac pain by nifedipine. *Br. Med. J.*, **1**, 1181–2

86. Debaiseux, J.C., Theroux, P., Waters, D.D. and Mazgala, H.F. (1980). Haemodynamic effects of a single oral dose of nifedipine following acute myocardial infarction. *Chest*, **78**, 574–9

87. Theroux, P., Waters, D.D., Debaiseux, J.C., Szlacheie, J., Mizgala, H.F. and Bourassa, M.G. (1980). Hemodynamic effects of calcium ion antagonists after an acute myocardial infarction. *Clin. Invest. Med.*, **3**, 81–5

88. Morledge, J. (1973). Effects of perhexiline maleate in angina pectoris: double blind clinical evaluation with ECG treadmill exercise testing. *Postgrad. Med. J.*, **49**, 64–7

89. Hudak, W.J., Lewis, R.E., Lucas, R.W. and Kuhn, W.L. (1973). Review of the cardiovascular pharmacology of perhexilene. *Postgrad. Med. J.*, Suppl. **16**, 16–25

90. Opie, L.H. (1980) Drugs and the heart. III. Calcium antagonists. *Lancet*, **1**, 806–9

91. Neumann, M. and Luisada, A.A. (1966). Double-blind evaluation of orally administered iproveratil in patients with angina pectoris. *Am. J. Med. Sci.*, **251**, 552–6

92. Pine, M.B., Citron, P.D., Bailly, D.J., Butman, S., Plasencia, G.D., Landa, D.W. and Wong, R.K. (1982). Verapamil versus placebo in relieving stable angina pectoris. *Circulation*, **65**, 17–22

93. Sandler, G., Clayton, G.A. and Thornicroft, S.C. (1968). Clinical evaluation of verapamil in angina pectoris. *Br. Med. J.*, **3**, 224–7

94. Aritman, K. and Ryden, L. (1982). Comparison of metoprolol and verapamil in the treatment of angina pectoris. *Am. J. Cardiol.*, **49**, 821–7

95. De Ponti, C., Mauri, F., Gilberto, G.R. and Caru, B. (1979). Comparative effects of nifedipine, verapamil, isosorbide dinitrate and propranolol on exercise-induced angina pectoris. *Eur. J. Cardiol.*, **10**, 47–58

96. Frishman, W.H., Klein, N.A., Strom, J.A., Willems, H., Lejeintel, Th., Pollack, S., Doyle, R., Kirsten, E. and Sonnenblick, E.H. (1982). Superiority of verapamil to propranolol in stable angina pectoris. A double-blind randomised crossover trial. *Circulation*, **65**, (Suppl. 1), 51–9

97. Subramanian, V.B., Lahiri, A., Bowles, M.J., Davies, A.B. and Raftery, E.B. (1981). Long term antianginal action of verapamil assessed by quantitated serial treadmill exercise test. *Am. J. Cardiol.*, **48**, 529–35

98. Subramanian, V.B., Bowles, M.J., Davies, A.B. and Raftery, E.B. (1981). Combined therapy with verapamil and propranolol in chronic stable angina. *Am. J. Cardiol.*, **49**, 125–32

99. Dunschede, H.B. and Grundie, P. (1975). Ergebnisse einer Feldprufung des koronartherapeutikums Adalat. *Med. Welt*, **26**, 1847–50

100. Folle, L.E., Ortiz, A., Artucio, R. and Dighiero, J. (1976). Efficacy of adalat in

angina pectoris patients in controlled clinical trial compared with placebo. In Iatene A.D. and Lichtlen, P. (eds.) *New Therapy of Ischaemic Heart Disease*, pp. 200-6. (Amsterdam: Excerpta Medica)

101. Moskowitz, R.M., Piccina, P.A., Nacarelli, G.V. and Zelis, R. (1979). Nifedipine therapy for stable angina pectoris: Preliminary results of effects on angina frequency and treadmill exercise response. *Am. J. Cardiol.*, **44**, 811-16

102. Mueller, H.S. and Chanine, R.A. (1981). Interim report of multicenter doubleblind placebo controlled studies of nifedipine in chronic stable angina. *Am. J. Med.*, **71**, 645-57

103. Ekelund, L.G. and Oro, L. (1979). Antianginal efficacy of nifedipine with and without a beta blocker, studied with exercise test. A double blind randomised sub-acute study. *Clin. Cardiol.*, **2**, 203-11

104. Dargie, H.J., Lynch, P.G., Krikler, D.M., Harris, L. and Krikler, S. (1981). Nifedipine and propranolol. A beneficial drug interaction. *Am. J. Med.*, **71**, 676-82

105. Pool, P.E. and Seagren, S.C. (1982). Long term efficacy of diltiazem in chronic stable angina associated with atherosclerosis. Effect on treadmill exercise. *Am. J. Cardiol.*, **49**, 573-7

106. Strauss, W.E., McIntyre, K.M., Parisi, A.F. and Shapiro, W. (1982). Safety and efficacy of diltiazem hydrochloride for the treatment of stable angina pectoris. Report of a co-operative clinical trial. *Am. J. Cardiol.*, **49**, 560-66

107. Subramanian, V.B., Bowles, M.J., Khurmi, N.S., Davies, A.B. and Raftery, A.B. (1982). Comparison of the antianginal efficacy of four calcium ion antagonists with propranolol. (Abstr.) *Am. J. Cardiol.*, **49**, 929

108. Parodi, O., Maseri, A. and Simonetti, I. (1979). Management of unstable angina at rest by verapamil. A double-blind cross over study in coronary care unit. *Br. Heart J.*, **41**, 167-74

109. Hugenholtz, P.G., Michels, H.R., Serruys, P.W. and Brower, R.W. (1981). Nifedipine in the treatment of unstable angina, coronary spasm and myocardial ischemia. *Am. J. Cardiol.*, **47**, 163-73

110. André-Fouet, X., Viallet, M., Gayet, C., Thizy, J.F., Wilner, C. and Pont, M. (1981). Diltiazem versus propranolol. A randomised trial in unstable angina. (Abstr.) *Circulation*, **64**, (Suppl. IV), 293

111. Gerstenblith, G., Onyang, P., Achuff, S., Bulkley, B., Becker, L.C., Mellitus, E.D., Boughman, K.L., Weiss, J.L., Flaherty, J.T., Kallman, C.H., Llewellyn, M. and Weisfeldt, M.L. (1982). Nifedipine in unstable angina: A double-blind randomised trial. *N. Engl. J. Med.*, **306**, 885-9

112. Johnson, S.M., Mauritson, D.R., Willerson, J.T., Hillis, L.D., Erck, B.J. and Brown, S.B. (1981). Comparison of verapamil and nifedipine in the treatment of variant angina pectoris. Preliminary observations in 10 patients. *Am. J. Cardiol.*, **47**, 1295-1300

113. Previtali, M., Salerno, J.A., Tavazzi, L., Ray, M., Medici, A., Chimienti, M., Spechia, G. and Bobba, P. (1980). Treatment of angina at rest with nifedipine. A short-term controlled study. *Am. J. Cardiol.*, **45**, 825-30

114. Tiefenbrunian, R.J., Sobel, B.E., Gowka, S., McKnight, R.C. and Ludbrook, P.A. (1981). Nifedipine blockade of ergonovine induced coronary arterial spasm: angiographic documentation. *Am. J. Cardiol.*, **48**, 184-7.

115. Severi, S., Davies, A., Maseri, A., Marzullo, P. and L'Abbate, A. (1980). Long term prognosis of 'variant' angina with medical treatment. *Am. J. Cardiol.*, **46**, 226-32

116. Kinura, E. and Kishida, H. (1981). Treatment of variant angina with drugs. A survey of 11 cardiology institutes in Japan. *Circulation*, **63**, 844-8

117. Waters, D.D., Theroux, P., Szlachcic, J. and Dauwe, F. (1981). Provocative testing with ergonovine to assess the efficacy of treatment with nifedipine, diltiazem and verapamil in variant angina. *Am. J. Cardiol.*, **48**, 123-30

118. Yasue, H., Nagao, M., Omote, S., Takvzawa, A., Muva, K., and Tanaka, S. (1978). Coronary arterial spasm and Prinzmetal's variant form of angina induced by hyperventilation and tris buffer infusion. *Circulation*, **58**, 56-62

119. Pilcher, J., Chandrasekhar, K.P., Russell, R.J., Boyce, M.J., Pierce, T.H. and Ikram, H. (1973). Long term assessment of perhexiline maleate in angina pectoris. *Postgrad. Med. J.*, **49**, Suppl. 3, 115-18
120. Weissberg, P.L. (1982). Therapeutic Progress - Review V. Treatment of angina. *J. Clin. Hosp. Pharm.*, **7**, 145-53
121. Eichelbaum, M., Ende, M. and Remberg, G. (1979). The metabolism of ^{14}C-verapamil in man. *Drug Metab. Disp.*, **7**, 145-8
122. Ludbrook, P.A., Tiefenbrum, A.J., Reed, F.R. and Burton, E.S. (1982). Acute haemodynamic responses to sublingual nifedipine: dependence on left ventricular function. *Circulation*, **65**, 489-98
123. McAllister, R.G. (1982) Clinical pharmacology of slow channel blocking agents. *Prog. Cardiovasc. Dis.*, **25**, 83-102
124. Sing, R.J., Esler, B. and McAllister, R.G. (1980). Intravenous verapamil for termination of re-entrant supraventricular tachycardias. Intracardiac studies correlated with plasma verapamil concentration. *Ann. Intern. Med.*, **93**, 682-9
125. Dominic, J., McAllister, R.G., Kuo, C.S., Reddy, C.P. and Surawicz, B. (1979). Verapamil plasma levels and ventricular rate response in patients with atrial fibrillation and flutter. *Clin. Pharmacol. Ther.*, **26**, 710-14
126. Hoster, F.A. (1975). Pharmacokinetics of nifedipine ^{14}C in man. In Lochner, W., Braasch, W. and Kroneberg, G. (eds) *Second International Adalat Symposium*, pp. 124-7. (New York: Springer)
127. Pederson, O.L., Christensen, N.J. and Ranisch, K.D. (1980). Comparison of acute effects of nifedipine in normotensive and hypertensive man. *J. Cardiovasc. Pharmacol.*, **2**, 357-66
128. Antman, E., Muller, J., Goldberg, S., MacAlpin, R., Rubenfire, M., Tabatznik, B., Liang, C.-S., Heupler, F. and Achuff, S. (1980). Nifedipine therapy for coronary-artery spasm. Experience in 127 patients. *N. Engl. J. Med.*, **302**, 1269-73
129. Bertrand, M.E., Leblanche, J.M. and Tilmant, P.Y. (1981). Treatment of Prinzmetal's variant angina. Role of medical treatment with nifedipine and surgical coronary revascularization combined with plexectomy. *Am. J. Cardiol.*, **47**, 174-8
130. Shah, R.R., Oates, N.S., Idle, S.R., Smith, R.L. and Lockhart, J.D.F. (1982). Impaired oxidation of debrisoquine in patients with perhexiline neuropathy. *Br. Med. J.*, **284**, 295-9
131. Krikler, D. (1974). Verapamil in cardiology. *Eur. J. Cardiol.*, **2**, 3-10
132. Lang, R., Klein, H.O., Weiss, E., Libhaber, C. and Kaplinsky, E. (1980). Effect of verapamil on blood level and renal clearance of digoxin. *Circulation*, **62** (Suppl. II), 83
133. Ebner, F. and Dunschede, H.B. (1976). Haemodynamic therapeutic mechanism of action and clinical findings of Adalat use based on world wide clinical trials. In Jatine, A.D. and Lichthen, P.R. (eds). *3rd International Adalat Symposium*, pp. 283-300. (Amsterdam: Excerpta Medica)
134. Pitt, B., Elliot, E.C. and Gregg, D.E. (1967). Adrenergic receptor activity in the coronary arteries of the unanaesthetized dog. *Circ. Res.*, **21**, 75-84
135. McRaven, D.R., Mark, A.L., Abboud, F.M. and Mayer, H.E. (1971). Responses of coronary vessels to adrenergic stimuli. *J. Clin. Invest.*, **50**, 773-8
136. Kelley, K.O. and Feigel, E.O. (1978). Segmental alpha receptor mediated vasoconstriction in the canine coronary circulation. *Clin. Res.*, **43**, 908-17
137. Yasue, H. (1980). Pathophysiology and treatment of coronary arterial spasm. *Chest*, **78**, 216-23
138. Levene, D.L. and Freeman, M.R. (1976). Alpha adrenoceptor mediated coronary arterial spasm. *J. Am. Med. Assoc.*, **236**, 1018-22
139. Gould, L.A., Reddy, C.V.R. and Gomprecht, R.F. (1973). Oral phentolamine in angina pectoris. *Jpn. Heart J.*, **14**, 393-7
140. Tzivoni, D., Keren, A., Benhorin, J., Gottlieb, S., Atlas, D. and Stern, S. (1982). Prazosin therapy for refractory variant angina. *Am. Heart J.*, **105**, 262-6

141. Lubbe, W.F. and White, D.A. (1978). Labetalol in hypertensive patients with angina pectoris: beneficial effect of combined alpha and beta blockade. *Clin. Sci. Mol. Med.*, **55** (Suppl. 4), 283S-286S
142. Halprin, S., Frishman, W., Kirschner, M. and Strom, J. (1980). Clinical pharmacology of new beta adrenergic blocking drugs. Part II. Effect of oral labetalol in patients with both angina pectoris and hypertension: a preliminary experience. *Am. Heart J.*, **99**, 388-96
143. Besterman, E.M.M. and Spencer, M. (1979). Open evaluation of labetalol in the treatment of angina pectoris occurring in hypertensive patients. *Br. J. Clin. Pharmacol.*, **8**, 2055-95
144. Silke, B., Nelson, G.I.C., Ahija, R.C. and Taylor, S.H. (1982). Comparative haemodynamic dose response effects of propranolol and labetalol in coronary heart disease. *Br. Heart J.*, **48**, 364-71
145. Frishman, W.H., Strom, J.A., Kirschner, M., Poland, M., Klein, N., Halprin, S., Le Jemtel, T.H., Kram, M. and Sonnenblick, E.H. (1981). Labetalol therapy in patients with systemic hypertension and angina pectoris. Effects of combined alpha and beta adrenoceptor blockade. *Am. J. Cardiol.*, **48**, 917-28
146. McNeill, J.J. and Lous, W.J. (1979). A double-blind cross over comparison of pindolol, metoprolol, atenolol and labetalol in mild to moderate hypertension. *Br. J. Clin. Pharmacol.*, **8**, 163S-166S
147. Hoffman, B.B. and Lefkowitz, R.J. (1980). Alpha-adrenergic receptor subtypes. *N. Engl. J. Med.*, **302**, 1390-6
148. Simoons, M.L., Tummers, J., Van Meurs-Van Woezik, H. and Van Dornburg, R. (1982). Alinidine, a new agent which lowers heart rate in patients with angina pectoris. *Eur. Heart J.*, **3**, 542-5
149. Daly, K., Bergman, G., Rothman, M., Atkinson, L., Jackson, G. and Jewitt, D.E. (1982). Beneficial effect of adding nifedipine to beta adrenergic blocking therapy in angina pectoris. *Eur. Heart J.*, **3**, 42-6
150. Krikler, D.M., Harris, L. and Rowland, E. (1982). Calcium channel blockers and beta blockers: Advantages and disadvantages of combination therapy in stable angina pectoris. *Am. Heart J.*, **104**, 702-8
151. Takaro, T., Hultgren, H.N., Detre, K.M. and Peduzzi, P. (1982). The Veterans Administration Co-operative Study of Stable Angina: current status. *Circulation*, **65**, Suppl. 2, II-60-67
152. European Coronary Surgery Study Group (1982). Prospective randomised study of coronary artery bypass surgery in stable angina pectoris: a progress report on survival. *Circulation*, **65**, Suppl. 2, II-67-71

3
Primary and secondary prevention of coronary artery disease by drug therapy

N.S. BABER

INTRODUCTION

Ischaemic heart disease is the commonest cause of death in developed countries, and is among the most frequent causes of morbidity. This remains true despite the decline in cardiovascular mortality during the last two decades in certain countries of the world. Since 1968, declining trends have been observed in some industrialized countries, such as the United States, Australia and Finland[1,2]. Other countries, notably England and Wales, have not shown a decline until 1979 when a cautious downward trend appeared[3]. Recent papers from Sweden indicate an increase in coronary mortality[4,5].

It is not certain whether these changes are due to a decline in incidence of coronary arterial disease (i.e. primary prevention) or to improvement in prognosis. There is substantial evidence for a decline in incidence.

First, the reduction in mortality and coronary incidence was apparent before there were substantial alterations in preventive measures. Second, in Sweden, the rise in coronary mortality is not commensurate with a rise in the main risk factors; cigarette smoking decreased in both the Göteborg[4] and the Stockholm[5] surveys. Third, risk factor intervention studies such as the WHO European Coronary Prevention Study[6], the North Karelia–Kuopio Study[2,7] and the American Multiple Risk Factor Intervention Trial[8] have indicated that reductions in risk factors are not associated with a reduction in the incidence of, or mortality from, coronary artery disease. Even in the most recent report from Finland[9] reductions in coronary mortality were seen equally in North Karelia where an active intervention programme began in 1972, and in Kuopio and Vaasa, counties where no intensive health education programme was instituted.

Fourth, a survey of patient records from the Mayo clinic[10,11] between 1950 and 1975 indicated that the fall in coronary heart disease incidence preceded the fall in mortality by about 10 years. Although this is a small study and not necessarily applicable to the rest of the USA, it does seem unlikely that the early fall in incidence could have coincided with any major changes in clinical practice.

On the other hand, WHO figures indicate a high correlation between attack rates of acute myocardial infarction and mortality rates from acute myocardial infarction[12], suggesting that differences between countries in coronary heart disease mortalities are unlikely to be due to differences in case fatality.

It seems unlikely that drug therapy has made a major contribution to decline in incidence of, or mortality from, coronary artery disease within a community. This is not to deny the value of correct therapy for the individual at risk, and the debate on mass strategies for a large number of people exposed to a low risk[1,3], as compared with selective policy of screening for individuals at high risk continues. As it is impossible to allot the changes in incidence of coronary disease in the community, with any certainty, to a particular drug therapy, the only other source of information on the efficacy of an intervention is the controlled clinical trial. However, there are a number of major concerns in interpreting the results of clinical studies: (1) the sample under study must be representative of the community to which the results will be extrapolated, (2) the study must be large enough to detect a clinically useful effect and (3) multiple risk factor intervention trials, in which drug therapy is only one part of the strategy, add a further complication in deciding what part a drug plays in reducing incidence of, or mortality from, coronary arterial disease.

There have been many recent reviews on different aspects of primary and secondary prevention. In particular, the role of β-adrenoceptor blocking agents in myocardial infarction has received close attention[14-16], because this class of drugs, among all others that have been tested for secondary prevention, has emerged as the most promising. May *et al.* published two comprehensive reviews of drug trials in secondary prevention[17-18]. In the first review, the authors concentrated on those trials which began after recovery from infarction and extended beyond the time of hospital discharge. The second paper was concerned with early intervention trials, with follow-up periods usually ending at hospital discharge, or less than 3 months' duration. Total mortality was used as the primary response variable, based on all randomized patients. The authors concluded that no single drug intervention has been conclusively shown to reduce mortality in the acute phase of myocardial infarction.

In the later intervention, long term, studies they concluded that benefit from β-blockade in the first 12–18 months following myocardial infarction has been demonstrated, and two other intervention, anticoagulants and platelet-active drugs gave promising but inconsistent results.

This present review will include studies reported up to the month of

May 1984. Primary drug prevention of ischaemic heart disease will be defined as the use of a drug (or drugs) in a patient population prior to the clinical manifestation of ischaemic heart disease, in the expectation of a reduction in morbidity or mortality. Secondary drug preventation of ischaemic heart disease will be defined as the use of a drug (or drugs) in a patient population who have clinical evidence of ischaemic heart disease, such as angina pectoris, myocardial infarction or the survival of sudden death in the expectation of a reduction in morbidity or mortality. It is of interest to note that the current vogue in prevention studies is to report total mortality, regardless of cause. This has two advantages. First, it avoids the problem of differential withdrawal from the two treatment groups. Second, it gives a practical and simple end point which requires no causative explanation. But it has two major disadvantages. First, total mortality reporting, by ignoring cause of death, loses information on possible modes of action of the agents under test. Second, it is justifiably argued that a drug cannot be expected to be effective when it is not being taken or is not active at the time of a new event. There is no resolution to this issue at present, and both views have their protagonists and antagonists.

Figure 3.1 is a schematic representation of the perceived factors that produce the clinical manifestation of ischaemic heart disease, and which are amenable to drug intervention. There are however some difficulties with the classification into primary and secondary preven-

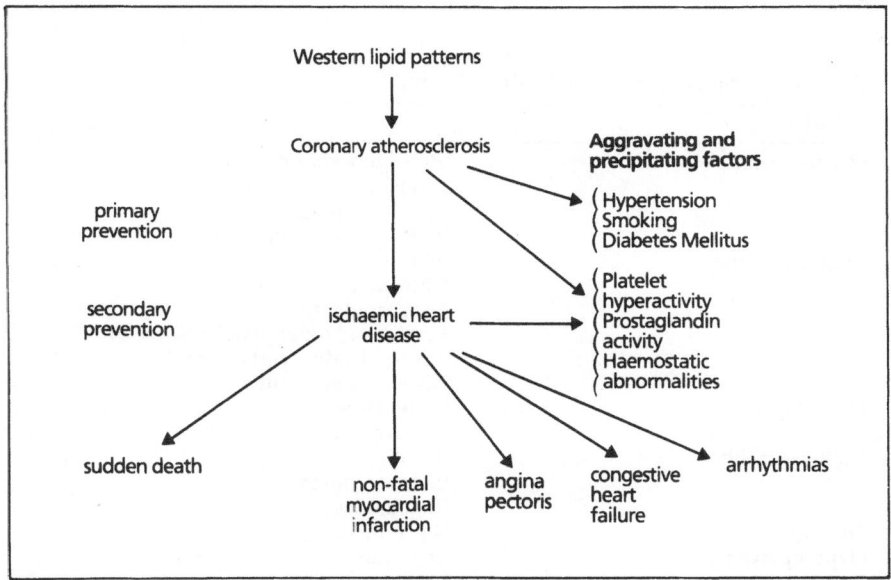

Figure 3.1 Schematic representation of aggravating and precipitating factors of coronary atherosclerosis and ischaemic heart disease, and clinical outcome amenable to drug therapy

tion by the definition previously given. Sudden death occurs in patients with severe ischaemic heart disease, but who frequently do not have evidence of a recent myocardial infarction or a history of angina pectoris. A drug trial in survivors of a sudden death is then, in most instances, a primary preventive medicine.

Drug intervention studies which begin in the first few hours after the onset of chest pain, and continue with long term therapy, have to be interpreted with respect to the consequences of the first evolving ischaemic event, and to the effects on a further event. Different processes of prevention may be operating in the two clinical situations. However, the distinction into primary and secondary prevention is maintained to aid in study classification.

Table 3.1 lists the primary prevention risk categories and the drugs which have been used in the treatment of the respective conditions.

Table 3.2 lists the secondary prevention risk categories in which treatment has been initiated in the first few hours or days after myocardial infarction, and been maintained for no longer than 3 months.

Table 3.3 lists the secondary prevention risk categories in which treatment has been maintained for longer than 3 months and was usually, but not invariably, initiated after recovery from the infarction.

Each drug regimen or policy will be considered separately and most emphasis will be given to studies which are prospective and randomized with a placebo or positive control, and with a total sample size of at least 100. These criteria are chosen for two reasons – first to avoid

Table 3.1 Primary prevention by drug therapy

Risk category	Drug or policy tested
Hypertension	*Pre-β-blocker drug therapy
	β-Blockers $\pm$ other drugs
	*Calcium antagonists
	Multi-intervention trials
Angina pectoris	*Nitrates
	β-Blockers
	Anticoagulants
	Aspirin and other platelet-active drugs
	*Prostaglandin synthetase inhibitors
	*Calcium antagonists
Heart failure	Vasodilators
	*Inotropic agents
Diabetes mellitus	*Insulin
	*Sulphonylureas
	*Biguanides
Obesity	No studies
Hyperlipidaemia	Clofibrate
	Cholestyramine
	Multi-intervention trial
Hyperfibrinogenaemia	No studies

*No information available

Table 3.2 Secondary prevention by drug therapy: short duration treatment (<3 months)

To reduce arrhythmias
  quinidine
  lignocaine
  procainamide
  mexiletine
  disopyramide
  verapamil
  *α-blockers

  nifedipine
  β-blockers
  bretylium
  phenytoin
  *amiodarone
  glucose–potassium–insulin

To reduce myocardial injury
  (a) *Reduction in oxygen requirements*
    nitrates
    vasodilators
    glucose–potassium–insulin

    calcium-antagonists
    β-blockers

  (b) *Increase oxygen supply*
    platelet active drugs
    hyaluronidase
    fibrinolytic (thrombolytics)
    anticoagulants

    *mannitol
    *hypertonic glucose
    *prostacyclin
    *thromboxane A$_2$ inhibitors

  (c) *Enhancing aerobic metabolism*
    glucose–potassium–insulin
  (d) *Reducing autolysis*
    *corticosteroids
    *non-steroidal anti-inflammatory drugs
    *chlorpromazine
    *ATP precursors

*No definitive studies

Table 3.3 Secondary prevention by drug therapy: long duration treatment (>3 months)

Antiarrhythmics
  phenytoin
  mexiletine
  aprinidine
  tocainide
Lipid-lowering drugs
  clofibrate
  oestrogen
  nicotinic acid
Platelet active agents
  aspirin
  dipyridamole
  sulphinpyrazone
Calcium antagonists
  verapamil
  nifedipine
Vasodilators
  captopril
  hydralazine
β-Blockers

treatment allocation bias and second, to give prominence to trials of sufficient size to discern a clinically important effect. Total mortality will be presented wherever possible, as the primary response variable for the reasons discussed above. Some studies publish cause-specific mortality only, but total mortality will be presented if the data are available from other sources. When there are important discrepancies between total and cause-specific or 'on treatment' mortality, a particular comment will be made.

Some of the newer agents have not been adequately tested in controlled trials, and the publications relate to intermediate response variables related to a proposed mode of action of the drug and not to mortality. These studies will be given less weighting.

Anticoagulants will not be considered, as they are discussed in Chapter 5.

PRIMARY PREVENTION

Antihypertensive drugs

Hypertension is one of the strongest risk factors for coronary heart disease[19]. Proof of a causal relationship is generally accepted only when an intervention trial in which control of the risk factor has occurred is followed by a lowering of the incidence of disease. Intervention trials in hypertension have repeatedly confirmed that treatment reduces the incidence of stroke and congestive heart failure[19,20]. In six large placebo controlled trials of hypertension[19-25] only one showed a strong trend towards lowering of coronary heart disease mortality[23]. The largest clinical trial, the Hypertension Detection and Follow-up Programme[26], in hypertension did not employ a placebo group, but claimed benefit in regard to coronary heart disease mortality.

There are a number of explanations for an inability to demonstrate a causal relationship between hypertension and coronary heart disease incidence and mortality[27]. Recent attention has been directed to a possible deleterious role of antihypertensive agents, particularly thiazide diuretics, through changes in lipid metabolism, carbohydrate intolerance, and arrhythmogenic consequences of hypokalaemia. Whether these potentially adverse effects of thiazide diuretics are clinically important or not, there is no convincing evidence that agents other than thiazide diuretics reduce the incidence of myocardial infarction or sudden death.

Two small uncontrolled studies with propranolol suggested substantial reductions in infarction rate and death from myocardial infarction[28,29]. More recently Berglund[30] reported a significant reduction in incidence of non-fatal myocardial infarction and death from ischaemic heart disease in hypertensive patients receiving β-blockers among their therapy, compared with a non-β-blocker antihypertensive regimen.

Beevers et al.[31], in a retrospective survey of 920 patients receiving various antihypertensive regimens, reported a significant trend for men and women whose regimen included a β-blocker to have fewer coronary episodes and strokes, compared with other regimens.

Several studies have shown that thiazide therapy is associated with hypokalaemia and significant ventricular arrhythmias[32], effects which may be offset by β-blockade[33,34].

The contribution made by the reduction in blood pressure to the overall results of recent multiple intervention programmes is difficult to assess.

In the Multiple Risk Factor Intervention Trial[8] in which reduction of hypertension, smoking habits, and hypercholesterolaemia were studied, there was no difference in the total mortality or in the incidence of deaths from coronary heart disease, in those patients receiving 'special intervention' compared with the 'usual care' group. Thiazide diuretics were the most frequently prescribed antihypertensive agents and β-blockers used only infrequently.

At present, it is unclear whether thiazide diuretics are harmful or whether β-blockers are particularly beneficial in reducing the incidence of myocardial infarction in hypertensive patients. Three large trials[35-37] are comparing the effects of thiazide and β-blockers and their results are awaited with interest.

Drug treatment of angina pectoris

There is no convincing evidence that any of the currently available treatments for angina pectoris reduces the incidence of myocardial infarction or sudden death.

Lambert[38] conducted a retrospective survey of 217 patients with angina pectoris, and reported that the infarction rate in those receiving β-blockers was 5.8% compared with 19.3% on other treatments. The rate of fatal infarction was also lower by one third (2.5% versus 9.5%) in the group receiving β-blockers. He confirmed these observations in a second non-randomized survey of 246 patients, 144 of whom received β-blockers, and 102 other treatments. The infarction rate was 3.7% in the β-blocker group and 20.9% in the other group. The rate of fatality was 1.4% versus 10.4% respectively.

There have been no prospective randomized studies to confirm these observations, but the work of Lambert together with the convincing evidence that β-blockers prolong life *after* myocardial infarction (*see below*), make it mandatory to compare new antianginal regimens against β-blockers in prophylactic studies.

There is one important study in threatened infarction in men in which a significant reduction in the incidence of myocardial infarction by treatment with aspirin was demonstrated[39] (*see* section on Platelet Active Drugs secondary prevention).

Heart failure therapy

There are no controlled trials of the effect of therapy in patients with mild or moderate heart failure secondary to ischaemic heart disease. The prognosis from severe chronic congestive heart failure is extremely poor, with mortality rates on conventional therapy ranging from 40% to 80% in the initial 1 or 2 years of follow-up[40].

Two studies have been published which provide preliminary data on survival in these patients. The Captopril Multicentre Research Group[41] randomly allocated 91 patients with New York Heart Association functional class III (54%) or II, to receive captopril, up to 50 mg three times a day, or placebo, in addition to their current therapeutic regimen. Fifty-six per cent of patients treated with captopril and 33% of patients treated with placebo had ischaemic heart disease as the cause of heart failure. After 3 months' treatment, four patients died in the placebo group and none in the captopril group. Functional and exercise improvement was significantly greater in the group receiving additional captopril treatment.

Packer et al.[42], in a non-randomized study, treated 175 patients with severe congestive heart failure with either hydralazine (120 patients) or captopril (76 patients); 21 patients received both drugs at different times. The survival rates were similar in the two groups after 1 year (53% captopril versus 46% hydralazine). Clinical improvement was greater with captopril.

There are no long term controlled studies with inotropic agents. A recent trial with oral prenalterol in eight patients suggested that beneficial effects on cardiac function are not maintained after 4 weeks[43].

Lipid lowering drugs

Drug-induced changes in serum lipids have been directed towards triglycerides, and low and high density cholesterol. Serum triglycerides are probably not an important risk factor in the genesis of ischaemic heart disease. Experimental coronary atherosclerosis cannot generally be produced in animals by raising serum triglycerides. Epidemiological studies are inconsistent, but many populations with very high rates of coronary disease and high serum cholesterols have low triglyceride levels. There seems to be general agreement that there is no independent contribution of triglycerides to ischaemic heart disease risk, when a correction is made for serum cholesterol and diabetes mellitus[44]. The 'lipid hypothesis' refers to cholesterol, and there is a well-established association between elevated serum cholesterol and an increased risk of developing coronary heart disease. The risk of developing ischaemic heart disease in association with raised serum cholesterol concentrations is proportionately greater for young adults than for older persons, but the association is not linear.

Figure 3.2 shows Ahrens'[45] graphic portrayal of the hypothesis which

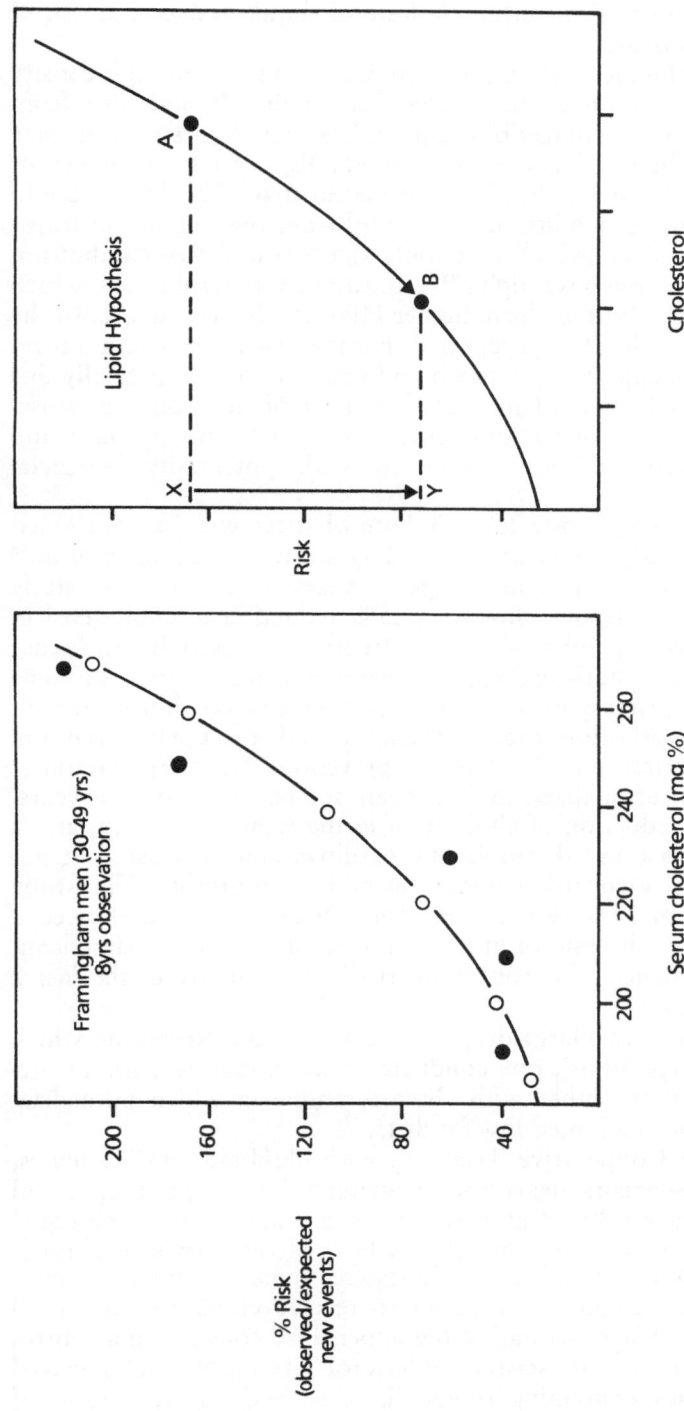

Figure 3.2 *Left*: Relation between serum cholesterol levels in men (30–49 years) and their relative risks of coronary heart disease (●) and a curve of 'best fit' to the data (○) from Framingham data. *Right*: The Lipid Hypothesis proposes that lowering serum cholesterol levels from A to B reduces the relative risk from X to Y

suggests that reduction of serum cholesterol should reduce the risk of coronary heart disease.

A recent development has been a renewal of interest in high-density lipoprotein cholesterol. In data from Framingham[46] and also from pooled data in other epidemiological studies there is a strong inverse relationship of high density lipoprotein (HDL) level to incidence of coronary heart disease. It has been suggested that HDL has a role in promoting the normal efflux of cholesterol from the cell and in trans-porting it to the liver, which is its only significant site of catabolism.

Babies and children have high HDL to total cholesterol ratios, which decrease with age. Women have higher HDL levels than men until the menopause, and it has been suggested that the relative protection from coronary disease enjoyed by women and children may be partially due to their high HDL. It is of interest that most of the 'common-sense' recommendations made by authorities concerned with primary and secondary prevention[47] are associated with potentially beneficial changes in HDL.

Three studies employing low cholesterol diets will be mentioned briefly. The mixed primary and secondary study by Mieftinen et al.[48] included 10612 subjects of mean age 50 years, in a cross-over study lasting 6 years: the results showed a 15% reduction in cholesterol in the treatment group, and a favourable trend in coronary heart disease and mortality, but statistical significance was achieved only in some subgroups. One primary prevention study[49] and two combined primary and secondary prevention studies[48,50] employed diet as the intervention.

The second primary and secondary prevention study by Dayton et al.[50] in 846 institutionalized males, mean age 66 years, over 8 years, showed a 20% reduction of cholesterol in the treatment group, and a significant decrease in atherosclerotic cardiovascular disease, but not in sudden death, myocardial infarction or total mortality. The study by Christakis[49] in 1277 subjects, aged 40–59 over 5 years, showed a 14% reduction in cholesterol in the treatment group, and a significant decrease in incidence of coronary heart disease, mainly in the last 2 years of the study.

There have been two large drug studies in primary prevention which test the 'lipid hypothesis', one conducted with clofibrate without die-tary control and the other with cholestyramine in which both drug and placebo groups adopted low fat diets.

In the WHO Cooperative Trial[51,52], with clofibrate, 15745 males, free of clinical ischaemic heart disease, living in Edinburgh, Prague and Budapest, and aged 30–59 at entry, were classified into three equal groups according to serum cholesterol. Half of the men in the upper third of the distribution of serum cholesterol (mean serum cholesterol 249 mg/dl) were assigned at random to receive clofibrate (Group I) taking 1.6 g/day. The other half of the upper third constituted a control group (Group II) (mean serum cholesterol 247 mg/dl) and received identical capsules containing olive oil. A second control group of

Table 3.4 Incidence of major ischaemic heart disease, non-fatal and fatal in WHO co-operative trial with clofibrate in men aged 30–59

| | Rates per 1000 per annum | | |
	Group I Clofibrate	Group II High cholesterol control	Group III Low cholesterol control
Number entered	5331	5296	5118
All major ischaemic heart disease	5.9*	7.4*	2.3†
Non-fatal myocardial infarction	4.6*	6.2*	1.7†
Fatal IHD	1.3	1.2	0.6
Sudden death	0.8	0.6	0.3

*$p < 0.05$ Groups I v. II
†$p < 0.01$ Non-fatal events Group III v. I and II

similar size (Group III) was chosen at random from the lowest third of the serum cholesterol distribution (181 mg/dl) and also received olive oil capsules. Investigators and participants were unaware of the groups to which individuals belonged. Subjects were in the study for a mean of 5.3 years and post-treatment surveillance lasted 4.3 years. No attempt was made to correct other risk factors for ischaemic heart disease.

A mean reduction of approximately 9% of the initial cholesterol levels was achieved in Group I. The incidence of non-fatal myocardial infarctions was reduced by 20% in Group I compared with Group II (4.6 versus 6.2 infarcts per 1000 subjects per year; $p < 0.05$), thus lending support to the 'lipid hypothesis'. There was no difference in fatal infarcts or in incidence of sudden death (death within 3 hours of onset of new symptoms) (Table 3.4). In general, the observed rates of major ischaemic heart disease for men in Group I, whose cholesterol fell during the trial, were substantially below the expected rates, whether their pretreatment cholesterols were low or high. The pattern is not so clear for men in Group II, but in both groups where cholesterol rose during the trial, the observed rates were higher than the expected. This again supports the 'lipid hypothesis'. Multivariate analysis showed that a 'best effect' subgroup of 872 men from Group I had a 34% reduction in events, compared with 23% in the remainder. This subgroup comprised men of mean age 46.5 years, mean cholesterol 258 mg/dl, who showed a reduction on treatment, and with systolic blood pressures over 135 mmHg, and who smoked. This group resembles more closely those who would be given clofibrate in clinical practice, and it is worth noting that the mean serum cholesterol in Group I men of 258 mg/dl before treatment does not represent a relative 'high risk'.

Unfortunately, these promising results have to be set against a greater crude total mortality in the clofibrate-treated group compared with Group II, though the age-standardized mortality rates are not significantly different between the three groups. Excluding deaths from 'other vascular causes' and from 'accidents' which are similar in Groups I and II, the number of deaths from other causes was 77 Group I, 47 Group II ($p < 0.05$) and 49 Group III. This increased mortality included deaths from malignancies of the liver, biliary and intestinal systems, though deaths from these conditions were commoner in Group III, making it possible that Group II had fortuitously low rates.

The total excess in mortality is equivalent to one man per 1000 per year in Group I compared with Group II. There is no plausible biological explanation for the result, which is not associated with a particular pathology, nor is it related to duration of exposure to the drug or concomitant increase in morbidity.

In conclusion, the results of the WHO Study[31, 52] suggest that clofibrate should be reserved for the treatment of defined hyperlipidaemias (particularly type III), especially when other risk factors are present. Treatment should only be maintained as long as the lipid reduction continues.

The Lipid Research Clinic programme[53] has reported on a 12-centre randomized double-blind study in 3806 asymptomatic men aged 35–59 (mean 48 years), in good health and free from any symptoms of coronary heart disease, but clearly at high risk by having Type II hyperlipoproteinaemia. They were studied over a minimum period of 7 years, and their mean baseline concentration of plasma cholesterol was 292 mg/dl and of low density lipoprotein (LDL) cholesterol 216 mg/dl. Four months before randomization and throughout the trial, they were given a diet in which the polyunsaturated: saturated ratio was increased. In addition the bile acid sequestrant, cholestyramine, was given at a dose of 24 g/day (six packs) to one group and a biologically inert silica mixture to the control group. The average consumption in both groups was about four packs a day (23% took less than two daily). No other drugs were prescribed, and no specific advice was given on smoking, exercise or weight.

The lowering of the plasma concentration of cholesterol was half (-14%) that predicted (-28%) and almost all occurred in LDL cholesterol. The decrease in plasma cholesterol in the control group was as predicted (4.9%), achieving an overall decrement in the treated group of 8.5% for plasma cholesterol and 12.6% for LDL cholesterol. High density lipoprotein showed a small increase of 2.8% by 7 years in the treatment group compared with the control group.

There was only a 7% reduction in total mortality (3.7% placebo, 3.6% cholestyramine), but a 19% reduction in the incidence of definite coronary heart disease and/or definite non-fatal myocardial infarction ($p < 0.05$), the primary end point of the study. There was a 24% reduction in coronary heart disease death rate (9.8% placebo, 8.1% cholestyramine) and 19% reduction in definite non-fatal myocardial infarction (8.4% placebo, 6.8% cholestyramine). The reduction in incidence of deaths from coronary heart disease was not manifest until 2 years after this study started, and was progressive.

There was an increase in deaths from accidents and violence in the cholestyramine-treated group. There were 21 incident and eight fatal cases of cancer in the gastrointestinal tract in the cholestyramine group, compared with 11 incident and one fatal case in the control group.

In conclusion, this trial has given clear evidence that reducing very high concentrations of cholesterol and LDL reduces the incidence of coronary heart disease, in high risk men. The cholesterol was lowered by half the predicted degree. Moreover, such a study requires a high degree of motivation over a long period in taking a bulky preparation.

Comment on primary prevention trials with lipid lowering drugs

The gain in knowledge for the vast amount of work expended is not very impressive, and the harder the end points, the less conclusive are the results. It would be envisaged that reduction in serum cholesterol, before the onset of clinical ischaemic heart disease, would be more likely to influence the course of coronary atherosclerosis than when myocardial infarction has occurred or angina pectoris is present. The fact that the trial results do not lend unequivocal support to the hypothesis may be related to the fact that many patients included were treated in the absence of defined hypercholesterolaemia and did not demonstrate a reduction in serum cholesterol. The multifactorial trials[6,8] have not shown that the inclusion of a cholesterol-lowering diet produces substantial reductions in mortality or morbidity in healthy men at risk. Added to this, the long term risks of drug treatment must be carefully scrutinized.

The results of the two major trials with clofibrate and cholestyramine indicate that the men at highest risk from high cholesterol concentrations have a 20% reduction in incidence of coronary heart disease when these levels are reduced by 9% in the WHO study and by 14% in the cholestyramine trial. In the former trial this reduction was confined to non-fatal myocardial infarction. Caution must be exercised in extrapolating these results to subjects with more modest elevations of cholesterol.

SECONDARY PREVENTION STUDIES

Short term studies

Antiarrhythmics (excluding β-adrenoceptor blocking agents)

Following acute myocardial infarction, death generally results from two pathophysiological processes. In the period early after infarction, electrical processes, in particular primary ventricular fibrillation (fibrillation unassociated with heart failure or cardiogenic shock), account for the largest percentage of deaths. Later deaths from acute

Table 3.5 Short-term antiarrhythmic therapy: design

Trial	Type of control	Type of blind	Number randomized	Entry window	Intervention(s)	Length of follow-up
Quinidine						
Holmberg and Bergman[65]	Placebo	DB	104	<24 h	quinidine p.o. 1200 mg/day	14 days
Jones et al.[66]	Placebo	DB	246	<24 h	quinidine p.o 1200 mg/day for 3 days	14 days
Procainamide						
Reynell[67]	Usual treatment	Open	106	<96 h	procainamide 2–4 g/day for 2–3 weeks	Hospital discharge*
Koch-Weser et al.[68]	Placebo	DB	110	<72 h	procainamide 1 g stat. + 2–4 g/day	7 days
Disopyramide						
Jennings et al.[73]	Placebo	DB	180	<48 h	disopyramide 100 mg stat. + 400 mg/day for time in CCU	Hospital discharge*
Nicholls et al.[74]	Placebo injection + capsules	DB	199	<24 h	disopyramide 100 mg i.v. stat. + 400 mg/day p.o.	Hospital discharge*
Wilcox et al.[75]	Placebo	DB	316	<24 h	disopyramide 450 mg/day	42 days
UK Rhythmodan Multicentre Study Group[76]	Placebo	DB	1985	<24 h	disopyramide 300 mg stat. + 40 mg/day for up to 14 days	14 days
Lignocaine						
Bennett et al.[78]	Usual treatment	Open	610	<48 h	lignocaine 50 mg i.v. stat. + 0.5–1.0 mg/min for 48 h	Hospital discharge*
Pitt et al.[79]	5% dextrose infusion	Open	222	<24 h	lignocaine 75–100 mg i.v. stat. + 2.5 mg/min for 48 h	Hospital discharge*
Darby et al.[80]	Usual treatment	Open	322	<48 h	lignocaine 200 mg i.m. stat. + 2 mg/min. i.v. for 48 h	Hospital discharge*
O'Brien et al.[81]	5% dextrose infusion	DB	300	on hosp.* admission	lignocaine 75 mg i.v. stat. + 2.5 mg/min for 48 h	2 days
Lie et al.[82]	5% glucose infusion	DB	225	<6 h	lignocaine 100 mg i.v. stat. + 3 mg/min for 48 h	CCU* discharge
Valentine et al.[83]	Saline	DB	364	<12 h	lignocaine 300 mg i.m. stat.	30 days
Lie et al.[84]	Saline	DB	321	<6 h	lignocaine 300 mg i.m. stat.	Hospital discharge*
Koster et al.[85]	No treatment	DB	1447	pre-hosp. admission	lignocaine 400 mg i.v.	Not given
Campbell et al.[86]	Placebo	DB	763	<6 h	tocainide 500 mg i.v. 600 mg oral	48 h
Bell et al.[87]	Placebo	DB	216	<36 h	mexiletine 400 mg stat. 600 mg/day	6 weeks

* Insufficient details given

92

Table 3.6 Short term antiarrhythmics therapy: results

Trial	Control Number randomized	Control No. of deaths	Per cent mortality	Number randomized	Intervention No. of deaths	Per cent mortality	p-Value*
Quinidine							
Holmberg and Bergman	55	4	7.3	49	9	18.4	0.16
Jones et al.†	58	6	10.3	45	4	8.9	1.0
Procainamide							
Reynell	55	5	9.1	51	5	9.8	1.0
Koch-Weser et al.†	33	3	9.1	37	3	8.1	1.0
Disopyramide							
Jennings et al.†	49	5	10.2	46	2	4.3	0.48
Nicholls et al.	99	12	12.1	100	10	10.0	0.80
Wilcox et al.	158	10	6.3	158	14	8.9	0.52
UK Rhythmodan Multicentre Study Group	990	55	5.6	995	72	7.2	0.14
Lignocaine							
Bennett et al.†	125	8	6.4	249	25	10.0	0.33
Pitt et al.	114	16	14.0	108	9	8.3	0.26
Darby et al.†	100	11	11.0	103	12	11.7	1.0
O'Brien et al.	146	4	2.7	154	11	7.1	0.14
Lie et al.†	105	10	9.5	107	8	7.5	0.77
Valentine et al.	157	18	11.5	207	26	12.6	0.88
Lie et al.†	153	6	3.9	157	5	3.2	0.97
Koster et al.	741	8	1.1	706	3	0.4	0.22
Tocainide							
Campbell et al.	379	8	2.1	384	7	1.9	0.98
Mexiletine							
Bell et al.	713	20	17.7	103	12	11.7	0.25

*p = Value computed for χ^2 test comparing the proportion of deaths in each group
†Incomplete reporting

myocardial infarction may also be electrical, but most frequently occur in association with extensive myocardial necrosis (heart failure and cardiogenic shock). A significant fraction of these episodes of secondary ventricular fibrillation occur from 24 hours to 1 week after the onset of infarction and is associated with diminishing pump function. Continuous monitoring in coronary care units has made possible the prompt recognition and treatment of serious arrhythmias, although a significant proportion may start before hospital admission. Enthusiasm for treatment with antiarrhythmic agents in the coronary care unit ranges from recommendations to treat all suspected cases of infarction with prophylactic lignocaine[54] to a high degree of scepticism about its value in treating warning arrhythmias[55].

There is a plethora of antiarrhythmic agents which have been studied in short and long term studies after myocardial infarction. Most of these are effective in suppressing various rhythm disturbances, but their benefit with regard to mortality when used prophylactically is much less convincing. There are a number of reasons for this.

Firstly, most reported studies are small in size or have a low placebo mortality. Secondly, many studies have failed to take account of the relationship between blood concentration and antiarrhythmic effect[54,56,57].

Thirdly, the conditions predisposing to any particular arrhythmia probably change during the evolution of myocardial infarction, and the electrophysiological properties of one drug may not be appropriate throughout. It is unrealistic to expect that any one agent will prove effective in suppressing severe arrhythmias in all patients. Fourthly, adverse effects are common, and many patients are withdrawn from studies.

Seventeen studies with quinidine, procainamide, disopyramide, lignocaine, tocainide and mexiletine meet the criteria for inclusion in this review (Tables 3.5 and 3.6). β-Blockers are regarded as a separate entity. In none of the studies was there a convincing attempt to titrate dose against antiarrhythmic effect. Some of the studies with lignocaine used increasing or repeated administrations if warning ventricular arrhythmias were not significantly suppressed.

Many studies with newer agents are being conducted, particularly with the Class I antiarrhythmic agents such as flecainide, encainide, lorcainide and tocainide, and with amiodarone. The author is not aware of any trials with these drugs which meet the review criteria.

QUINIDINE

Quinidine has been used for the treatment of supraventricular and ventricular arrhythmias for over 50 years. Its use is attended by occasional instances of sudden cardiac death. It is difficult to distinguish quinidine toxicity from failure to control the pre-existing arrhythmias in these circumstances, but it is recognized that the presence of the long Q–T syndrome and digitalis therapy increase the chance of severe ventricular arrhythmias with quinidine[58]. The therapeutic ratio of quinidine is low, and gastrointestinal upsets are common, especially when the drug is first introduced.

Early reports[59,60] and some later ones[61] advocated its use to prevent ventricular arrhythmias following myocardial infarction. Later studies[62-64] did not support this view. The two trials which meet the review criteria do not allow definite conclusions to be drawn.

Holmberg and Bergman[65] reported a double-blind study in 104 postinfarction patients. Treatment with quinidine or placebo started within 24 h of admission to hospital and continued for 2 weeks. Overall arrhythmia frequency, especially the incidence of ventricular premature beats, was reduced by quinidine, but the difference was not statistically significant. The mortality was twice as high in the intervention group as in the control group (nine versus four).

Jones et al.[66] randomized 246 patients suspected of having an uncomplicated myocardial infarction within the previous 24 h to either quinidine or placebo tablets. Of these patients, 143 were subsequently withdrawn from the study as they did not satisfy the criteria for diagnosis of myocardial infarction. The remaining 103 were monitored on therapy for a total of 3 days, and outcome was determined 11 days later, at the time of hospital discharge. Quinidine significantly reduced the incidence of ventricular tachycardia and ventricular premature beats, but there was no difference in mortality either for the first 72-hour period or at the end of hospitalization (four versus six deaths).

PROCAINAMIDE

Procainamide has a similar spectrum of antiarrhythmic activity to that of quinidine, and can be given parenterally or orally. Acute intervention with procainamide is frequently reserved for patients who fail to respond to quinidine. For chronic oral therapy, procainamide is inconvenient because the short half-life dictates that the drug must be given every 3-4 h to maintain an effective plasma level. Gastrointestinal symptoms are less frequent than with quinidine, but agranulocytosis is a well-documented complication in the early weeks of treatment.

Reynell[67] conducted an open study in 106 patients randomized within 4 days of the onset of myocardial infarction. Two different dosage schedules of procainamide were evaluated – 0.5 mg four times a day from the end of the first week after infarction until the end of the fourth week, or alternatively in a second phase of the trial, 1 mg four times a day.

By the time of hospital discharge, there was no evidence that the drug at either dose reduced mortality (five deaths in each group) or the incidence of ventricular arrhythmias. Koch-Weser and his colleagues[68] reported the results of a placebo controlled trial in 110 patients admitted within 72 h of their infarction. Patients allocated to procainamide received a loading dose of 1 g followed by 250, 375 or 500 mg every 3 h, depending on bodyweight. Results from 70 patients in whom a myocardial infarction was confirmed are reported. Procainamide significantly decreased all forms of ventricular arrhythmias compared with the control group, an effect which was more apparent as the duration of therapy increased. After 7 days, the mortality was the same in both groups (three deaths in each group).

DISOPYRAMIDE

This drug is not chemically related to other antiarrhythmic drugs, but is similar in activity to quinidine or procainamide. It is available for oral and parenteral administration.

Zainal et al.[69] report a study in 58 postinfarction patients randomized to disopyramide or placebo. There was a drug-associated significant reduction in mortality, incidence of infarct extension, ventricular tachycardia and ventricular fibrillation. However, the trial received considerable criticism[70-72] and three subsequent studies in which the prophylactic value of disopyramide with regard to mortality has been tested, were equivocal.

Jennings et al.[73] randomized 180 postinfarction patients to disopyramide or matching placebo, whilst patients were in the Coronary Care Unit (CCU). The maximum time between onset of symptoms and randomization was 48 h, but the median time for both groups was 8 h. Eighty-five patients were not considered in the analysis; myocardial infarction was not confirmed in 70, and the e.c.g. recordings were faulty in 15 others. Twice as many patients receiving placebo as were treated with disopyramide required supplementary antiarrhythmic therapy whilst in the CCU (42 versus 21). This highly significant difference was mainly accounted for by the higher incidence of ventricular arrhythmias in the placebo group. Five patients on placebo and two in the intervention group died by the time of hospital discharge. This difference is not statistically significant.

The study by Nicholls et al.[74] was also double-blind and randomized. 199 patients admitted within 24 h of their infarction received a loading dose of 100 mg disopyramide intravenously followed by oral treatment for 10 days, or received placebo. At the time of discharge there was no significant difference in total mortality between the disopyramide and placebo groups (ten versus 12 deaths).

Wilcox et al.[75] randomized 473 patients with suspected myocardial infarction within 24 h of the onset of symptoms to oral disopyramide, oxprenolol or placebo. Ninety per cent of patients in each group began treatment within 12 h of symptoms. Treatment stopped at 6 weeks, at which time there was no significant difference in total mortality between the disopyramide and placebo groups (14 versus ten deaths). There were non-significant reductions in the incidence of ventricular arrhythmias in the disopyramide group. The oxprenolol results are given in the section on β-blockers.

The UK "Rhythmodan" Multicentre Study Group[76] randomized 1985 patients who entered hospital with a suspected myocardial infarction, to oral disopyramide (300 mg loading dose, then 100 mg four times a day) or placebo. Treatment was started within 24 h of onset of symptoms (mean time 9 h) and continued until hospital discharge or 14 days, whichever was sooner. Of these patients, 995 received disopyramide and 990 received placebo. The total mortality was 7.2% and 5.6%. Patients who had proven infarction (687 on disopyramide and 716 on placebo) did not have a reduced mortality with treatment (9.5% versus 7.4%). Reinfarction rate was not altered by disopyramide. The incidence of congestive heart failure was similar in the two groups, but the mortality was higher in patients with conduction defects treated with disopyramide (63%) compared with placebo (26%).

LIGNOCAINE

There are numerous reports on the use of lignocaine in the prophylactic treatment of acute myocardial infarction. Unlike procainamide and quinidine, lignocaine has little effect on supraventricular arrhythmias, but is generally accepted as the drug of first choice in the suppression of ventricular arrhythmias. It acts rapidly when given parenterally and has a short duration of action which enables its effect to be titrated. Bioavailability is poor after oral administration because of high first pass metabolism, making it unsuitable for chronic therapy.

Many of the studies with lignocaine use ventricular fibrillation as the primary end point and reviews of the studies stress the value of lignocaine in preventing ventricular fibrillation in younger patients who are enrolled early and who have no evidence of cardiogenic shock or congestive heart failure[77]. Unfortunately, mortality data are incomplete in a number of these trials.

Reverting to the review criteria of 100 patients randomized to intervention or control with mortality reported as a major end point, the trials with lignocaine can be divided into two groups. Five trials randomized patients at various times after entry to hospital. Three trials have reported results in which prophylactic treatment was given in the prehospital phase.

The hospital-based studies include three open[78-80] and two double-blind trials[76,77]. The first open study was reported by Bennett et al.[78] in which 610 patients were randomized to one of three groups within 48 h of onset of symptoms of suspected infarction. Groups one and two received 50 mg of lignocaine intravenously, followed by a 48 h infusion at a rate of 0.5 mg/min in one group and 1 mg/min in the other. The control group did not receive lignocaine.

Two hundred and ninety-nine patients were withdrawn from the study, 236 of them because the initial diagnosis of myocardial infarction was not confirmed and the rest due to complications, especially atrioventricular block and pulmonary oedema. There was no significant difference in the incidence of these complications between intervention and control groups. Lignocaine therapy at either infusion rate did not significantly reduce the incidence of ventricular premature beats, ventricular tachyarrhythmias or total mortality.

A second study from the same centre was reported by Darby et al.[80] in a similar population. The initial loading dose of lignocaine was given by intravenous injection followed by an intravenous infusion at the rate of 2 mg/min. There were no significant differences in the incidence of ventricular extrasystoles and in mortality at the time of hospital discharge, in the intervention and control groups (12 versus 11 deaths). Ventricular tachycardia and fibrillation were actually more common in the lignocaine-treated group, but this difference was not statistically significant.

Pitt et al.[79] randomly allocated 222 patients within 10 h of symptoms to lignocaine infusion (2.5 mg/min or control). There was a reduction in the incidence of ventricular tachyarrhythmias and fewer deaths in the lignocaine group (nine versus 16) but neither difference was significant.

The two double-blind hospital-based trials failed to show a significant reduction in mortality following treatment with lignocaine. O'Brien et al.[81] gave 75 mg lignocaine intravenously followed by a maintenance infusion of 2.5 mg/min for 48 h to 154 patients, 146 acting as controls. The incidence of ventricular tachycardia and fibrillation was not reduced in the treatment group and the mortality on lignocaine exceeded that in the control group (11 versus four deaths).

Lie et al.[82] randomized 225 patients under 70 years of age with uncomplicated infarcts to lignocaine infusion (3 mg/min) or glucose for 48 h. Eleven patients experienced ventricular fibrillation and six ventricular tachycardia in the control group, compared with 0 and two in the lignocaine group. This difference was significant for ventricular fibrillation ($p < 0.002$), but the mortality was similar in the intervention and control groups (eight versus ten). There was a high incidence of unwanted effects (15%) on lignocaine, especially in the older patients.

Three studies have been reported in which lignocaine has been administered very early after the onset of symptoms by medical or paramedical staff. Valentine et al.[83] organized a study in which 374 patients with suspected myocardial infarction were randomly allocated to treatment with 300 mg intramuscular lignocaine or placebo, administered by family physicians. Ten patients died before injection, and in 95 patients the presumptive diagnosis of myocardial infarction proved to be incorrect. Of the remaining 269 patients, 156 received lignocaine and 113 placebo. This unequal division is unlikely to be due to chance, and bias in assignment must be considered a likely possibility. There were three deaths in the lignocaine-treated group and eight in the control group in the first 2 hours of injection. However, the total mortality after 30 days did not bear out the earlier results (26 deaths in the lignocaine group and 18 in the placebo group). The second study was reported by Lie et al.[84] in 310 patients randomized to intramuscular lignocaine or placebo. There was no effect on early mortality or at the time of hospital discharge. The authors reasoned that the lig-nocaine blood concentrations were at the lower end of the therapeutic range for the suppression of ventricular premature beats and that lar-ger doses would be required. Koster et al.[85] have reported the preli-minary findings of a large randomized trial in the prehospital phase. One thousand four hundred and forty-seven patients were given 400 mg intramuscular lignocaine or a dummy injection by paramedical staff before transfer to hospital. Of these, 706 received lignocaine and 741 were controls. Four hundred and thirty-four (30%) of patients proved subsequently to have an acute myocardial infarction. Three patients died in the treated group and eight in the control group, all within 1 h of injection and none from primary ventricular fibrillation, There was one case of primary ventricular fibrillation in the treated group and five in the control group.

TOCAINIDE
One study which meets the criteria for review has been reported with tocainide, a structural analogue of lignocaine, but with a longer half-life and high oral bioavailability. Campbell et al.[86] reported the results of a multicentre trial in which 791 patients were randomly allocated to receive combined intravenous and oral tocainide or to placebo within 6 h of the onset of chest pain. Seven hundred and sixty-three subsequently proved to meet the entry criteria, of whom 384 received tocainide. The study lasted for 48 h, at the end of which there were eight deaths in the placebo group and seven in the tocainide group. Eleven patients experienced ventricular fibrillation on placebo and six on tocainide. Significantly fewer patients were withdrawn from tocain-ide treatment with other serious ventricular arrhythmias. Tocainide was well tolerated in this study.

MEXILETINE
Mexiletine is an orally active Class I antiarrhythmic agent with similar properties to lignocaine. Bell et al.[87] reported a study in 216 patients randomized to treatment with oral mexiletine (single dose 400 mg followed by 200 mg three times a day) or placebo within 36 h of the onset of symptoms. Treatment was initiated by general practitioners. Fifty-nine patients subsequently proved not to have a myocardial in-farction. The total mortality at 6 weeks was 20 in the placebo group and 12 in the mexiletine group. This difference was not significant. There were seven sudden deaths in the placebo groups and four in the mexiletine group (not significant). The frequency of ventricular fibrilla-tion was significantly reduced in the mexiletine group, but there was only one case of ventricular fibrillation.

SUMMARY
In summary, six antiarrhythmic drugs have been evaluated in 17 trials which meet the review criteria. All the agents have been reported to

Table 3.7 Drugs to reduce myocardial injury. Miscellaneous: design

Trial	Type of control	Type of blind	Number randomized	Entry window	Intervention(s)	Length of follow-up
Hyaluronidase						
Maroko et al.[146]	Usual treatment	Open	111	<8h	hyaluronidase 500 µg i.v./kg per 6h for 48h	Hospital discharge
Flint et al.[148]	Placebo	Open	483	<6h	hyaluronidase 200 000 iu i.v. on admission	6 months
Henderson et al.[149]	Placebo	Open	192	<12h	hyaluronidase 200 000 iu i.v. on admission	2 weeks
Nitrates						
Lis et al.[98]	Placebo	DB	140	<12h	nitroglycerin 10 µg/min in 2h for 24h according to BP response	4 months
Flaherty et al.[94]	Placebo	DB	104	<12h	nitroglycerin infusion 5 µg/min according to BP response for 48h	3 months
Nitroprusside						
Durrer et al.[101]	Glucose	DB	328	<12h	nitroprusside infusion 15 µg/min according to BP response for 24h oral + isosorbide dinitrate 20 mg/day for 6 days	4 weeks
Cohn et al.[102]	Placebo	DB	812	<24h	nitroprusside 10 µg/min infusion according to response for 48h	13 weeks
Glucose–potassium insulin						
Mittra[106]	Usual treatment	Open	170	<48h	20 µg insulin s.c. daily + oral potassium and glucose	14 days
Pentecost et al.[107]	Usual treatment	Open	241	<48h	48 h infusion of GIK	Hospital discharge*
Medical Research Council[108]	Usual treatment	Open	986	<48h	20 µg insulin s.c. daily + oral potassium and glucose for 14 days	28 days
Rogers et al.[109]	Usual treatment	Open	190	<12h	50 µg insulin, 300 g glucose, 80 mEq/l potassium at 1.5 ml/kg per h for 2 days	

* Incomplete reporting

100

Table 3.8 Drugs to reduce myocardial injury. Miscellaneous: results

Trial	Central			Intervention			p-Value*
	Number randomized	No. of deaths	Per cent mortality	Number randomized	No. of deaths	Per cent mortality	
Hyaluronidase							
Maroko et al.	57	11	19.3	54	8	14.8	0.71
Flint et al.	242	45	18.5	239	27	11.3	0.025
Henderson et al.	81	7	8.6	84	1	11.9	0.06
Nitrates							
Lis et al.	76	10	13.2	64	5	7.8	0.22
Flaherty et al.	48	11	22.9	56	11	19.6	0.43
Nitroprusside							
Durrer et al.	165	20	12.1	163	9	5.5	<0.05
Cohn et al.	405	77	19.0	407	69	17.0	0.25
Glucose–potassium insulin							
Mittra	85	24	28.2	85	10	11.8	0.01
Pentecost et al.*	100	16	16.0	100	15	15.0	1.0
Medical Research Council*	488	115	23.6	480	103	21.5	0.48
Rogers*	94	?	0	96	?	0	—

* Incomplete reporting

suppress ventricular arrhythmias in the acute phase of myocardial infarction. Lignocaine and, to a lessser extent, tocainide reduce the incidence of ventricular fibrillation. None of these trials, however, has demonstrated a reduction in short term mortality to accompany these antiarrhythmic effects.

Drugs to reduce myocardial injury (see Tables 3.7 and 3.8)

Drugs to be considered in this class may reduce oxygen requirements, or increase oxygen supply to the ischaemic myocardium, or reduce, or postpone autolysis. Some of these agents have several effects; for example, β-blockers reduce oxygen demand by decreasing the work of the heart, but they are also antiarrhythmic and may have other important effects on platelet function and prostaglandin production.

DRUGS REDUCING OXYGEN REQUIREMENTS

Nitrates. Nitrates have many pharmacological effects which would recommend them as agents to reduce mortality for myocardial infarction, and it is surprising that no formal studies have been conducted.

The trinitrates, in the form of nitroglycerin, the dinitrates and mononitrates have established places in the treatment of angina pectoris. Until recently, nitroglycerin has been avoided in the treatment of pain caused by myocardial infarction, because of the belief that the arterial hypotension and reflex tachycardia so induced might extend the ischaemic process. Studies in single vessel ischaemia in dogs by Epstein et al.[88] have indicated that nitroglycerin reduces the extent of ST segment elevation, reduces the amount of myocardial creatine kinase loss and reduces the morphological extent of infarction as well as improving survival. These effects were enhanced when the rise in heart rate and hypotension were offset by co-administration of the α-agonist, methoxamine.

These observations were confirmed in experimentally induced multivessel disease[89]. Electrophysiological evidence of ischaemia was prevented provided hypotension and reflex tachycardia were minimized.

Kent et al.[90] were able to demonstrate that nitroglycerin raises the ventricular fibrillation threshold following experimentally induced ischaemia in dogs, an effect which was augmented by the addition of methoxamine, which also raised systemic pressure. The same group[91] confirmed that the decrease in ventricular fibrillation threshold during ischaemia was reversed by nitroglycerin, and was associated with a significant reduction in the incidence of death due to ventricular fibrillation.

Nitroglycerin administered alone consistently reduces left ventricular filling pressure, and left ventricular volume. Thus myocardial wall tension and myocardial oxygen requirements would diminish.

Canine experiments have also shown that nitroglycerin can reduce resistance to flow in coronary collateral vessels thereby improving flow to the ischaemia myocardium[92].

These experiments illustrate the opposing effects of nitroglycerin-induced reduction in arterial pressure reduction in ischaemic injury and suggest that the net effect on the balance of myocardial requirements and delivery may be variable and unpredictable.

In man, several groups have demonstrated that nitroglycerin can reduce ischaemic injury during acute myocardial infarction[93,94] and that left ventricular filling pressure was reduced. It has also been observed that these beneficial effects can be demonstrated in patients with acute myocardial ischaemia in the absence of haemodynamic evidence of left ventricular failure[93,95].

Jaffe et al.[96] reported that intravenous glyceryl trinitrate administered to 43 patients within 10 h of the onset of symptoms significantly reduced enzymatically determined infarct size compared with a control group of 42, but only in patients with inferior infarcts. There were more ventricular arrhythmias in treated patients, but this difference was not statistically significant. There was a significant drop in systolic blood pressure, but no clinical evidence of heart failure. Flaherty et al.[97] were unable to show that intravenous nitroglycerin administered to 56 patients within 12 h of onset of symptoms resulted in a reduction in infarct size as determined by creatine kinase release or precordial R wave preservation, except in those patients admittted early to the trial (under 10 h). This subset also had a lower incidence of congestive heart failure. However, by 3 months, 11 of the 56 patients in the treated group had died, compared with 11 of 48 in the placebo group.

In a study of 140 patients admitted within 12 h of onset of symptoms, Lis et al.[98] randomly allocated 64 patients to receive a 48 h infusion of nitroglycerin and 76 received the vehicle placebo. Patients with systolic blood pressure above 130 or below 95 mmHg were excluded, as were those with heart rates below 50 beats/min, or above 130 beats/min.

The 4 month mortality was 7.8% in the treatment (five patients) group, compared with 13.2% in the placebo group (ten patients). This is not statistically significant. There was a significant reduction in the analgesic intake in the treatment group. Eighty-three per cent of patients who received nitroglycerin were able to resume normal activity by 3 months compared with 60% in the placebo group.

Nitroprusside. Sodium nitroprusside infusions have been shown to improve acute left ventricular function in experimental[99] and clinical myocardial infarction[100], by raising cardiac output and reducing filling pressure.

Two studies on mortality have been reported which meet the criteria of this review. Durrer et al.[101] randomized 328 patients to receive an infusion of nitroprusside, followed by isosorbide dinitrate or to 5% glucose. At 1 week, five of the 163 treated patients died, compared with ten of the controls ($p < 0.05$). Peak creatine kinase activity, incidence of cardiogenic shock and clinical signs of left ventricular failure were significantly reduced in the nitroprusside group.

Cohn et al.[102] randomly allocated 812 men within 24 h of onset of symptoms and with a left ventricular filling pressure of at least 12 mmHg, to receive an infusion of nitroprusside or placebo for 48 h. By 3 weeks, 47 died in the nitroprusside group, compared with 42 in the placebo group. After 13 weeks, the number of deaths was 69 in the nitroprusside group and 77 in the placebo group. These differences are not significantly different. Patients receiving treatment within 9 h of onset of pain had a higher mortality than those beginning later.

Glucose-potassium-insulin. Sodi-Pallares and his co-workers in 1961[103] suggested that an infusion of potassium combined with glucose and insulin (G.I.K.) might stabilize the membrane potential of anoxic myocardial cells, and prevent intracellular potassium loss. A reversal of this process could possibly prevent electrical instability and subsequent generation of ventricular arrhythmias. More recent work suggests that G.I.K. depresses circulating free fatty acid concentration which are known to be toxic to membranes and to provide glucose as an alternative source of energy by glycolytic production of adenosine triphosphate. This would reduce oxygen demand and possibly limit infarct size.

Studies on myocardial performance have not given consistent findings. Whitlow et al.[104] treated 13 patients with suspected acute myocardial infarction within 12 h of onset of symptoms for 48 h with G.I.K. and compared the results in 15 control patients. Treatment resulted in significant improvements in global and infarct zone ejection fractions, and in decreases in end-diastolic pressures. Sundstedt et al.[105] in a randomized study of 50 patients with suspected infarction within 6 h of onset were unable to demonstrate differences in cumulative creatine kinase or myoglobin release between treatment and control groups, and the frequency of ventricular extrasystoles was the same.

Four studies, in which mortality was a major end point, have been reported. All are randomized, but of open design. Mittra[106] randomized 170 patients within 48 h of the onset of chest pain to receive G.I.K. by either subcutaneous insulin and oral potassium and glucose, or a control group who received routine care. All subjects received anticoagulants. By 14 days of treatment, there were ten deaths in the G.I.K. group, and 24 in the control group ($p < 0.05$).

Pentecost et al.[107] randomized 200 patients to receive G.I.K. infusion for 2 days or a control group. Treatment was initiated within 48 h of onset of symptoms. There was no difference in the mortality of the two groups by the time of hospital discharge, usually 4 weeks (15 intervention versus 16 control group).

The Medical Research Council Trial[108] undertook a multicentre trial in 986 patients, randomized to 10 units of insulin twice a day, with oral glucose and potassium, or to routine medical care. In addition, some centres administered oral starch placebo tablets. Anticoagulants were given only when necessary. Intervention was given for 14 days, and mortality determined at 28 days. There was no significant difference in total mortality (G.I.K. 103 deaths; control 115 deaths).

Rogers et al.[109] randomly allocated 190 patients with chest pain of 12 h duration to receive G.I.K. infusion for 48 h, or to a control group. No patients died within the group whilst in hospital. Acute myocardial infarction was confirmed enzymatically in 64% of the G.I.K. treated patients, compared with 77% of the control group ($p < 0.06$). In patients who subsequently developed acute myocardial infarction, the mortality was 6.6% (4/61) in the intervention group and 12.5% (9/92) in the control group. This was not significant. No significant differences in ventricular function between the two groups were demonstrated at hospital discharge.

Calcium-channel blocking agents. Many calcium channel blocking drugs are undergoing clinical trials in hypertension and angina pectoris, and most experience has been gained with verapamil, diltiazem and nifedipine. Verapamil and nifedipine have been shown to protect against experimentally-induced myocardial ischaemia[110], and to reduce infarction size after experimental coronary artery occlusion[111]. They have also been shown to reduce release of creatine phosphokinase in patients with acute myocardial infarction after intravenous administration[112]. Nifedipine has been shown to have antiarrhythmic activity in an isolated rat heart model[113] but has minimal electrophysiological effects in man[114].

There are two reports on the effect of early intervention with nifedipine in man. The Norwegian Nifedipine Group[115] randomized 227 patients with suspected myocardial infarction within 12 h at onset to placebo or to sublingual followed by oral nifedipine. Ten patients died in each group within the first 6 weeks, and there was no difference in calculated infarct size from enzyme release data. Muller et al.[116] reported a similar study in 171 patients with threatened infarction randomized to receive oral nifedipine or placebo within 5 h of onset of pain. There was no reduction in infarct size, and the 2 week mortality was 8% nifedipine, 0% placebo ($p < 0.05$) and at 6 months 10% and 9% (not significant) respectively.

DRUGS INCREASING OXYGEN SUPPLY

Platelet active drugs. It is probably incorrect to consider aspirin, sulphinpyrazone and dipyridamole under this title as the mechanisms underlying their beneficial (and undesirable) effects are almost certainly not entirely through modification of platelet activity. Their biochemical actions are complex, and the relevance of each to observed clinical effects, ill-understood.

Aspirin induces a functional defect in platelets, demonstrable clinically by a prolonged bleeding time through inactivation of the enzyme cyclo-oxygenase, thereby eliminating the synthesis of thromboxane A_2 (TXA_2), a potent platelet aggregator. Released thromboxane A_2 also produces vasoconstriction as part of the response to vascular injury. In addition, aspirin inhibits prostacyclin (PGI_2) the major cyclo-oxygenase product in vascular endothelium. The main action of PGI_2 is to inhibit platelet aggregation and induce vasodilatation, generally desirable properties in patients with coronary arterial disease. Hence an 'aspirin dilemma' arose, as inhibition of vascular prostacyclin was seen to be potentially deleterious; the dilemma was invoked to explain the inconclusive results of some clinical trials. Low dose (about 150 mg daily) aspirin was recommended, on the premise that vessel prostacyclin synthesis is less sensitive to aspirin inhibition than is platelet TXA_2 production. Since the cyclo-oxygenase enzyme in endothelium, but not in platelets, can be resynthesized, production can resume between doses of aspirin. Efforts to solve the 'aspirin dilemma' and offer explanations for variable trial results have not been wholly satisfactory[117].

The development of selective thromboxane A_2 synthetase enzyme inhibitors have provided a way to a clearer understanding of the 'aspirin dilemma', and clinical trials in myocardial ischaemia are under way.

Dipyridamole has been used in several clinical studies. It has a variety of pharmacological effects with uncertain importance in clinical practice. It does inhibit platelet function, but in doses considerably higher than those required for coronary dilatation[118]. It is a phosphodiesterase inhibitor, thus potentiating the breakdown of adenosine triphosphate into cyclic adenosine monophosphate, a nucleotide which blocks platelet function. It has subsequently been shown that dipyridamole potentiates endogenous prostacyclin activity, and stimulates prostacyclin release from blood vessels[119]. It also inhibits thromboxane A_2 generation by platelets[120] and improves platelet survival[121]. The Persantin–Aspirin Reinfarction Study Research Group[122] tested the combination of dipyridamole and doses of aspirin high enough to prevent vascular PGI_2 generation. The result has indicated that aspirin alone produced a greater reduction in mortality than the combination, and recent data have suggested that aspirin may negate the potentially beneficial effects of dipyridamole on vascular PGI_2 synthesis[119]. Dipyridamole alone may reduce the capacity of the vascular endothelium to produce PGI_2[123].

Sulphinpyrazone was initially used as an uricosuric agent, but both it and its metabolites can inhibit platelet cyclo-oxygenase[124,125]. It has also been shown to reduce the susceptibility of endothelium to damage[126] but it does not affect endothelial cell synthesis of prostacyclin at doses which block the platelet enzyme[127]. Sulphinpyrazone has been reported to have antiarrhythmic activity in animals[128] but not in man[129]. This group also reported a persistent and significant rise in serum urea and creatinine. Other workers have also reported renal impairment following treatment with sulphinpyrazone[130,131].

Many other drugs have antiplatelet activity. Clofibrate has been shown to reduce platelet retention in patients with ischaemic heart disease, to suppress collagen-induced platelet aggregation and to prolong platelet survival in man[132,133]. In particular the β-adrenoceptor blocking drugs have antiplatelet activity. *In vitro* studies on human and animal platelets suggest that inhibition of catecholamine-induced platelet aggregation is via the β_2- rather than the β_1-receptor[134,135] and that propranolol can inhibit the release and action of thromboxane A_2[136]. Practolol, acebutolol and oxprenolol appear to be less effective in these *in vitro* models of aggregation[135,137], and aspirin in combination with propranolol is more effective than propranolol alone[138]. Other workers have suggested that antiplatelet effects of propranolol are due to membrane stabilization[139], and occur only at high doses, possibly through inhibition of platelet thromboxane A_2 synthesis[140]. However, 80 mg/day propranolol was sufficient to reverse abnormal platelet aggregability and raise platelet aggregation threshold of adenosine diphosphate (ADP) in patients with angina pectoris[141]. Green et al.[142], studying patients from the Beta Blocker Heart Attack Trial, have reported that following oral doses of 40–320 mg/day, propranolol had no effect on platelet-collagen affinity, or factor VIII coagulant activity, but significantly reduced circulating platelet aggregates.

It thus appears that there may be at least two actions of propranolol on platelet function, one at a high concentration possibly mediated through the (+)-isomer and involving inhibition of thromboxane synthesis. At lower doses of propranolol circulating platelets may become refractory to ADP and tend to aggregate less.

Two short term trials which satisfy the criteria for this review have been conducted (Tables 3.9 and 3.10). One study used aspirin, the other dipyridamole, and both were of 1 month duration, were double-blind and placebo controlled. Gent et al.[143] randomly allocated 103 patients to receive dipyridamole 100 mg four times a day or placebo within 14 days of myocardial infarction, 75% within 3 days. Other treatment for the complications of myocardial infarction was administered as required. Treatment was continued for 28 days. Seventeen patients were withdrawn from analysis because of insufficient evidence to support the diagnosis of myocardial infarction, drug-related side-effects or incomplete follow-up. There were eight deaths in the dipyridamole group and three in the control group.

Elwood and Williams[144] studied the effects of a single dose (300 mg) aspirin given to patients with a suspected myocardial infarction on their first contact with a doctor. Mortality was determined at 1 month. A total of 2530 patients were admitted, but in 825, the initial diagnosis of myocardial infarction was not confirmed. The analysis based on the remaining patients indicated no benefit from a single dose of aspirin, with 159 deaths in the aspirin group and 172 in the placebo group.

In the short term study by Wilcox et al.[129] with sulphinpyrazone,

Table 3.9 Short term studies with platelet active agents: design

Trial	Type control	Type of blind	Number randomized	Entry window	Intervention(s)	Length of follow-up
Gent et al.[143]	Placebo	DB	120	<14 days	dipyridamole (400 mg/day)	28 days
Elwood and Williams[144]	Placebo	DB	2530	h–days	ASA* (300 mg stat.)	28 days

*ASA = acetylsalicylic acid or aspirin

Table 3.10 Short term studies with platelet active agents: results

Trial	Control			Intervention			p-Value*
	Number randomized	Control No. of deaths	Per cent mortality	Number randomized	Intervention No. of deaths	Per cent mortality	p-Value*
Gent et al.†	52	3	5.8	51	8	15.7	0.19
Elwood and Williams†	1281	172	13.4	1249	159	12.7	0.65

* p = Value computed for χ² test comparing the proportion of deaths in each group
† Incomplete reporting

108

designed to test the antiarrhythmic effects of this drug, there were eight deaths in the treatment group and one in the control group ($p < 0.05$).

Hyaluronidase (see Tables 3.7 and 3.8). Hyaluronidase, or intravenous GL enzyme, has been shown to reduce the extent of experimentally-induced myocardial necrosis[145] and preliminary studies in man reported reductions in precordial ST elevation[146,147]. Flint *et al.*[148] assessed the benefit of intravenous hyaluronidase in 483 patients enrolled within 6 hours of the onset of chest pain. A single injection of 200 000 iu or placebo was given immediately on hospital admission. At 4 days, there were ten deaths in the enzyme treated group, and 18 in the placebo group. At 6 months, there were 27 deaths (11.3%) in the hyaluronidase group and 45 (18.5%) in the placebo group ($p = 0.025$).

Henderson *et al.*[149] reported the results of a randomized trial in 142 patients admitted within 12 h of onset of chest pain; 165 patients were subsequently diagnosed as having definite or possible myocardial infarction. By 2 weeks, one of the 84 hyaluronidase treated patients had died, compared with seven of the 81 placebo group. At 120 days, the figures were 7.2% versus 13.9%.

Thrombolytic agents. Streptokinase and urokinase have both been investigated in clinical trials as thrombolytic agents, though all recent work with intracoronary administrations has been carried out with streptokinase. Both act on the endogenous fibrinolytic system by promoting conversion of inactive plasminogen to the proteolytic enzyme plasmin[151]. The latter degrades fibrin and other plasma proteins before being inactivated by various naturally occurring inhibitors[152]. Coronary thrombosis has been re-established as an immediate precursor in the early phases of the clinical syndrome of evolving myocardial infarction[147, 153]. Complete cessation of blood flow to canine myocardium results in initiation of necrosis in approximately 20 min[147, 153]; and transmural necrosis in dogs is complete between 3 and 6 h[148, 154].

Coronary thrombolysis requires 3–7 h of treatment in experimental studies[149, 155], and early investigators concluded that clot lysis time far exceeded the ischaemic time tolerance for myocardial necrosis and acute infarcts[149, 156]. This led to important delays of 12–72 h after the onset of chest pain in the administration of streptokinase for acute myocardial infarction in all 11 European trials. Indeed, prevention of secondary thrombi was the primary objective of these studies[151, 157].

More recent experimental work has emphasized that canine myocardium remains viable for 3–6 h or longer after ligation[147, 153] and that the 'wave front' of necrosis appears to extend from the subendocardium outward to the subepicardium, which is a region more likely to receive a continual blood supply through communications from the subepicardial vessels downstream to the acute obstruction. This favours a longer interval before necrosis of the subepicardial zone. Streptokinase thrombolysis usually occurs promptly within 20–60 min in both animals[158], and humans[153,159] with acute myocardial infarction. Thus, there appears to be a therapeutic window of several hours between the onset of coronary thrombosis and the occurrence of irreversible myocardial necrosis, during which ischaemic myocardium may be preserved by coronary reperfusion.

There are many studies with both intravenous and intracoronary thrombolytic administration in which the end point has been recanalization or a measurement of ventricular function. The recent success with intracoronary streptokinase in these terms has redirected attention back to the potential benefits of systemic thrombolytic therapy administered promptly after the onset of acute infarction. Saltrups et al.[160] studied 24 patients randomly allocated to intracoronary or intravenous streptokinase within 3 h of onset of first-transmural myocardial infarction. Intravenous administration resulted in reperfusion in three of 11 patients, whilst intracoronary administration resulted in reperfusion in ten of 11 patients.

Berte et al.[161] studied 28 similar patients, and noted recanalization in 11 of 15 treated by the intracoronary route, and in eight of 13 treated by the intravenous route. Taylor et al.[162] in a sequential study of 126 patients showed that recanalization was successful in 48/63 and 53/63 respectively in the patients treated with streptokinase by the intracoronary and intravenous routes. Larger comparative trials are required, and the relative advantages and disadvantages of the two routes of administration carefully reviewed[163].

Thirteen trials in which intravenous streptokinase was administered meet the criteria for this paper. They have already been extensively reviewed[16,164,165]. Stampfer et al.[165] pooled results from eight trials which were randomized and controlled with a placebo or anticoagulant group. They concluded that there was a 20% reduction in the total mortality at 6 weeks among patients treated with streptokinase compared with the control groups ($p = 0.01$). The details of these 13 trials are given in Tables 3.11 and 3.12. Only two trials investigated the use of urokinase[167,168]; the remaining 11[168-179] gave streptokinase as an initial loading dose (250 000–1 250 000 units) followed by an intravenous infusion at a rate of 100 000–150 000 units/h for between 12 and 72 h, although in the Frankfurt study[172], infusion only lasted for 3 h. Some studies employed variable rather than fixed doses of the intervention.

In most studies, the control group also received an intravenous infusion, most commonly of heparin initially, followed by oral anticoagulation. Follow-up in each study was either until hospital discharge or for approximately 6 weeks. In four studies, follow-up was extended to 6 or 12 months, but without long term thrombolytic intervention. The results at these further time points did not alter the initial conclusions. The total number of patients randomized in these studies ranged from 107 to 776. Intervention was always started within 72 h of the onset of acute myocardial infarction symptoms, and in six trials was started within 12 h.

Table 3.11 Intravenous thrombolytic agents: design

Trial	Control	Type of blind	Number randomized	Entry window	Intervention Initial	Maintenance	Duration of infusion	Length of follow-up
1st European[168]	heparin	SB	192	<72h	†SK1250	100/h	72h	Hospital discharge*
2md European[169]	heparin	DB	764	<24h	SK 250	100/h	24h	Hospital discharge*
Finnish[170]	glucose	Open	426	<72h	SK 600	variable	up to 48h	42 days
Italian[171]	heparin	Open	321	<12h	SK 250	150/h	12h	40 days
Frankfurt[172]	laevulose	DB	206	<12h	SK 250	500/3h	3h	Hospital discharge*
French[166]	heparin	Open	120	<24h	UK fixed	fixed	24h	30 days
Australian[173]	heparin	Open	534	<24h	SK 250	100/h	18h	Hospital discharge*
Streptokinase Myocardial Infarction Trial (SMIT)[174]	heparin or glucose	DB	107	<24h	SK 250	100/h	24h	21 days
European Collaborative[167]	glucose	Open	341	<12h	UK variable	variable	18h	21 days
United Kingdom[175]	none	Open	660	<24h	SK 250	100/h	24h	42 days
North German[176]	heparin	Open	483	<12h	SK 250	100/h	16h	42 days
Austrian[177]	none	Open	728	<12h	SK 500	750/4h 1500/16h	20h	40 days
European Cooperative[178,179]	glucose	Open	315	<12h	SK 250	100/h	24h	21 days

* Insufficient details given
† Units in thousands; SK = streptokinase UK = urokinase

Table 3.12 Short term intravenous thrombolytic agents: results

Trial	Control Number randomized	Control No. of deaths	Per cent mortality	Number randomized	Intervention No. of deaths	Per cent mortality	p-Value*
1st European†	84	15	17.9	83	20	24.1	0.42
2nd European†	357	94	26.3	373	69	18.5	0.014
Finnish	207	17	8.2	219	22	10.0	0.63
Italian	157	18	11.5	164	19	11.6	1.0
Frankfurt	104	29	27.9	102	13	12.7	0.012
French	60	8	13.3	60	2	3.3	0.10
Australian	263	22	8.4	271	17	6.3	0.45
SMIT	54	3	5.6	53	7	13.2	0.30
European Collaborative	169	24	14.2	172	29	16.9	0.60
United Kingdom†	293	44	15.0	302	43	14.2	0.88
North German	234	51	21.8	249	63	25.3	0.42
Austrian	376	65	17.3	352	37	10.5	0.012
European Cooperative	159	30	18.9	156	18	11.5	0.10

*p-Value computed for χ^2 test comparing the proportion of deaths in each group
†Incomplete reporting

Seven of the 13 trials initiated therapy in the coronary care unit, and evaluated in-hospital mortality. Five gave equivolcal results[167,171,173–175].

The small French study[166] used a fixed dose of urokinase, and yielded a result which was not statistically significant (two versus eight deaths). The European Cooperative trial[178,179] randomized 315 high and medium risk patients, as determined by e.c.g. and haemodynamic criteria. The mortality rates at 6 months favoured intervention but were not statistically significant (18 versus 30 deaths).

The six remaining trials evaluated patients admitted to general wards only, or a mixture of patients from general wards and the coronary care unit.

In the first European Working Party study[168], there was no reduction in mortality (20 streptokinase deaths versus 15 control deaths). In their second trial[169], there was a statistically significant difference ($p < 0.014$) in favour of streptokinase (69 versus 94 deaths), but this includes eight deaths in the heparin group occurring after randomization, but before treatment could be started.

The Frankfurt[172] and Austrian[177] studies also suggested that streptokinase prolonged life in survivors of myocardial infarction. The Frankfurt study[172] was the second trial from this group, the first reporting an equivocal result on an open comparison of streptokinase with anticoagulants. In the double-blind trial, there was a greater than 50% reduction in mortality ($p < 0.05$) by intervention at the time of hospital discharge (13 deaths streptokinase; 29 deaths control). In the Austrian study[177] there was also a significant reduction ($p < 0.05$) in total mortality after 40 days follow-up (37 deaths streptokinase; 65 deaths control).

The remaining two trials, from Finland[170] and North Germany[176] studied assorted CCU and general ward patients. Both yielded inconclusive findings. The North German trial, in common with five of the other 12 trials, yielded a result with more deaths in the intervention compared with the control group (63 versus 51 deaths).

After reviewing these 13 trials in over 5000 patients, the question of whether the acute administration of intravenous thrombolysis agents reduces mortality remains unanswered. There is a trend in favour of the intervention in seven trials, but there is a statistically significant difference in only three. Another problem is whether the results apply to current clinical practice with these agents, as in two of these studies the control group mortality rate was over 26%.

The value of intracoronary streptokinase has been reviewed by Furberg[180]. Only three of the eight trials discussed meet the criteria for this review.

Kennedy et al.[181] studied 250 patients in a multicentre trial of 14 hospitals. Patients were eligible for enrolment up to 12 h after the onset of chest pain, and mean time of randomization was 4.5 h. After an initial coronary angiogram, 134 patients received streptokinase, and six received standard care on the coronary care unit. The unequal

Table 3.13 Mortality data from eight randomized controlled trials of intracoronary streptokinase

Trial	Mean follow-up time	Mortality Streptokinase (n)	Control (n)
Khaja et al.	9.6 months	1/20	4/20
Anderson et al.	In hospital	1/24	4/26
Leiboff et al.	11 months	4/22	2/18
Simoons et al.[182]	10 months	10/86	11/87
Verani et al.	6 weeks	4/29	2/35
Theroux et al.	12 months	4/10	3/8
Rentrop et al.	4 months	13/57	6/54
Kennedy et al.[181]	30 days	5/134	13/116
Total		42/382	45/364
Percentage		11%	12.4%
Difference in percentage		11%	12.4%
		11% (p = 0.64)	

After Furberg (1984)[180]

114

Table 3.14 Long term antiarrhythmics studies: design

Trial	Type control	Type of blind	Number randomized	Entry window	Intervention(s)	Length of follow-up
Collaborative Group	Low-dose	DB	568	At hospital discharge	phenytoin (300–400 mg/day)	12 months
Australia/Britain[183] Peter et al.[184]	phenytoin Usual care	Open	150	Before CCU discharge	phenytoin (variable to maintain serum levels of 40–80 mol/l)	24 months
Ryden et al.[185]	Placebo	DB	162	<2 days	tocainide (750 mg i.v. stat. + 1200 mg/day)	6 months
Bastian et al.[186]	Placebo	DB	146	7–10 days	tocainide (1200 mg/day)	6 months
Chamberlain et al.[187]	Placebo	DB	344	6–14 days	mexiletine (600–750 mg/day)	4 months (3 months intervention)
IMPACT[188]	Placebo	DB	630	3–25 days	mexiletine (720 mg/day)	12 months
Ghent–Rotterdam Study[189]	Placebo	DB	305	<14 days	aprindine (100–200 mg/day)	12 months

Table 3.15 Long term antiarrhythmics: results

Trial	Number randomized	Control No. of deaths	Per cent mortality	Number randomized	Intervention No. of deaths	Per cent mortality	p-Value*
Collaborative Group Australia/Britain	285	23	8.1	283	26	9.2	0.75
Peter et al.	76	14	18.4	74	18	24.3	0.50
Ryden et al.†	56	5	8.9	56	5	8.9	1.00
Bastian et al.	74	3	4.1	72	4	5.6	0.97
Chamberlain et al.	163	19	11.7	181	24	13.3	0.78
IMPACT	313	15	4.8	317	24	7.6	0.18
Ghent–Rotterdam Study	152	19	12.5	153	12	7.8	0.25

* p-Value computed for χ^2 test comparing the proportion of deaths in each group
† Incomplete reporting

randomization is curious and unexplained by the authors. The total mortality at 30 days was 3.7% in the streptokinase group and 11.2% in the control group ($p < 0.02$). By 6 months, the mortalities were 14.7% in the control group and 3.7% in the intervention group ($p < 0.0025$).

The second trial conducted by Simoons et al.[182] is still (1984) continuing. The interim report indicates that 173 patients have been randomly allocated to receive intracoronary streptokinase or conventional therapy (86 streptokinase and 87 control). By 10 months, ten had died in the streptokinase group and 11 in the control group.

The third trial[180] of sufficient size for inclusion is also from an interim report. 111 patients were randomly allocated to streptokinase (57) or control therapy (54). By 4 months 13 had died in the treatment group and six in the control group.

In the remaining five small trials reviewed by Furberg[180], the number of deaths is too low to draw any conclusions.

The eight studies are summarized in Table 3.13.

The overall percentage difference of 11% in favour of treatment is not significant ($p = 0.64$), and larger controlled trials are required before a decision about the usefulness of intracoronary streptokinase can be made.

Long-term studies

Antiarrhythmic drugs (excluding β-blockers) (Tables 3.14 and 3.15)

There are seven long term studies in which antiarrhythmic agents have been administered for 3 months or more, to prevent death in postinfarction patients.

The drugs to be evaluated are phenytoin, tocainide, mexiletine and aprindine. Six of the seven trials were double-blind[183-189], and one was open[183]. Patients were admitted within 25 days of their infarction or prior to hospital discharge. In only one study, with aprindine[189], were patients selected according to the presence of ventricular arrhythmias and the dosage of aprindine was adjusted in an attempt to control arrhythmias and avoid side-effects.

Total mortality was selected as the end point in two of the studies; the other five evaluated arrhythmic suppression, but data for mortality are available. In none of the studies is there a statistically significant difference in total mortality between the control and intervention groups. In five there is a trend that appears to indicate that antiarrhythmics may actually be detrimental. The study with aprindine makes an important observation. In 14 patients who had had a 24 h electrocardiogram prior to documented ventricular fibrillation after the first month of follow-up, all but one still showed the presence of complex ventricular arrhythmias, implying that the risk of death in those in whom it had disappeared (spontaneously or as a result of treatment) was improved for sudden death.

The recent results of IMPACT[188], a study with mexiletine, has been published in outline. Despite a significant reduction in some forms of complex ventricular arrhythmias after 1 and 4 months of treatment with mexiletine, compared with placebo, there is a non-significant increase in total mortality (7.6% versus 4.8%), cardiovascular deaths (6.6% versus 4.5%), and sudden death (2.2% versus 1.3%) with mexiletine. These findings are in line with those of Chamberlain et al.[187] although it should be noted that patients in this study were at higher risk.

COMMENT ON RESULTS
In these seven clinical studies of antiarrhythmic agents in over 2000 postinfarction patients, there is no evidence that antiarrhythmic therapy prolongs life in an unselected group, despite an effective reduction in the incidence of ventricular arrhythmias in five of the studies. In five of the studies there was a trend towards higher mortality in the intervention group.

Two other approaches to select high risk patients and individual treatment have been evaluated. Myerburg et al.[190] have titrated the dose of quinidine and procainamide to estimated therapeutic levels and maintained treatment for 12 months. In 16 patients with chronic ventricular arrhythmias who survived prehospital cardiac arrest, eight survived for longer than 1 year and eight had recurrent arrests. The survivors had stable therapeutic blood concentrations of the antiarrhythmic agent, but the recurrent cardiac arrest group did not. However, there was no correlation between suppression of arrhythmias, therapeutic concentration and recurrence of cardiac arrest.

Grayboys et al.[191] titrated the dose of the antiarrhythmic agent to abolish malignant arrhythmias and maintained that dose. In a non-randomized, open study of 123 patients, 98 had a successful abolition of their malignant arrhythmias, and 25 did not. The annual incidence of sudden death was 2.3% over 32 months in those successfully controlled, compared with 17 deaths in those uncontrolled over 19 months follow-up. This approach has been confirmed in another non-randomized trial of 50 patients with coronary arterial disease and complex ventricular arrhythmias, studied over a mean observation period of 16 months and treated with single or combined Class I, II and III antiarrhythmic agents[192]. Thirty-nine patients were considered responders, and three died, compared with five deaths in the 11 non-responders ($p < 0.01$).

Both of these designs require testing in a prospective, randomized trial, but the logistic problems are formidable.

Lipid lowering drugs (Tables 3.16 and 3.17)

There are seven trials which meet the criteria of the review, in which lipid lowering drugs have been studied. Two other studies employed diet alone, and these will be briefly summarized first.

Table 3.16 Long term studies with lipid lowering drugs: design

Trial	Type control	Type of blind	Number randomized	Entry window	Intervention(s)	Length of follow-up
Oslo Diet–Heart Study[193,194]	'Usual care'	Open	412	1–2 y	diet	60 months
Medical Research Council[195]	'Usual care'	Open	421	2–13 weeks	diet	11 y (2–81 months)*
Oliver and Boyd[196]	Placebo	SB	100	3–4 months	oestradiol (0.2 mg/day)	60 months
Stamler et al.[197]	Placebo	DB	275†	>2 months	oestrogen (10 mg/day)‡	58 months
Coronary Drug Project[198-201]	Placebo	DB	8341	>3 months	oestrogen (2.5 mg/day)	56 months
					oestrogen (5.0 mg/day)	21 months
					dextrothyroxine (6.0 mg/day)	36 months
					clofibrate (1800 mg/day)	74 months
					nicotinic acid (3000 mg/day)	74 months
Veterans Administration Drug–Lipid Cooperative[202]	Placebo	DB	570	1–16 months	oestrogen (1.25 mg/day)	60 months
					nicotinic acid (4000 mg/day)	
					nicotinic acid (4000 mg/day) + oestrogen (1.25 mg/day)	
					dextrothyroxine (4 mg/day)	
					dextrothyroxine (4 mg/day) + oestrogen (1.25 mg/day)	
Physicians of Newcastle upon Tyne Region[203]	Placebo	DB	497§	>6 weeks	clofibrate (1500–2000 mg/day)	43 months
Scottish Society of Physicians[204]	Placebo	DB	523	8–16 weeks	clofibrate (1600–2000 mg/day)	40 months (9–48 months)*
Carlson et al.[207,208]	Diet	Open	558	4 months	clofibrate (2000 mg/day) + nicotinic acid (3000 mg/day) + diet	

* Insufficient details given
† Includes 12 non-MI patients
‡ During the first year of the study, an oestrogen androgen group was abandoned and combined with the oestrogen group
§ Includes 202 non-MI patients

Table 3.17 Lipid lowering drugs: results

Trial	Number randomized	Control No. of deaths	Per cent mortality	Number randomized	Intervention No. of deaths	Per cent mortality	p-Value*
Oslo Diet–Heart Study							
(0–5 y)	206	55	26.7	206	41	19.9	0.13
(0–11 y)	206	108	52.4	206	101	49.0	0.55
Oliver and Boyd	50	12	24.0	50	17	34.0	0.39
Stamler et al.	119	—	33.8	156	—	23.6	0.094
Medical Research Council	207	31	15.0	214	28	13.1	0.68
Coronary Drug Project (CDP)	2789	525	18.8	1101	219	19.9 (2.5 mg oestrogen)	0.47
	2789	230	8.2	1119	108	9.7 (5 mg oestrogen)	0.18
	2715	339	12.5	1083†	160	14.8 (dextro-thyroxine)	0.067
	2789	709	25.4	1103	281	25.5 (clofibrate)	1.00
	2789	709	25.4	1119	273	24.4 (nicotinic ...)	0.53

Table (continued)

Trial	n	Deaths	Mortality (%)	n	Deaths	Mortality (%)	p*
Drug–Lipid Cooperative				77	24	31.2 (oestrogen)	0.82
				68	21	30.9 (nicotinic acid)	0.87
				74	17	23.0 (nicotinic acid + oestrogen)	0.46
						29.9 (dextro-thyroxine)	0.99
						11.1 (dextro-thyroxine + oestrogen)	0.019§
ΔPhysicians of the Newcastle upon Tyne Region‡	253	48	19.0	244	27		
ΔScottish Society of Physicians	367	35	9.5	350	34	9.7	1.00
Carlson et al.‡	279	26	9.3	279	24	8.6	0.88

*p-Values computed for χ^2 test comparing the proportion of deaths in each group
†Dextrothyroxine analysis excludes 27 dextrothyroxine patients and 74 placebo patients with frequent ventricular ectopic beats at entry
‡Primary end point is cardiac mortality (sudden death plus fatal MI plus congestive heart failure)
§Not statistically significant after continuity correction of Fisher's extract test
ΔExcluding patients with 'angina only' at entry

In the Olso Diet–Heart Study[193,194], 412 men, aged 30–64 years, were randomized 1–2 years after a first myocardial infarction to a diet low in saturated fats and cholesterol, and high in polyunsaturated fats, or to a control group. Trial entry mean serum cholesterol values were 296 mg/dl in both groups and fell by 17.6% in the treatment group and by 3.7% in the control group over the first 5 years. A 25% reduction in total mortality was noted in the intervention group at the end of 5 years, but this was not statistically significant. The combined incidence of both fatal and non-fatal reinfarctions and of major coronary heart disease relapses was, however, significantly reduced in the diet group. At the 11 year follow-up there was no difference between the two groups in total coronary heart disease or cardiovascular deaths, but there was again a statistically significant reduction in fatal myocardial infarction in the diet group (57 control versus 32 diet; $p < 0.004$). Total mortality difference at 11 years had fallen to 6%.

The Medical Research Council trial[195] conducted a study in which the intervention group received 85 mg/day of highly unsaturated soya bean oil in replacement of saturated fats, and the control group ate their customary diet. Male subjects under 60 years of age who had survived their first myocardial infarction were selected and were followed up for approximately 5 years. Initial mean serum cholesterol levels of 272 mg/dl were reduced by 12% in the test diet group and by 6% in the contrast group. There were no significant differences in fatal or non-fatal reinfarction rates between the two groups, and recurrence was not related to initial or to change in cholesterol levels. Total mortality was approximately the same in both groups.

OESTROGEN

The oestrogen trials of Oliver and Boyd[196], Stamler et al.[197] and the Coronary Drug Project[198] were the first in this category to be reported. Oliver and Boyd[196] used ethinyl oestradiol, while the others evaluated conjugated equine oestrogen at three different dosage levels.

All studies reported difficulties in adherence to the protocol because of breast tenderness or changes in libido. More significantly, both oestrogen regimens in the Coronary Drug Project[199–201] had to be terminated prematurely, because of adverse cardiovascular effects. The 5 mg/day oestrogen group was terminated after an average follow-up of 21 months, due to an excess of non-fatal reinfarctions, pulmonary embolism, and thrombophlebitis, compared with the placebo group. No beneficial effect on mortality was noted. The lower oestrogen group was followed for an average of 56 months before being terminated because of a higher total mortality in the treatment group. In addition, there were trends suggesting an excess of venous thromboembolism and mortality from malignant disease, particularly lung cancer.

The trial by Stamler et al.[197] reported no significant difference in survival between the oestrogen and placebo groups. There was an apparent benefit in the oestrogen group when patients who started oestrogen within 3 months of their most recent infarction, or within 2 months of admission to the study, were excluded.

Overall the studies with oestrogen therapy indicate no significant difference in total mortality compared with placebo-treated groups.

DEXTROTHYROXINE

Two of the reviewed studies utilized dextrothyroxine[199,202]. In the Coronary Drug Project[199], a total of 1119 men were randomized to 6 mg/day dextrothyroxine or placebo, and were followed for an average of 36 months before treatment was stopped prematurely. Twenty-seven patients in the dextrothyroxine group had frequent ectopic ventricular beats in the baseline resting e.c.g. and were discontinued after an average 21 months follow-up because of a higher mortality rate than a similar group of patients (74) receiving placebo. For the remaining 1083 patients receiving dextrothyroxine, total mortality was 18.4% higher than in the placebo group at 36 months. This never achieved statistical significance, but the difference in mortality between the groups increased progressively with time.

Deaths from coronary and all cardiovascular causes were also more common in the dextrothyroxine group, as was the incidence of recurrent myocardial infarction.

The Veterans Administration Drug–Lipid Cooperative Study[202] evaluated the long term efficacy of oestrogen, dextrothyroxine and nicotinic acid. Five hundred and seventy men who had sustained one or more myocardial infarctions were randomly allocated to placebo, oestrogen (2.25 mg/day), nicotinic acid, dextrothyroxine (4 mg/day), nicotinic acid with oestrogen or dextrothyroxine with oestrogen. As in the Coronary Drug Project, none of the regimens reduced total mortality.

CLOFIBRATE

The effect of clofibrate after myocardial infarction has been studied in four trials which meet the criteria for this review. The Coronary Drug Project[198,201] randomized 1103 men to a fixed dose of 1.8 g/day clofibrate. There was an average follow-up of 74 months. Total mortality in the clofibrate and placebo groups was almost identical and no subgroups were identified in which a beneficial effect was found. Coronary death alone or in combination with definite non-fatal myocardial infarction, if specified as an end point, was lower in the clofibrate group, although the differences were not statistically significant. However, the clofibrate group, when compared with the placebo group did experience a greater incidence of thromboembolism, angina pectoris, intermittent claudication, cardiac arrhythmias and non-fatal cardiovascular events. The incidence of gallstones was also increased twofold in the clofibrate-treated group.

The Newcastle[203] and Scottish studies[204] compared the effects of clofibrate and placebo in patients with coronary heart disease manifest as angina with or without myocardial infarction. The trials have similar design features and have been reviewed together by Dewar and Oliver[205], and by Rahlfs and Bedall[206]. However, there are several important differences in the group of patients admitted to the trial. The placebo group mortality rate was greater in the Newcastle compared with the Scottish study (5.34/1200 patient months versus 2.97/1200 patient months). Many more patients in the Newcastle study had multiple infarcts. In the Newcastle study, both groups with high initial serum cholesterol levels had more events, but this was not observed in the Scottish study. Thus Newcastle patients appeared to be at higher risk. The Newcastle study[203] comprised 497 patients of both sexes who were randomly assigned to receive clofibrate 1.5–2.0 g/day or to corn-oil capsules, and were followed for an average of 43 months. Forty-nine patients were prescribed additional anticoagulants in a single-blind manner and are included in the analysis. Total mortality is not reported, but there is a significant reduction in cardiac mortality ($p < 0.02$) and a striking reduction in the number of sudden deaths ($p < 0.05$) in the clofibrate treated group. This difference is particularly impressive for patients who entered the study in the 'angina only' or 'angina plus myocardial infarction' groups. There were fewer non-fatal myocardial infarctions in the clofibrate group ($p < 0.055$).

The Research Committee of the Scottish Society of Physicians[204] randomized 523 men and women to receive 1.6–2.0 g/day clofibrate or placebo. They were followed for approximately 40 months. A hundred and fifty-one patients received additional anticoagulant treatment. There was no difference in cardiac mortality between the clofibrate and placebo groups, but, as in the Newcastle study, there was a reduction in cardiac mortality (62%) and non-fatal infarction in those patients with pre-existing angina pectoris. There were more fatal infarcts in men in the 'infarct only' group treated with clofibrate compared with placebo (16% clofibrate versus 12% placebo). There was a significant reduction in sudden death ($p < 0.02$) in the angina pectoris ($\pm$ myocardial infarction) group.

In conclusion, the trials concur in showing that clofibrate is beneficial in those who present with angina and who continue to have angina after myocardial infarction. Clofibrate was well tolerated in both studies.

Carlson et al.[207] and Rosenheimer and Carlson [208] reported on a study in which 558 survivors of myocardial infarction were randomly allocated to diet alone, or diet with clofibrate (2 g/day) plus niacin (3 g/day). The design was open, and treatment was initiated 4 months after myocardial infarction. After a follow-up time of about 48 months (treatment time is not precisely specified) there was no difference in the total mortality between the groups, but a 50% reduction in non-fatal reinfarction ($p < 0.01$), and mean serum cholesterol was reduced by 15–20%.

Table 3.18 Long term studies with platelet active drugs: design

Trial	Type control	Type of blind	Number randomized	Entry window	Intervention(s)	Mean length of follow-up
Elwood and Sweetman[210]	Placebo	DB	1239	<6 months	ASA* (300 mg/day)	12 months
Coronary Drug Project Aspirin Study (CDPA)[211]	Placebo	DB	1529	week–year	ASA (972 mg/day)	22 months
German–Austrian Multicentre Prospective Clinical Trial[212,213]	Placebo	DB	626	28–42 days	ASA (1500 mg/day)	24 months
Elwood and Williams[214]	Placebo	DB	1725	Days–week	ASA (900 mg/day)	12 months
Aspirin Myocardial Infarction Study (AMIS)[215]	Placebo	DB	4524	2–60 months	ASA (1000 mg/day)	40 months
Persantine Aspirin Reinfarction Study (PARIS)[122]	Placebo	DB	2026	2–60 months	ASA (972 mg/day) + ASA (972 mg/day) + dipyrimadole (225 mg/day)	41 months
Anturane Reinfarction Trial (ART)[216–219]	Placebo	DB	1629	23–35 days	Sulphinpyrazone (800 mg/day)	16 months
Anturane Reinfarction Italian Study[220]	Placebo	DB	727	15–25 days	Sulphinpyrazone (800 mg/day)	19 months

*ASA = acetylsalicylic acid or aspirin

Table 3.19 Long term study with platelet active drugs: results

Trial	Control Number randomized	Control No. of deaths	Per cent mortality	Intervention Number randomized	Intervention No. of deaths	Per cent mortality	p-Value*
Elwood and Sweetman	624	61	9.8 (18.5)§	615	47	7.6 (12.2)	0.22
Coronary Drug Project	771	64	8.3	758	44	5.8	0.071
Aspirin Study (CDPA)	309	22	7.1	317	13	4.1	0.14
German–Austrian Multicentre Prospective Clinical Trial†‡							
Elwood and Williams	878	127	14.5	847	103	12.2	0.18
Aspirin Myocardial Indfarction Study (AMIS)	2257	219	9.7	2267	246	10.8	0.22
Persantine Aspirin Reinfarction Study (PARIS)	406	52	12.8	(ASA) 810	85	10.5	0.27
				(ASA+810 dipyridamole)	87	10.7	0.33
Anturane Reinfarction Trial (ART)	816	89	10.9	813	74	9.1	0.26
Anturane Reinfarction Italian Study	362	29	8.0	365	38	10.4	0.31

* p-Values computed for χ^2 test comparing the proportion of deaths in each group
† Incomplete reporting
‡ Primary end point is sudden death plus fatal MI
§ Numbers in parentheses refer to life table mortality at 24 months

COMMENT ON SECONDARY PREVENTION STUDIES WITH LIPID LOWERING DRUGS

Shaper[209] pointed out that the risk of recurrence of coronary heart disease event cannot usefully be assessed by the usual coronary heart disease risk factors. Recovery from and prognosis after a major episode is more reliably assessed by the clinical course, such as presence or absence of heart failure, serious ventricular arrhythmias, age and degree of persistent ischaemia.

No strong case can be made for the routine use of cholesterol-lowering drugs for patients with angina pectoris or myocardial infarction. The overall impression on reviewing the secondary prevention lipid-lowering trials together, is that life is not prolonged in the postinfarction group studied. Positive trends or statistically significant results are (in most cases) seen only when several end points are combined, or when certain subgroups of patients are excluded. The most convincing results come from the studies with clofibrate with a particular effect on case-specific mortality and non-fatal myocardial infarction.

As with the primary prevention studies with lipid lowering drugs, a variety of adverse effects were associated with the use of several of the drugs employed, which detracts from long term use of these agents.

Platelet active drugs

Eight studies, six with aspirin[122, 210–215] and two with sulphinpyrazone[216–221], meet the criteria of this review (Tables 3.18 and 3.19). All trials were double-blind, and placebo controlled, with random allocation to active intervention or placebo. The six aspirin trials employed daily doses varying from 300 to 1500 mg, and one[122] of those studies incorporated a second intervention group receiving aspirin and dipyridamole. The German–Austrian trial also included a second intervention group that was treated with phenprocoumon, an anticoagulant. The two sulphinpyrazone trials used 400 mg twice a day.

The population studied was large compared with many trials with other interventions and the variation in size reflects the response variables chosen and the anticipated benefit of the intervention. The first trial by Elwood and co-workers[210] and the CDPA[211] enrolled men only, whilst in the remaining six studies the proportion of females ranged from 10% to 20%.

Chosen trial end points also varied from trial to trial. Elwood[210], AMIS[215] and CDPA[211] selected total mortality for analysis, the German–Austrian investigators[212,213], preferred a combined end point of sudden death and fatal myocardial infarction, and the Anturane Reinfarction trial[216–219] organizers chose cardiac mortality. The Italian Anturane trial[220] organizers selected fatal and non-fatal myocardial reinfarction as the primary end point, whilst PARIS[122] had three end points, including total mortality.

Three of the studies analysed fewer patients than had been randomized. Where possible, all randomized patients are included in the analysis presented in Tables 3.18 and 3.19. In particular, the results from the Anturane trial for all randomized patients, published separately from the main report[219], is included in this review.

None of the trials in which aspirin was the active intervention demonstrated a statistically significant difference between intervention and control groups for total mortality. But in all of these studies except AMIS, which was the largest, a trend in favour of the drug was reported.

Several reviewers[221,222] have concluded that reliable information can be expected when the results of all six trials are pooled. When this is done, about one sixth of deaths are preventable. Support for the view that the reduction in cardiovascular mortality is real comes from the highly significant reduction in cardiovascular morbidity. However, this must be balanced against the statistically non-significant reduction in the incidence of recurrent non-fatal myocardial infarction reported in two studies[122,215]. It must also be noted that 10–20% of patients reported dyspepsia, nausea or vomiting in studies involving doses of 1000 mg/day aspirin or greater. One per cent reported melaena and 0.1% haematemesis.

A recent study of the effects of aspirin in men with unstable angina pectoris may be compared with those in patients after myocardial infarction. Lewis et al.[39] randomly allocated 1266 men with unstable angina pectoris to receive 324 mg aspirin in buffered solution (625 men) or placebo (641 men).

After 12 weeks of treatment, total mortality was 21 in the placebo group (3.3%) and ten in the intervention group (1.6%) – $p = 0.054$. There were statistically significant reductions in acute myocardial infarction or death (57%; $p = 0.0005$) and in fatal and non-fatal myocardial infarction. Although treatment was stopped at 3 months, by 1 year the mean mortality was 5.5% in the aspirin group and 9.6% in the placebo group ($p = 0.008$). The results were not affected by concurrent use of β-blocking drugs[223], and the incidence and severity of angina was not affected.

In conclusion, none of the aspirin trials has unequivocally shown a significant reduction in total mortality in patients who have survived an infarction, but pooled results suggest a small but useful effect of 15–20%. It remains to be elucidated which patients should be selected, and what dose is appropriate. In contrast, the results in men with unstable angina are promising and need to be confirmed. It may be that low dose aspirin will be more effective before or during ischaemic episodes than following thrombosis. This is supported by the significant benefits from aspirin therapy in patients with transient cerebral ischaemic attacks[224–226].

The two studies with sulphinpyrazone[216–220] are similar in design, but have not produced consistent results.

After two reanalyses[212,213], the controversy which surrounds the American study involves the eligibility of patients at the time of randomization, the patients who should be included in the analysis according to time of death after drug withdrawal, and the effect of mode of death on the results. Accepting total mortality on all randomized patients (as shown in Table 3.19) then there is no significant difference between the treatment and placebo for the whole study. Using the same criterion for effect on survival in the first 6 months, there is a statistically non-significant ($p < 0.118$) reduction in the sulphinpyrazone group (32%). A less rigorous analysis, but one suggested by Temple and Pledger[219], compared the effects of treatment and placebo on all cardiac deaths in all randomized patients, excluding only deaths occurring more than 7 days from the last dose of medication. It was anticipated that no pharmacological effect of the drug could be expected after 1 week. This analysis revealed a 45% reduction in mortality by sulphinpyrazone at 6 months of treatment ($p < 0.055$).

However, the reanalysis did continue to support the statistically significant reduction in incidence of sudden death ($p < 0.01$) in the first 6 months, regardless of how the analysis was conducted (64%–74%).

The Italian Anturane trial[220] was conducted in 1727 patients. The design was similar to the American study, except that patients were withdrawn if a 'thromboembolic event' occurred. After a mean follow-up time of 19.2 months, there were 29 deaths in the control group and 38 in the treatment group; there was no significant difference in the number of sudden deaths in the two groups. There was a significant and cumulative reduction in the incidence of reinfarction (15 sulphinpyrazone versus 34 placebo) and all thromboembolic events (16 sulphinpyrazone versus 42 placebo, $p < 0.001$).

It may be concluded that sulphinpyrazone does have a beneficial effect in patients who have survived a myocardial infarction, but its cause-specific effects are inconsistent and may not result entirely from differences in patient selection.

Calcium-channel blocking drugs

There is only one published study of a calcium-channel blocking drug in survivors of myocardial infarction. The Danish Study Group[227] randomized 3497 patients under the age of 75 years on admission to the coronary care unit with suspicion of myocardial infarction. 3918 had been excluded from randomization because of heart failure, heart block, severe disabling disease or treatment with β-blockers or calcium-channel blockers. Treatment was given as 0.1 mg/kg verapamil intravenously and 120 mg orally on admission, followed by 120 mg t.d.s. or matching placebo.

Treatment was maintained for 6 months for patients who subsequently prove to have myocardial infarction. Of 1436 patients with acute myocardial infarction, 717 received verapamil and 719 placebo.

At 6 months, 92 (12.8%) patients in the verapamil group had died, compared with 100 patients (13.9%) in the placebo group. This difference is not significant. By 12 months the figures were 15.2% and 16.4% respectively. The reinfarction rate was similar in the two groups (7% verapamil, 8.3% placebo at 6 months).

Heart failure as a reason for withdrawal was similar (55 verapamil and 43 placebo), but the incidence of heart failure was significantly higher with verapamil (187 versus 142; $p < 0.005$). Second and third degree heart block was a reason for withdrawal in 117 patients on verapamil and 54 on placebo ($p < 0.01$).

The incidence of patients with second and third degree atrioventricular block was also significantly higher on verapamil therapy (115 verapamil, 50 placebo, $p < 0.001$). Of those patients who receive treatment initially, but who were withdrawn when myocardial infarction was not confirmed, 7.3% died in the verapamil group and 6.8% in the placebo group.

Retrospective subgroup analyses demonstrated a benefit for patients over 65 years of age and for those who were randomized late (6–24 h) after the onset of symptoms.

Two multicentre trials with nifedipine are under way (SPRINT and TRENT) and results are awaited with interest.

β-ADRENOCEPTOR BLOCKING DRUGS (SHORT AND LONG-TERM STUDIES)

These agents have undergone extensive clinical evaluation over the last 20 years for their beneficial effects on the process of and outcome from myocardial ischaemia.

About 60 clinical trials have been completed, involving a total of some 30000 patients. The objectives of these studies have included effects of β-blockers on mortality, reinfarction, arrhythmias, measures of infarct size, chest pain and cardiac function. Eleven different β-blockers (including labetolol, a combined non-selective β-blocker and α-antagonist) have been studied. Their effects on mortality and morbidity in survivors of acute infarction, and in patients with threatened and evolving infarcts, have been the subject of several major reviews, to which the reader is referred for further information[14–18].

For this review, it is necessary to separate the clinical studies into those which assess the role of β-blockers in the months and years after recovery from infarction, from those which begin treatment during the evolution of the infarction. Unfortunately, the latter group of studies is complicated by three factors: (1) some trials do not begin early enough after the onset of chest pain to influence the evolution of the impending infarct, (2) some trials involve the use of early intravenous β-blockade with or without a loading oral dose, and terminate treatment at 21–28 days, and (3) some trials continue long term β-blockade up to 1 year.

No trials of sufficient size have been reported which study the effect of early, short term treatment only, on long term mortality. This is an important issue particularly in view of the fact that the results of three trials in which early intravenous β-blockade followed by chronic oral β-blockade[222-224,228-230] have been conducted, have shown that mortality at 1 week is not affected by β-blockade.

Tables 3.20 and 3.21 refer to the results of trials in which treatment was initiated early after onset of chest pain and the mortalities are given at the *end of the trial*. Tables 3.22 and 3.23 refer to trials in which oral treatment was initiated after recovery from infarction and maintained for months or years.

It may be stated at the outset that the pooled results from all available randomized controlled trials of treatment after recovery from infarction show a highly significant ($p < 0.00001$) reduction in total mortality of 21%, whilst the pooled results from the early intervention trials of intravenous and/or oral β-blockade have shown a non-significant reduction of about 8% in total mortality.

In line with other studies presented in this review, only trials which meet the stated criteria will be selected. The reader is referred to the review by Yusuf *et al.*[16] for information on all available β-blocker trials. However, it should be noted that the exclusion of a limited number of small studies with few end points will not affect the direction of the pooled result, and have only marginal influence on its magnitude.

Early intervention trials

Twenty trials[75, 222-242] meet the criteria for this review. Their designs are given in Table 3.20 and the effects on total mortality in Table 3.21. The studies fall into four classes: (1) oral administration up to 1 month, (2) intravenous followed by short term oral administration, (3) intravenous followed by long term oral administration and (4) acute and long term oral administration.

None of the studies in which treatment was initiated orally have shown a reduction in mortality, whether the analysis is conducted at the end of the trial, or after 1 week of treatment. Whilst this may be due to small sample size and insufficient power to detect a small but useful effect, it is more likely that β-blockade cannot be established rapidly enough to halt the evolving ischaemic process, unless initiated intravenously. Rutherford *et al.*[249] showed that oral β-blockade even instituted early after onset of chest pain, leads to a considerable delay in achieving adequate β-blockade. In contrast, studies by Sleight *et al.*[250] and Ramsdale *et al.*[251] have shown that marked reductions in heart rate occurred within 15 minutes of the onset of injection.

It has now been clearly established that β-blockade must be initiated within the first 12 hours, after onset of chest pain, if the enzyme release and electrocardiographic changes associated with infarction

Table 3.20 β-Blockers: design of intravenous and/or oral early intervention trials

Trial	Type control	Type of blind	Number randomized	Entry window	Intervention(s)	Length of follow-up (length of time treatment was given)
(a) Oral administration up to 1 month						
Balcon et al.[231]	Placebo	DB	155	<24 h	propranolol (80 mg/day)	28 days
Clausen et al.[232]	No β-blocker	Open	130	<24 h	propranolol (40 mg/day)	22 days
Multi-centre Study[233]	Placebo	DB	226	<48 h	propranolol (80 mg/day)	28 days
Barber et al.[234]	Placebo	DB	107	<24 h	propranolol (160 mg/day)	28 days
Norris et al.[235]	Placebo	DB	536	<3 days	propranolol (80 mg/day)	21 days
Briant and Norris[236]	Placebo	DB	172	on hospital admission	alprenolol (400 mg/day)	3 days
Lombardo et al.[237]	Placebo	DB	260	<24 h	oxprenolol (120 mg/day)	21 days
Fuccella[238]	Placebo	DB	257	<48 h	oxprenolol (120 mg/day)	21 days
(b) Intravenous followed by short term oral administration						
Evemy and Pentecost[239]	No β-blocker	Open	128	<24 h	practolol (15 mg i.v. stat.–400 mg/day for 2 days)	28 days
Johansson[240]	Saline i.v. stat + placebo	Open	130	on hospital admission	oral timolol for 10 days	
Yusuf et al.[241]	No β-blocker	Open	477	<12 h	hospital discharge	24 h
International Collaborative Study Group[242]	Placebo	DB	144	<5 h	timolol infusion for 2 weeks – oral timolol (no details)	
Brown et al.[243]	No treatment	SB	735	<4 h	propranolol 0.1 mg/kg i.v. + 320 mg over 27 h	Hospital discharge

132

Hjalmarson et al.[230]	Placebo	DB	1395	<48 h	metoprolol (15 mg i.v. stat. + 200 mg/day p.o. for 90 days)	90 days
Andersen et al.[228]	Placebo	DB	480	medián time 6 h	alprenolol 5–10 mg i.v. – 400 mg orally/day	1 year
McIlmoyle et al.[229] Boyle et al.[245]	Placebo	DB	391	2–4 h	metoprolol 15 mg i.v. – 200 mg orally 1 day	1 year
(d) Oral administration followed by long term oral administration						
Wilcox et al.[246*]	Placebo	DB	261	<24 h	propranolol (120 mg/day for 6 weeks then 80 mg twice a day)	1 year
Wilcox et al.[246*]	Placebo	DB	256	<24 h	atenolol 10 mg/day for 1 y	1 year
Barber et al.[247]	Placebo	DB	448	up to several days; median time 3 h	practolol (600 mg/day)	2 years
Wilcox et al.[75]	Placebo	DB	315	<24 h	oxprenolol (120 mg/day)	42 days
CPRG[248]	Placebo	DB	313	<72 h (mean 2.1 days)	oxprenolol (80 mg/day)	56 days

* Same study

Table 3.21 β-Blockers: results of intravenous and/or oral treatment

Trial	Control Number randomized	Control No. of deaths	Control Per cent mortality	Intervention Number randomized	Intervention No. of deaths	Intervention Per cent mortality	p-Value*
Balcon et al.*	58	15	25.9	56	16	28.6	0.91
Clausen et al.	64	16	25.0	66	18	27.3	0.92
Multi-centre study*	111	12	10.8	114	15	13.2	0.74
Barber et al.	53	12	22.6	54	10	18.5	0.77
Norris et al.*	228	24	10.5	226	31	13.7	0.37
Briant and Norris	57	4	7.0	62	5	8.1	1.00
Lombardo et al.	127	11	8.5	133	8	6.2	0.28
Fuccella*	114	9	8.0	106	15	14.0	0.19
Evemy and Pentecost*	48	4	8.3	46	7	15.2	0.47
Johansson	45	5	11.1	40	5	12.5	1.00
Yusuf et al.†	233	13	8.0	244	4	2.0	<0.05
International Collaboration Study	71	8	11.2	73	6	8.2	0.37
Brown et al.	371	14	3.8	364	15	4.1	0.48
Hjalmarson et al.‡	697	62	8.9	698	40	5.7	0.03
Andersen et al.‡	242	64	26.4	238	61	25.6	0.46
McIlmoyle et al.‡	187	23	12.2	204	22	10.8	0.38
Wilcox et al.§	129	19	14.7	259	36	13.9	0.47
Barber et al.	226	52	23.0	222	48	21.6	0.41
Wilcox et al.	158	10	6.3	157	14	8.9	0.26
CPRG	136	5	3.7	177	9	5.1	0.38

* Incomplete reporting
† Long term data not available. This is the only study to show a significant reduction in early mortality
‡ Mortality at 1 week in these intravenous studies was not reduced by β-blockers
§ The two β-blocker groups have been added together

134

are to be influenced. This has been convincingly demonstrated for propranolol[246,252,253], atenolol[241], metoprolol[229,254,255], alprenolol[244], sotalol[256], and timolol[242].

It is further confirmed by a significant reduction in the number of patients with 'threatened' infarction treated with a β-blocker, continuing to myocardial infarction, compared with a control group. This has been demonstrated for propranolol[257], in a study in which 55% of the treated patients developed infarction compared with 96% of the controls, and for atenolol[241,258] in which 49% of the treated patients developed infarction compared with 66% of the controls. The pooled results indicate that β-blockade can reduce the odds of full development of myocardial infarction by about half ($p < 0.001$).

It is perhaps surprising then that only two of the seven trials in which treatment was initiated intravenously have shown a significant reduction in total mortality. But even these two trials are inconsistent. In the study by Yusuf et al.[241] in 477 patients there was a significant reduction in total mortality at the time of hospital discharge (6.0% placebo versus 2.0% atenolol; $p < 0.05$). In the study by Hjalmarson et al.[230] in 1395 patients, the 7 day mortality was not reduced by intravenous and oral metoprolol (3% in each group) but mortality at 1 year was significantly reduced (8.9% placebo versus 5.7%; $p < 0.03$). The median time to randomization in this study was 11.1 h after the onset of chest pain, and most authorities now regard this study as providing further evidence for the value of long term β-blockade.

The other two early intervention intravenous studies with long term follow-up are equivocal[228,229,245]. Further data from two large early intervention studies with intravenous atenolol and metoprolol are eagerly awaited.

The study by Yusuf et al.[241] indicated a significant reduction in early morbidity with atenolol compared with placebo: other early interventions treated with intravenous β-blockers are equivocal despite the beneficial effects on other end points. At least two studies with atenolol[259] and metoprolol[260] have demonstrated significant reductions in the frequency of ventricular arrhythmias on ambulatory electrocardiographic taping recorded in the first 24 h of the evolving infarct. Yusuf et al.[241] also showed a reduction in non-fatal cardiac arrest (10/233 contol versus 3/244 atenolol) and Ryden et al.[260] reported a significant reduction in ventricular fibrillation during hospitalization (17/698 control versus 6/697 metoprolol). More recently, Brown et al.[243] in their study with propranolol (PREMIS) have reported a reduction in the frequency of ventricular fibrillation during hospitalization from 14/371 (3.8%) controls to 2/364 (0.5%) in the treated group.

Three controlled studies have reported significant prevention and relief of anginal pain after myocardial infarction – one with propranolol[261], one with metoprolol[262], and one with atenolol[251]. The latter authors also reported a parallel reduction in cardiac work, suggesting a decrease in oxygen demand.

The pioneering studies by Mueller *et al.*[263] and Gold *et al.*[261] indicated that intravenous propranolol administered immediately after infarction decreased cardiac output, mean arterial pressure and heart rate, but with little overall change in pulmonary wedge pressure. Earlier Bay *et al.*[264] reported that intravenous propranolol after infarction would lead to significant increase in wedge pressure, and Lehman[265] reported similar findings when intravenous β-blockade was given 12 h after the onset of chest pain. Yusuf *et al.*[16] have reviewed 22 early intervention studies of β-blockers, nine with intravenous administration. Eight per cent of patients developed evidence of heart failure compared with 6.6% of controls (*see below*).

In conclusion, early intravenous or intravenous followed by oral β-blockade has been shown to produce useful effects in suppressing arrhythmias, reducing infarct size, in preventing extension of threatened infarction, and in reducing chest pain. However, only one study with atenolol has shown a significant reduction in early mortality. This may indicate that the overall effect on mortality is less substantial than that achieved with late oral intervention, but results of large studies with atenolol and metoprolol are awaited.

Late intervention trials

Twelve studies[260-272] with oral treatment meet the criteria for this review. Their designs and results are given in Tables 3.22 and 3.23. As already mentioned, the pooled results show a highly significant reduction in total mortality of 21% ($p < 0.00001$). Two trials (BHAT[274], Norwegian Multi-Centre Study Group[271]) have demonstrated that propranolol and timolol, respectively, reduce the total mortality by 20%–30%. A further study with practolol[267,268] showed a trend for reduction in total mortality ($p < 0.09$), and the long term results of the study by Hjalmarson *et al.*[230] with intravenous followed by oral metoprolol have also shown a significant reduction in total mortality ($p < 0.03$).

The important results from these trials raise many issues which may never be completely resolved. Is the difference between the 'positive' trials and the equivocal or 'negative' trials due to differences in sample size, patient selection (the placebo mortality varied from 5% to 18%), pharmacological properties, dose or a combination of these factors? With the possible exception of the European Infarct Study (EIS) with slow-release oxprenolol[278], the results of all those trials have 95% confidence limits which include a 20% reduction in total mortality.

The result from EIS indicated a difference of 30.5% in cumulative mortality rates against oxprenolol, but this was not statistically significant ($p = 0.14$). The pooled reduction in mortality from all 12 studies of 21% have confidence limits ranging from a 12% reduction to a 28% reduction. This pooled reduction of 21% is also contained within the 95% confidence limits of each individual trial except EIS, which appears to suggest that the results of EIS are systematically different.

Table 3.22 β-Blockers: design of late intervention long term oral studies

Trial	Type control	Type of blind	Number randomized	Entry time	Intervention	Mean length of follow-up (months)
Wilhelmsson et al.[266]	Placebo	DB	230	1–3 weeks after hospital discharge	alprenolol (400 mg/day)	24
Multi-centre International Study[267,268]	Placebo	DB	3053	7–28 days	practolol (400 mg/day)	14
Baber et al.[269]	Placebo	DB	720	2–14 days	propranolol (120 mg/day)	9
Rehnquist et al.[270]	Placebo	DB	111	hospital discharge	metoprolol (200 mg/day)	12
Norwegian Multi-centre Study Group[271]	Placebo	DB	1884	7–28 days	timolol (20 mg/day)	17
Taylor et al.[272]	Placebo	DB	1103	1–14 months	oxprenolol (80 mg/day)	48
Hansteen et al.[273]	Placebo	DB	560	4–6 days	propranolol (160 mg/day)	12
BHAT[274]	Placebo	DB	3837	5–21 days	propranolol (180–240 mg/day)	24
Julian[275]	Placebo	DB	1456	5–14 days	sotalol (320 mg/day)	12
Australian/Swedish[276]	Placebo	DB	529	1–21 days	pindolol (15 mg/day)	24
Manger Cats[277]	Placebo	DB	583	<1 week post-discharge	metoprolol (200 mg/day)	12
European Infarct Study[278]	Placebo	DB	1741	14–36 days	oxprenolol-SR (320 mg/day)	12

137

Table 3.23 β-Blockers: results of late intervention long term oral studies

Trial	Number randomized	Control No. of deaths	Per cent mortality	Number randomized	Intervention No. of deaths	Per cent mortality	p-Value
Wilhelmsson et al.	116	14	12.1	114	7	6.1	0.18
Multi-centre	1520	127	8.4	1533	102	6.7	0.09
International Study							
Baber et al.	365	27	7.4	355	28	7.9	0.92
Rehnquist et al.	52	6	11.5	59	4	6.8	0.29
Norwegian Multi-centre Study Group	939	152	17.5	945	98	10.6	0.0003
Taylor et al.	471	48	10.1	632	60	9.5	0.38
Hansteen et al.	282	37	13.1	278	25	8.9	0.13
BHAT	1921	188	9.5	1916	138	7.0	0.005
Julian	583	52	8.9	873	64	7.3	0.27
Australian/Swedish	266	47	17.6	263	45	17.1	0.48
Manger Cats	293	16	5.5	290	9	3.1	0.16
European Infarct	883	45	5.1	858	57	6.6	0.18

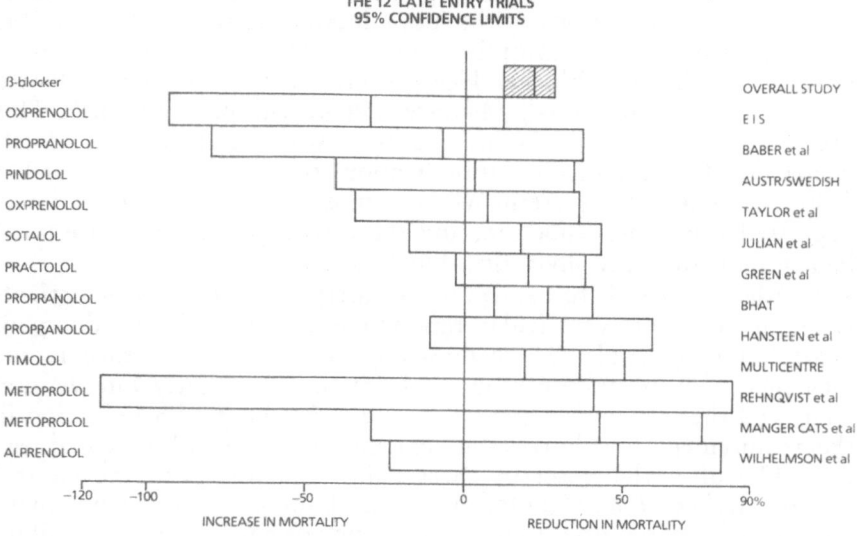

Figure 3.3 Results of 12 late intervention oral β-blockers studies. Difference in mortality rates and 95% confidence limits

However, there is no statistical evidence to support this; a significance test for heterogenicity of the treatment effect among the 12 studies gives a non-significant result $(p > 0.1)$ (Lewis, J.A., personal communication). The result could have been expected by chance, as argued by Yusuf et al.[16] and Wilhelmsen[278].

However, other explanations are possible. Taylor et al.[279] have suggested there may be a dose response to oxprenolol and that 320 mg/day used in EIS was in excess of the optimal dose. There is some support for this from the study with sotalol[275]. However, there are no studies which have directly compared different doses, and such retrospective analysis must be regarded with caution.

It should be noted that the most impressive results have come from trials with non-selective β-blockers without intrinsic sympathomimetic activity. This ancillary property was developed in the expectation that less cardiac depression would occur, but its value must be seriously questioned.

Subgroup analyses have been conducted in all these 12 trials, in an attempt to identify prognostic risk factors which will determine response to β-blockade. Much has been written about the validity of retrospective analysis, and the chance findings which may arise[15, 281-283].

Prognostic indices of harm or benefit in a particular subgroup from one study have not been confirmed by subsequent trials[228,267,268].

The most consistent findings suggest that patients with electrical or mechanical complications of the index infarct are those who have the greatest reduction in mortality with β-blockade. This has been observed in the Beta Blocker Heart Attack Trial[283], in the trial with timolol[271] and in the study by Hansteen et al. with propranolol[273]. This presents the physician with a paradox, as severe depression of left ventricular function is a contraindication to β-blockade[16,284]. Further work is required to ascertain whether those patients with moderately depressed ventricular function, and those with positive exercise tests, benefit most from prophylactic β-blockade.

Another approach to ascertain the safety of β-blockers in patients with impaired left ventricular function is to study the incidence of heart failure in trials. There does appear to be a difference in the incidence of heart failure reported from the acute early intervention trials and the late oral studies. Yusuf et al.[241] reported a reduction in the requirement for diuretics in patients given atenolol treated less than 12 h after the onset of chest pain compared with the control group. Herlitz et al.[285] noted a similar finding in their study with metoprolol and reported that the frequency of congestive heart failure was the same in the intervention (27%) and control groups (30%).

In two later intervention trials, BHAT[274], and in the Norwegian Multi-Centre Trial with timolol[271], there were more withdrawals for heart failure in the treatment groups. The subgroup analysis from BHAT[283] indicates a higher incidence of heart failure in those patients with mechanical complications in the acute phase prior to randomization compared with patients receiving placebo.

It may be that early β-blockade if administered cautiously may limit infarct size at a time when a large mass of reversibly ischaemic myocardium can be salvaged. After infarction is complete, the negative inotropic effect may predominate, with an increased risk of precipitation of heart failure. However, as there is a close relation between history of heart failure and subsequent sudden death, the potential for a greater absolute reduction in mortality by β-blockade in patients with moderate failure, managed conventionally, must be seriously considered.

The mode of action of β-blockers in prolonging life after myocardial infarction remains controversial, but it has become apparent that both antiarrhythmic and anti-ischaemic properties are important. Sudden death is most frequently due to ventricular fibrillation. It is variously defined in studies from 'instantaneous' to within '2 hours of symptoms', but effects of β-blockers on its incidence would support an antiarrhythmic mode of action.

An overview of 13 studies which report sudden death separately from non-sudden death, indicates a 30% reduction by β-blockade ($p < 0.00001$), with 95% confidence limits of 19%–40%[16]. Non-sudden death reduction is about 12% and not significant.

An antiarrhythmic effect of β-blockers is further supported by the studies of Rossi *et al.*[259] with atenolol, and Ryden *et al.*[260] with metoprolol. Twenty-four hour ambulatory electrocardiographic recordings in BHAT also support an antiarrhythmic effect of propranolol[286].

An anti-ischaemic effect of long term β-blockers is supported by a reduction by about one quarter of the non-fatal reinfarction rate, from the pooling of results of 18 trials[16]. There is an overall reinfarction rate of 7.5% in the control group and 5.7% in the treatment group (*p* < 0.0001). Three individual studies demonstrated a significant reduction in non-fatal reinfarction[241] with practolol[247], metoprolol[230] and timolol[16].

In summary, the late intervention studies taken together have indicated that life may be prolonged in a substantial number of patients after recovery from infarction. The overall reduction in mortality is about 20% with an absolute reduction from approximately 10% to 8%. There is no substantial evidence that this is drug specific; but it would be prudent to recommend the use of a β-blocker which has, in its own right, been shown to have a significant effect. Benefit appears to be greatest in those with mechanical and electrical damage, and future clinical research will be directed to identifying these patients.

CONCLUDING REMARKS

An enormous amount of time and money has been spent in evaluating drugs in the primary and secondary prevention of myocardial infarction and death. It must be said that, on the whole, the results are disappointing. The physician does not have enough information to choose prophylactic drug regimens to suit more than a few high risk patients, but perhaps this is not surprising in a multifactorial disease.

In primary prevention, the only drugs to receive extensive evaluation are clofibrate and cholestyramine. The favourable results are confined to the test group of men with high serum cholesterols, and the effect was on cause-specific coronary heart disease, with no significant reduction in total mortality. The most convincing results have come from the study of aspirin in unstable angina pectoris[39], and this requires confirmation.

In secondary prevention, antiarrhythmic drugs (excluding β-blockers) have been unimpressive, particularly in the long term trials, and there is considerable concern about adverse effects, including mortality, with some of these drugs. The lipid lowering drug studies have yielded positive trends, or significant results, but only when multiple end points are combined, or certain subgroups excluded. Aspirin in individual trials has not shown a reduction in total mortality, but the pooled results indicate a 15%–20% reduction. However, the correct dosage remains a problem. The first sulphinpyrazone study, following extensive reanalysis which has weakened confidence in the trial, unexpectedly showed a reduction in sudden death whilst the second study showed a significant reduction in the incidence of reinfarction. These results are impressive, but inconsistent, and other studies are required.

The first published trials with calcium antagonists are disappointing, and the results of vasodilators in patients with severe heart failure are too preliminary for comment. There are no controlled trials with inotropic drugs in chronic mild heart failure, and the two studies in heart failure following myocardial infarction are conflicting. In the acute phase of infarction, hyaluronidase administration has produced promising results, and appears relatively safe. Other large trials are under way. Comparative studies of intravenous versus intracoronary streptokinase indicate that results by the two routes could be comparable. Combined thrombolytic and antiarrhythmics or anti-ischaemic therapy is an attractive possibility for future studies, and the use of nitrates needs to be reassessed.

The β-blockers have emerged as of proven value for long term oral use after recovery from infarction, but the acute situation is complex. However, as with the platelet active agents, physicians are reluctant to extrapolate trial results to all their postinfarction patients. Those at hish risk yet with the greatest chance of benefit from β-blockade may be excluded, or may be offered coronary artery surgery.

If prophylaxis has not made a large impact on the incidence and consequences of coronary arterial disease, then some important principles have been learned. Trial design, and analysis, have improved considerably, though some investigators are still unwilling to allow their studies to finish before publishing the results. Pooling of results has allowed trials to be critically compared. The issue of disease-specific versus all-cause mortality is always under debate, and the mode of action of new agents is often illuminated by unexpected findings in large studies.

Not enough attention has been paid to dose-response studies and pharmacokinetics, or to the relationship between the effect of drugs on intermediate end points such as suppression of arrhythmias for antiarrhythmic agents, and mortality. It has also become clear that the expectation of the size of effect of some interventions is modest and the 20% reduction in total mortality achieved by β-blockade in survivors of myocardial infarction may not easily be obtained again.

Acknowledgements

My sincere thanks to Mrs Edith Husband and Mrs Shirley Thomason for their patient care in the preparation of this manuscript.

References

1. Rose, G. (1981). Strategy of prevention: lessons from cardiovascular disease. *Br. Med. J.*, **282**, 1847–51
2. Salonen, J.T., Puska, P., Kottle, T., Tuomilehto, J. and Nissinen, A. (1983). Decline in mortality from coronary heart disease in Finland from 1969 to 1979. *Br. Med. J.*, **286**, 1857–60

3. Marmot, M.G. (1984). Lifestyle and national and international trends in coronary heart disease mortality. *Postgrad. Med. J.*, **60**, 3–8
4. Welin, L., Larsson, B., Svärdsudd, K., Wilhelmsen, L. and Tibblin, G. (1983). Why is the incidence of ischaemic heart disease in Sweden increasing? *Lancet*, **1**, 1087–9
5. Alfredsson, L. and Ahlbom, A. (1983). Increasing incidence and mortality from myocardial infarction in Stockholm county. *Br. Med. J.*, **286**, 1931–3
6. World Health Organization European Collaborative Group (1983). Multifactorial trial in the prevention of coronary heart disease: 3. Incidence and mortality results. *Eur. Heart. J.*, **4**, 141–7
7. Puska, P., Tuomilehto, J., Salonen, J., Neittaanmäki, L., Maki, J., Virtamo, J., Nissinen, A., Koskela, K. and Takalo, T. (1979). Changes in coronary risk factors during comprehensive five year community programme to control cardiovascular diseases (North Karelia Project). *Br. Med. J.*, **2**, 1173–8
8. Multiple Risk Factor Intervention Trial (1982). *J. Am. Med. Assoc.*, **248**, 1465–77
9. Salonen, J.T., Puska, P. and Mustamiemi, H. (1979) Changes in morbidity and mortality during comprehensive community programme to control cardiovascular diseases during 1972–77 in North Karelia. *Br. Med. J.*, **2**, 1178–83
10. Connolly, D.C., Oxman, H.A., Nobrega, F.T., Kurland, L.J., Kennedy, M.A. and Elveback, L.R. (1981). Coronary heart disease in residents of Rochester, Minnesota 1950–75. I. Background and study design. *Mayo Clin. Proc.*, **56**, 661–4
11. Elveback, L.R., Connolly, D.C. and Kurland, L.J. (1981). Coronary heart disease in residents of Rochester, Minnesota. II. Mortality, incidence and survivorship. *Mayo Clin. Proc.*, **56**, 665–72
12. Pisa, Z. and Nemura, K. (1982). Trends of mortality from ischaemic heart disease and other cardiovascular diseases in 27 countries, 1968–1977. *World Health Stat. Q.*, **35**, 11–35
13. Oliver, M.F. (1983). Point of View: Should we not forget about mass control of coronary risk factors? *Lancet*, **2**, 37–8
14. Baber, N.S. (1981). Clinical experience with beta adrenoceptor blocking agents in myocardial ischaemia: A dilemma and a challenge. *Pharmacol. Ther.*, **13**, 285–320
15. Chamberlain D.A., (1983). Beta-adrenoceptor antagonists after myocardial infarction – where are we now? *Br. Heart. J.*, **49**, 105–10
16. Yusuf, S., Peto, R., Lewis, J., Collins, R. and Sleight, P. (1984). Beta blockade during and after myocardial infarction: An overview of the randomized trials. *Prog. Cardiovasc. Dis.* (In press)
17. May, G.S., Furberg, C.N., Eberlain, V.A. and Geran, B.J. (1983). Secondary prevention after myocardial infarction: a review of short term acute phase trials. *Prog. Cardiovasc. Dis.*, **XXV**, 335–59
18. May, G.S., Eberlain, K.A., Furberg, C.D., Passmani and de Mets, B.L. (1982). Secondary prevention after myocardial infarction: A review of long term trials. *Prog. Cardiovasc. Dis.* **XXIV**, 331–52
19. Kannel, W.B., Castelli, W.P. and Gordon, T. (1979). Cholesterol in the prevention of atherosclerotic diseases. *Ann. Intern. Med.*, **90**, 85–92
20. Veterans Administration Cooperative Study Group on Anti-hypertensive Agents (1967). Effects of treatment on morbidity in hypertension. I. Results in patients with diastolic blood pressures averaging 115 through 129 mm/Hg. *J. Am. Med. Assoc.*, **202**, 1028–34
21. Veterans Administration Cooperative Study Group on Anti-hypertensive agents (1970). Effects of treatment on morbidity in hypertension II. Results in patients with diastolic blood pressure averaging 90 through 114 mm/Hg. *J. Am. Med. Assoc.*, **213**, 1143–52
22. Smith, W.M. (1977). Treatment of mild hypertension: Results of a ten year intervention trial. *Circ. Res.*, **40** (Suppl. 1), 98–105

23. Morgan, T.O., Adams, W.R., Hodgson, M. and Gibbend, R.W. (1980). Failure of therapy to improve prognosis in elderly males with hypertension. *Med. J. Aust.*, **2**, 27–31

24. Management Committee (1980). The Australian Therapeutic Trial in mild hypertension. *Lancet*, **1**, 1261–7

25. Helgeland, A. (1980). Treatment of mild hypertension: a five year controlled drug trial: The Oslo Study. *Am. J. Med.*, **69**, 725–32

26. Hypertension, Detection and Follow-up Programme Cooperative Group (1979). Five year findings of the HDFP. I. Reduction in mortality of persons with high blood pressure, including mild hypertension. *J. Am. Med. Assoc.*, **242**, 2562–71

27. Ames, R.P. (1983). Metabolic disturbances increasing the risk of coronary heart disease during diuretic-based anti-hypertensive therapy: Lipid alterations and glucose intolerance. *Am. Heart J.*, **106**, 1207–15

28. Stewart, I.McD.G. (1976). Compared incidence of first myocardial infarction in hypertensive patients under treatment containing propranolol or excluding beta receptor blockade. *Clin. Sci. Mol. Med.*, **51**, 509s–11s

29. Lambert, D.M.D. (1976). Effect of propranolol on mortality in patients with angina. *Postgrad. Med. J.*, **52**, Suppl. 4, 57–60

30. Berglund, G., Wilhelmsen, L., Sannerstedt, R., Hansson, L., Andersson, O., Sivertsson, R., Wedel, H. and Wikstrand, J. (1978). Coronary heart disease after treatment of hypertension. *Lancet*, **1**, 1–5

31. Beevers, D.G., Johnson, J.H., Larkin, H. and Davies, P. (1983). Clinical evidence that beta adrenoceptor blockers prevent more cardiovascular complications than other anti-hypertensive drugs. *Drugs*, **25** (Suppl. 2), 326–30

32. Whelton, P.K., Brennan, P., Miall, W.E., Greenberg, G., Subramamian, B. and Raftery, E.B. (1982). Thiazide-associated cardiac arrhythmias. *Circulation*, **66**, Suppl. 2, 11–238

33. Carlsson, E., Fellenius, E., Lindborg, D. and Svensson, L. (1978). Beta-adrenoceptor blockers, plasma potassium and exercise. *Lancet*, **2**, 424–5

34. Struthers, A.D., Reid, J.L., Whitesmith, L. and Rodger, J.C. (1984). The effects of cardioselective and non-selective beta adrenoceptor blockade on haemodynamic and hypokalaemia response to intravenous adrenaline in man. (In press)

35. Medical Research Council Working Party on the treatment of myocardial infarction: potassium, glucose and insulin treatment for acute myocardial infarction (1968). *Lancet*, **2**, 1355–60

36. Wilhelmssen, L., Berglund, G., Elmfeldt, D. and Wedel, H. (1981). Beta blockers versus saluretics in hypertension. Comparison of total mortality, myocardial infarction and sudden death. Study design and early results on blood pressure reduction. *Prev. Med.*, **10**, 38–49

37. IPPPSH Collaborative Group (1980). The International Prospective Primary Prevention Study in Hypertension (IPPPSH) - objectives, design and preliminary date review. In Burley, D.M. and Birdwood, G.F. (eds.) *The Clinical Impact of Beta Adrenoceptor Blockade*, pp. 193–203. (Horsham: Ciba Laboratories).

38. Lambert, D.M.D. (1977). Long term effects of propranolol on morbidity and mortality in patients with angina pectoris. *Cardiovasc. Med.*, **2**, 253–60

39. Lewis, H.D., Davis, J.W., Archibald, D.G., Steinke, W.E., Smitherman, T.C., Doherty, J.E., Schnafer, H.W., le Winter, M.M., Linares, E., Pouget, J.M., Sabharwal, S.C., Chester, E. and De Mots, H. (1983). Protective effects of aspirin against acute myocardial infarction and death in men with unstable angina. *N. Engl. J. Med.*, **309**, 396–403

40. Chatterjee, K. and Parmley, W.W. (1983). Vasodilator therapy for acute myocardial infarction and chronic congestive heart failure. *J. Am. Coll. Cardiol.*, **1**, 133–53

41. Captopril Multicentre Research Group (1983). A placebo-controlled trial of captopril in refractory chronic congestive heart failure. *J. Am. Coll. Cardiol.*, **2**, 755–63

42. Packer, M., Lee, W.H., Bair, J., Medina, N., Yushak, M. (1984). Does vasodilator therapy alter prognosis in patients with severe chronic heart failure? Comparative effects of hydrallazine and captopril on clinical outcome and survival in 175 patients treated over 6 years. *J. Am. Coll. Cardiol.*, **3**, 561

43. Currie, P.J., Kelly, M.J., Middlebrook, K., Federman, J., Sainsbury, E., Ashley, J. and Pitt, A. (1984). Acute intravenous and sustained oral treatment with the beta₁ agonist prenalterol in patients with chronic severe cardiac failure. *Br. Heart J.*, **51**, 530–8

44. Hulley, S.B., Rosenman, R.H., Bawal, R.D. and Brand, C.J. (1980). Epidemiology as a guide to clinical decisions. The association between triglyceride and coronary heart disease. *N. Engl. J. Med.*, **302**, 1383–9

45. Ahrens, E.H. (1976). The management of hyperlidaemia: whether rather than how. *Ann. Intern. Med.*, **85**, 87–93

46. Gordon, T., Castelli, W.P., Hjartland, R.C., Kannel, W.B. and Dawber, T.R. (1977). High density lipoprotein as a protective factor against coronary heart disease. *Am. J. Med.*, **62**, 707–14

47. International Society and Federation of Cardiology Scientific Councils on Atherosclerosis, Epidemiology and Prevention and Rehabilitation (1981). Secondary prevention in survivors of myocardial infarction. *Br. Med. J.*, **282**, 894–6

48. Miehinen, M., Turpemen, O., Karvonen, M.J., Elosuo, R. and Paavilainen, E. (1972). Effect of cholesterol-lowering diet on mortality from coronary heart disease and other causes. *Lancet*, **2**, 835–8

49. Christakas, G., Rinzler, S.H. and Archer, M. (1966). The anti-coronary club. A dietary approach to the prevention of coronary heart disease. *Am. J. Public Health*, **56**, 299–314

50. Dayton, S., Pearce, M.L., Hashimoto, S., Dixon, W.J. and Tomiyesu, U. (1969). A controlled trial of a diet high in unsaturated fat. *Circulation*, II (Suppl.), 1–63

51. Report from the Committee of Principal Investigators (1978). A cooperative trial in the primary prevention of ischaemic heart disease using clofibrate. *Br. Heart J.*, **40**, 1069–1118

52. Committee of Principal Investigators Report for WHO Cooperative (1980). Trial on primary prevention of ischaemic heart disease using clofibrate to lower serum cholesterol: Mortality follow-up. *Lancet*, **2**, 379–84

53. Anonymous (1984). The Lipid Research Clinics coronary primary prevention trial results, I. reduction in incidence of coronary heart disease. *J. Am. Med. Assoc.*, **251**, 351–64

54. Harrison, D.C. and Berte, L.E. (1982). Should prophylactic anti-arrythmic drug therapy be used in acute myocardial infarction? *J. Am. Med. Assoc.*, **247**, 2019–21

55. Pentecost, B.L., De Giovanni, J.V., Lamb, P., Cadigan, P.J., Evemy, K.L. and Flint, E.J. (1981). Re-appraisal of lignocaine therapy in myocardial infarction. *Br. Heart J.*, **45**, 42–7

56. Woosley, R.L., Kornhauser, D., Smith, R., Reele, S., Higgins, S.B., Nies, A.S., Shand, D.G. and Oates, J.A. (1979). Suppression of chronic ventricular arrhythmias with propranolol. *Circulation*, **60**, 819–27

57. Myerburg, R.J., Kessler, K.M., Kiem, T., Pefkaros, K.C., Conde, C.A., Cooper, D. and Castellanos, A. (1981). Relationship between plasma levels of procainamide, suppression of premature ventricular complexes and prevention of recurrent ventricular tachycardia. *Circulation*, **64**, 280–90

58. Leahey, E.B. Jr., Reiffel, J.A., Drusin, R.E., Heissenbuttel, R.H., Lovejoy, W.P. and Bigger, J.T. (1978). A drug interaction between quinidine and digoxin. *J. Am. Med. Assoc.*, **240**, 533–4

59. Levine, S.A. (1932). The treatment of acute coronary thrombosis. *J. Am. Med. Assoc.*, **99**, 1737–40

60. Boone, J.A. and Pappas, A. (1956). Prophylactic use of quinidine following myocardial infarction. *S. Afr. Med. J.*, **49**, 169–171

61. Bloomfield, S.S., Romhilt, D.W., Chou, T. and Fowler, N.O. (1971). Quinidine for prophylaxis of arrhythmias in acute myocardial infarction. *N. Engl. J. Med.*, **285**, 979–86

62. Cutts, F.B. and Rapopart, B. (1952). The routine use of quinidine in acute myocardial infarction. *N. Engl. J. Med.*, **247**, 81–3

63. Begg, T.B. (1961). Prophylactic quinidine after myocardial infarction. *Br. Heart J.*, **23**, 415–20

64. Hvidt, S., Blatt, B. and Hvidt, R. (1962). The routine use of quinidine in myocardial infarction. *Acta Med. Scand.*, **172**, 567–71

65. Holmberg, S. and Bergman, H. (1967). Prophylactic quinidine in myocardial infarction: A double-blind study. *Acta Med. Scand.*, **181**, 297–304

66. Jones, D.J., Kostick, W.J. and Gunton, R.W. (1974). Prophylactic quinidine for prevention of arrhythmias after myocardial infarction. *Am. J. Cardiol.*, **33**, 655–60

67. Reynell, P.C. (1961). Prophylactic procainamide in myocardial infarction. *Br. Heart J.*, **23**, 421–5

68. Koch-Weser, J., Klein, S.W., Foo-Canto, L.L., Kastor, J.A. and De Sanctis, R.W. (1969). Antiarrhythmic prophylaxis with procainamide in acute myocardial infarction. *N. Engl. J. Med.*, **281**, 1253–60

69. Zainal, N., Carmichael, D.J.S., Griffiths, J.W. and Besterman, E.M.M. (1977). Oral disopyramide for the prevention of arrhythmias in patients with acute myocardial infarction admitted to open wards. *Lancet*, **2**, 887–9

70. Dollery, C.T., Krikler, D.M. and Shillingford, J.P. (1977). Disopyramide in myocardial infarction. *Lancet*, **2**, 1185

71. Pottage, A., Pickens, S. and Robron, R.H. (1977). Disopyramide in myocardial infarction. *Lancet*, **2**, 1362

72. Carmichael, D.J.S., Besterman, E.M.M. and Kidner, A.H. (1977). Disopyramide in myocardial infarction. *Lancet*, **2**, 1185–6

73. Jennings, G., Model, D.G., Jones, M.B.S., Turner, P.P., Besterman, E.M.M. and Kidner, P.H. (1976). Oral disopyramide in prophylaxis of arrhythmias following myocardial infarction. *Lancet*, **1**, 51–4

74. Nicholls, D.P., Haybyrne, T. and Barnes, P.C. (1980). Intravenous and oral disopyramide after myocardial infarction. *Lancet*, **2**, 936–8

75. Wilcox, R.G., Rowley, J.M., Hampton, J.R., Mitchell, J.R.A., Roland, J.M. and Banks, D.C. (1980). Randomized placebo-controlled trial comparing oxprenolol with disopyramide phosphate in immediate treatment of suspected myocardial infarction. *Lancet*, **2**, 765–9

76. UK Rhythmodan Multicentre Study Group (1984). Oral disopyramide after admission to hospital with suspected acute myocardial infarction. *Postgrad. Med. J.*, **60**, 98–108

77. De Silva, R.A., Hennekens, C.H., Lown, B. and Casscells, W. (1981). Lignocaine prophylaxis in acute myocardial infarction: An evaluation of randomized trials. *Lancet*, **2**, 855–8

78. Bennett, M.A., Wilner, J.M. and Pentecost, B.L. (1970). Controlled trial of lignocaine in prophylaxis of ventricular arrhythmia complicating myocardial infarction. *Lancet*, **2**, 909–11

79. Pitt, S., Lipp, H. and Anderson, S.T. (1971). Lignocaine given prophylactically to patients with acute myocardial infarction. *Lancet*, **1**, 612–16

80. Darby, S., Bennett, M.A. and Cruickshank, J.C. (1972). Trial of combined intramuscular and intravenous lignocaine in prophylaxis of ventricular tachyarrhythmias. *Lancet*, **1**, 817–19

81. O'Brien, K.P., Taylor, P.M. and Croxon, R.S. (1973). Prophylactic lidocaine in hospitalized patients with acute myocardial infarction. *Med. J. Aust.*, **2**, (Suppl.) 36–37

82. Lie, K.I., Wellens, H.J., Van Capelle, F.J. and Durrer, D. (1974). Lidocaine in the prevention of primary ventricular fibrillation: A double-blind randomized study of 212 consecutive patients. *N. Engl. J. Med.*, **291**, 1324–6

83. Valentine, P.A., Frew, J.L., Mashford, M.L. and Sloman, J.G. (1974). Lidocaine in the prevention of sudden death in the pre-hospital phase of acute infarction: a double-blind study. *N. Engl. J. Med.*, **291**, 1327-31

84. Lie, K.I., Liem, K.L., Louridtz, W.J., Janse, M.J., Willebrands, A.P. and Durrer, D. (1978). Efficacy of lidocaine in preventing primary ventricular fibrillation within 1 hour after a 300 mg intramuscular injection. A double-blind study of 300 hospitalized patients with acute myocardial infarction. *Am. J. Cardiol.*, **42**,

85. Koster, R.W. and Dunning, A.J. (1981). Pre-hospital prevention of ventricular fibrillation in acute myocardial infarction. *Circulation*, **64** (Suppl. V), 196(A)

86. Campbell, R.W.F., Hutton, I., Elton, R.A., Goodfellow, R.M. and Taylor, E. (1983). Prophylaxis of primary ventricular fibrillation with tocainide in acute myocardial infarction. *Br. Heart J.*, **49**, 557-63

87. Bell, J.A., Thomas, J.M., Isaacson, J.R., Snell, N.J. and Holt, D.W. (1982). A trial of prophylactic mexiletine in home coronary care. *Br. Heart J.*, **48**, 285-90

88. Epstein, S.E., Goldstein, R.E., Redwood, D.R., Kent, K.M. and Smith, E.R. (1973). The early phase of acute myocardial infarction: pharmacologic aspects of therapy. *Ann. Intern. Med.*, **78**, 918-36

89. Myers, R.E., Scherer, J.L., Goldstein, R.E., Kent, K.M. and Epstein, S.E. (1974). Nitroglycerine-induced reduction in acute myocardial ischaemia in dogs with pre-existing multi-vessel coronary occlusive disease. *Clin. Res.*, **22**, 292A

90 Kent, K.M., Smith, E.R., Redwood, D.R. and Epstein, S.E. (1974). Beneficial electrophyiological effects of nitroglycerine during acute myocardial infarction. *Am. J. Cardiol.*, **33**, 513-16

91. Borer, J.S., Kent, K.M., Goldstein, R.E. and Epstein, S.E. (1974). Nitroglycerine-induced reduction in the incidence of spontaneous ventricular fibrillation during coronary occlusion in dogs. *Am. J. Cardiol.*, **33**, 517-20

92. Becker, L.C., Fortuin, J.N. and Pitt, B. (1971). Effect of ischaemia and anti-anginal drugs on the distribution of radioactive microspheres in the canine left ventricle. *Circ. Res.*, **28**, 263-9

93. Awan, N.A., Amsterdam, E.A., Vera, Z., De Maria, A.N., Hiller, R.R. and Mason, D.T. (1976). Reduction of ischaemic injury by sublingual nitroglycerine in patients with acute myocardial infarction. *Circulation*, **54**, 761-5

94. Flaherty, J.T., Reid, P.R., Kelly, D.J., Taylor, D.R., Weisfeldt, M.L. and Pitt, D. (1975). Intravenous nitroglycerine in acute myocardial infarction. *Circulation*, **51**, 132-9

95. Epstein, S.E., Kent, K.M., Goldstein, R.E., Borer, J.S. and Redwood, D.R. (1975). Reduction of ischaemic injury by nitroglycerine during acute myocardial infarction. *N. Engl. J. Med.*, **292**, 29-35

96. Jaffe, A.S., Geltman, E.M., Tiefenbrunn, A.J., Ambos, H.D., Strauss, H.D., Sobel, B.E. and Roberts, R. (1983). Reduction of infarct size in patients with inferior infarction with glyceryl trinitrate: A randomized study. *Br. Heart J.*, **49**, 452-60

97. Flaherty, J.T., Becker, L.C., Bulkley, B.H. and Weiss, J.L. (1983). A randomized prospective trial of intravenous nitroglycerine in patients with acute myocardial infarction. *Circulation*, **68**, 576-88

98. Lis, Y., Bennett, D., Lambert, G. and Robson, D. (1984). A preliminary double-blind study of intravenous nitroglycerine in acute myocardial infarction. *Intensive Care Med.* (In press)

99. da Luz, P.L., Forrester, J.S. and Wyatt, J.L. (1975). Haemodynamic and meta-bolic effects of sodium nitroprusside on the performance and metabolism of regional ischaemic myocardium. *Circulation*, **52**, 400-407

100. Franciosa, J.B., Giuha, N.M. and Limas, C.J. (1972). Improved left ventricular function during nitroprusside infusion in acute myocardial infarction. *Lancet*, **2**, 650-7

101. Durrer, J.D., Lie, K.I., van Capelle, F.J.L. and Durrer, D. (1982). Effect of sodium nitroprusside on mortality in acute myocardial infarction. *N. Engl. J. Med.*, **306**, 1121-8

102. Cohn, J.N., Franciosa, M.D., Francis, G.S., Archibald, D., Tristani, F., Fletcher, R., Mantero, A., Cintron, G., Clarke, J., Hager, D., Saunders, R., Cobb, F., Smith, R., Loeb, H. and Settle, H. (1982). Effect of short term infusion of sodium nitroprusside on mortality rate in acute myocardial infarction complicated by left ventricular failure. N. Engl. J. Med., 306, 1129-35

103. Sodi-Pallares, D., De Micheli, A.A. and Fishleder, B.L. (1961). Effects d'un régime hyposode hyperpotassique et riche en eau sur l'évolution clinique et électrocardiographique de certaines cardiopathies. Acta Cardiol., 16, 166-200

104. Whitlow, P.L. and Rogers, W.J. (1983). Glucose-insulin potassium infusion in acute myocardial infarction. Am. J. Cardiol., 51, 1566-70

105. Sundstedt, C.D., Sylven, C. and Mogersen, L. (1981). Glucose-insulin potassium albumin infusion in the early phase of acute myocardial infarction - a controlled study. Acta. Med. Scand., 210, 67-71

106. Mittra, B. (1965). Potassium, glucose and insulin in treatment of myocardial infarction. Lancet, 2, 607-609

107. Pentecost, B.L., Mayne, N.M.C. and Lamb, P. (1968). Controlled trial of intravenous glucose and insulin in acute myocardial infarction. Lancet, 4, 946-8

108. Medical Research Council Working Party on the Treatment of Myocardial Infarction (1968). Potassium, glucose and insulin treatment for acute infarction. Lancet, 2, 1355-8

109. Rogers, J., McDaniel, H.G., Manlte, J.A. and Rackley, C.E. (1982). Glucose-insulin-potassium infusion in acute myocardial infarction - results of a prospective randomized study. Clin. Res., 30, 216A

110. Nayler, W.G., Ferrari, R. and Williams, A. (1980). Protective effect of pre-treatment with verapamil, nifedipine and propranolol on mitochondrial function, in ischaemic and reperfused myocardium. Am. J. Cardiol., 46, 242-8

111. Wende, W., Bleifeld, W., Meyer, J. and Stüchlen, H.W. (1975). Reduction of the size of acute experimental myocardial infarction by verapamil. Basic Res. Cardiol., 70, 198-208

112. Wolf, R., Habel, F., Witt, E., Nötges, F.E. and Hochrein, H. (1977). Wirkung von Verapamil auf die Hämodynamik und Grösse des akuten Myokardinfarkts. Herz, 2, 110-19

113. Lubbe, W.F., Millean, J.A. and Nguyen, T. (1983). Antiarrhythmic actions of nifedipine in acute myocardial ischaemia. Am. Heart J., 105, 331-3

114. Singh, B.N. (1983). The pharmacology of slow-channel blocking drugs. Cardiovasc. Rev. Rep., 4, 179-92

115. Norwegian Nifedipine Study Group (1984). Nifedipine in acute myocardial infarction: Fails to reduce infarct size in human trials. In International Symposium on Calcium Entry Blockers and Tissue Protection, Rome, March 15-16, p. 40

116. Muller, J.E., Morrison, J., Stone, P.H., Rude, R.E., Romer, B., Roberts, R., Pearle, D.L., Turi, Z.G., Schneider, J.F., Serfoe, D.H., Tate, C., Scheiner, E., Sobel, B.E., Hennekens, C.H. and Braunwald, E. (1984). Nifedipine therapy in patients with threatened and acute myocardial infarction: a randomized double-blind placebo-controlled comparison. Circulation, 69, 740-7

117. de Gaetano, G., Cerletti, C. and Berlete, V. (1982). Pharmacology of anti-platelet drugs and clinical trials on thrombosis prevention: A difficult task. Lancet, 2, 974-7

118. Emmons, P.R., Hampton, J.R., Harrison, M.J.G., Honour, A.J. and Mitchell, J.R.A. (1967). Effects of prostaglandin E_1 on platelet behaviour in vitro and in vivo. Br. Med. J., 2, 468-72

119. Mehta, J. and Mehta, P. (1982). Dipyridamole and aspirin in relation to platelet aggregation and vessel wall prostaglandin generation. J. Cardiovasc. Pharmacol., 231, 688-93

120. Mehta, P., Mehta, J. and Haralek, C. (1981). Dipyridamole inhibits thromboxane generation and promotes prostacyclin release. Circulation, 64, IV-284

121. Fuster, V. and Cheesbro, J.H. (1981). Anti-thrombotic therapy: Role of platelet

inhibitor drugs II. Pharmacologic effects of platelet-inhibitor drugs. *Mayo Clin. Proc.*, **56**, 185–95

122. The Persantin–Aspirin Reinfarction Trial Research Group (1980). Persantin and aspirin in coronary heart disease. *Circulation*, **62**, 449A-55A

123. Brotherton, A.F.A. and Hoak, J.C. (1982). Role of Ca^{2+} and cyclic AMP in the regulation of the production of prostacyclin by the vascular endothelium. *Proc. Natl. Acad. Sci. USA*, **79**, 495–9

124. Smythe, H.A., Ogryzlo, M.A., Murphy, E.A. and Mustard, J.F. (1965). The effect of sulphinyprazone (Anturan) on platelet economy and blood coagulation in man. *Can. Med. Assoc. J.*, **92**, 818–21

125. Buchanan, M.R., Rosenfeld, J. and Hirsch, J. (1978). The prolonged effect of sulphinpyrazone on collagen-induced platelet aggregation in vivo. *Thromb. Res.*, **13**, 883–6

126. Harker, L.A., Wall, R.T., Harlan, J.M. and Ross, R. (1978). Sulphinpyrazone prevention of homocysteine-induced endothelial cell injury and arteriosclerosis. *Clin. Res.*, **26**, 554A

127. Livio, M., Villa, S. and de Gaetano, G. (1980). Long-lasting inhibition of platelet prostaglandin but normal vascular prostacyclin generation following sulphinpyrazone administration to rats. *J. Pharm. Pharmacol.*, **32**, 718–19

128. Moschos, C.B., Escobinas, A.Z. and Jorgensen, O.B. (1980). Effects of sulphinpyrazone on ischaemic myocardium. In McGregor, M., Mustard, J.F. and Oliver, O. (eds) *Proceedings of an International Symposium*, Bermuda, Symposia Specialists, 175

129. Wilcox, R.G., Richardson, D., Hampton, J.R., Mitchell, J.R.A. and Banks, D.C. (1980). Sulphinpyrazone in acute myocardial infarction: Studies on cardiac rhythm and renal function. *Br. Med. J.*, **281**, 531–4

130. Boelart, J., Van Eeghem, P., Daniels, R., Mayner, A., Sraer, J.D., Kauritsky, O., David, S. and El Namos, M. (1980). The Anturane Reinfarction Trial. *N. Engl. J. Med.*, **303**, 49–52

131. Butler, A.L. (1981). Renal dysfunction due to Anturane. *N. Engl. J. Med.*, **305**, 106–107

132. Packham, M.A. and Mustard, J.F. (1977). Clinical pharmacology of platelets. *Blood*, **50**, 555–73

133. Weiss, H.J. (1976). Anti-platelet drugs: a new pharmacologic approach to the prevention of thrombosis. *Am. Heart J.*, **92**, 86–102

134. Kerry, R. and Scrutton, M.C. (1983). Platelet beta adrenoceptors. *Br. J. Pharmacol.*, **79**, 681–91

135. Weksler, B.B. and Pink, J. (1975). Propranolol as a modifier of platelet function by membrane action. *Clin. Res.* **23**, 284A

136. Siess, W., Scherer, B. and Weher, P.C. (1979). Propranolol inhibits release and action of thromboxane in platelets. *Sixth Scientific Meeting of International Society of Hypertenson, Gothenburg*, 1979, 310, (Abstr.)

137. Martin, M.A., Silas, J.H. and Smith, B.M. (1980). Effects of beta-adrenoceptor blockers on platelet function and seratonin, concentrations. *Br. J. Pharmacol.*, **70**, 161P-63P

138. Keber, I., Jerse, M., Keber, D. and Stegnar, M. (1979). The influence of combined treatment with propranolol and acetylsalicylic acid on platelet aggregation in coronary heart disease. *Br. J. Clin. Pharmacol.*, **7**, 287–91

139. Lee, G., Joye, J.A., Demaria, A.M., Low, R.I., Amsterdam, E.A. and Mason, D.T. (1980). Clinical pharmacology and therapeutic efficacy of anti-platelet drugs in coronary artery disease: evaluation of aspirin, sulphinpyrazone, dipyridamole and propranolol. *Advances in Heart Disease*, Clinical Cardiology Monographs **3**, 249–65

140. Campbell, W.R., Johnson, A.R., Callahan, K.S. and Graham, R.M. (1981). Anti-platelet activity of beta adrenergic antagonists: inhibition of thromboxane synthesis and platelet aggregation in patients receiving long term propranolol treatment. *Lancet*, **2**, 1382–4

141. Frishman, W.H., Weksler, B., Christodoulos, J.P., Smithen, C. and Killip, T. (1974). Reversal of abnormal platelet aggregability and change in exercise tolerance in patients with angina pectoris following oral propranolol. *Circulation*, 50, 887-96

142. Green, D., Rossi, E.C. and Haring, O. (1982). The beta blocker heart attack trial: Studies of platelets and factor VIII. *Thromb. Res.*, 28, 261-7

143. Gent, A.E., Brook, C.S.D., Foley, T.H. and Miller, T.N. (1968). Dipyridamole; A controlled trial of its effect in myocardial infarction. *Br. Med. J.*, 4, 366-8

144. Elwood, P.C., Cochrane, A.L., Burr, M.L., Sweetnam, A.M., Williams, G., Welsby, E., Hughes, S.J. and Renton, R. (1974). A randomized controlled trial of acetylsalicylic acid in the secondary prevention of mortality from myocardial infarction. *Br. Med. J.*, 1, 436-40

145. Maroko, P.R., Libby, P., Bloor, C.M., Sobel, B.E. and Braunwald, E. (1972). Reduction by hyaluronidase of myocardial necrosis following coronary artery occlusion. *Circulation*, 46, 430-37

146. Maroko, P.R., Hillis, L.D., Muller, J.E., Tavazzi, L., Heyndrickx, G., Ray, M., Chiarello, M., Distante, A., Askenazi, J., Salerno, J., Carpentier, J., Reshetnaya, N., Radkany, P., Libby, P., Raabe, D.S., Chezov, E.I., Babba, P. and Braunwald, E. (1977). Favourable effects of hyaluronidase on electrocardiographic evidence of necrosis in patients with acute myocardial infarction. *N. Engl. J. Med.*, 296, 898-903

147. Saltisi, S., Robinson, P.S., Collart, D.J., Webb-Peploe, M.M. and Croft, D.N. (1982). Effects of early administration of a highly purified hyaluronidase preparation (GL enzyme) on myocardial infarct size. *Lancet*, 1, 867-71

148. Flint, E.J., de Giovanni, J., Cadyon, P.J., Lamb, P. and Pentecost, B.L. (1982). Effect of GL enzyme (a highly purified form of hyaluronidase) on mortality after myocardial infarction. *Lancet*, 1, 871-4

149. Henderson, A., Campbell, R.W.F. and Julian, D.G. (1982). Effect of a highly purified hyaluronidase preparation (GL enzyme) on electrocardiographic changes in acute myocardial infarction. *Lancet*, 1, 874-6

150. Brogden, R.N., Speight, T.M. and Avery, G.S. (1973). Streptokinase, a review of its clinical pharmacology, mechanism of action and therapeutic uses. *Drugs*, 5, 357-445

151. Aoki, N., Maroc, M., Matsude, M. and Tachiya, K. (1971). Behaviour of alpha$_2$-plasmin inhibitor in fibrinolytic states. *J. Clin. Invest.*, 60, 361-9

152. De Wood, M.A., Spory, J., Nolske, R., Mouser, L.T., Burroughs, R., Golden, M.S. and Lang, H.T. (1980). Prevalence of total coronary occlusion during the early hours of transmural myocardial infarction. *N. Engl. J. Med.*, 303, 897-902

153. Reimer, K.A., Low, J.E., Rasmussen, M.M. and Jennings, R.B. (1977). The wavefront phenomenon of ischaemic cell death. I Myocardial infarct size vs. duration of coronary occlusion in dogs. *Circulation*, 56, 786-94

154. Constantini, C., Corday, E., Lang, T.W., Meerbaum, S., Brasch, J., Kaplein, L., Rubins, S., Gidd, H. and Osher, J. (1975). Revascularization after three hours of coronary arterial occlusion: effects on regional cardiac metabolic function and infarct size *Am. J. Cardiol.*, 36, 368-84

155. Ruegsegger, P., Nydick, I. and Hutter, R.C. (1959). Fibrinolytic (plasmic) therapy of experimental coronary thrombi with alteration of the evolution of myocardial infarction. *Circulation*, 19, 7-13

156 Ruegsegger, P., Nydick, I. and Abarquez, R. (1960). Effect of fibrinolytic (plasmin) therapy on physiopathology of myocardial infarction. *Am. J. Cardiol.*, 6, 519-24

157. Aber, C.P., Bass, N.M., Berry, C.L., Carson, P.H.M., Dobbs, R.J., Fox, K.M., Hamblin, J.J., Haydic, S.P., Howitt, G., MacIver, J.E., Portal, R.W., Raftery, E.D., Ronsell, R.H. and Stock, J.P.P. (1976). Streptokinase in acute myocardial infarction: A controlled multi-centre study in the United Kingdom. *Br. Med. J.*, 2, 1100-14

158. Ganz, W., Buchbinder, N., Marcus, H., Mondkar, A., Maddahi, J., Charuzi, Y.,

O'Connor, L., Shell, W., Fishloein, M. C., Kass, R., Miyamoto, A. and Swan, H. J. C. (1981). Intracoronary thrombolysis in evolving myocardial infarction. *Am. Heart J.*, **101**, 4–13

159. Rentrop, P., Blanke, H., Karsch, K. R., Kaiser, H., Köstering, H. and Leitz, K. (1981). Selective intra-coronary thrombolysis in acute myocardial infarction and unstable angina pectoris. *Circulation*, **63**, 307–17

160. Saltrups, A., Boxall, J. and Ho, B. (1984). Intra-coronary versus intravenous streptokinase in acute myocardial infarction. *Circulation*, **68** Suppl. III, 119A

161. Berte, L. E., Jutzy, K. R., Alderman, E. L., Miller, R. G., Friedman, J. P., Creger, W. P. and Elinstrom, M. (1984). Randomized comparison of intravenous and intra-coronary streptokinase in early post myocardial infarction. *Circulation*, **68** Suppl. III, 119A

162. Taylor, G. J., Mikell, H. W., Moses, J. T., Dove, J. E., Batchelder, A., Thull, J. A., Schneider, H. A. and Wellens, H. A. (1984). Intravenous and intracoronary streptokinase for MI. *Circulation*, **68** Suppl. III, 1254 A

163. Udall, J. A. (1983). Intravenous versus intra-coronary streptokinase therapy for acute myocardial infarction. *Cardiovascular Rev. Rep.*, **4**, 635–48

164. Duckert, F. (1979). Thrombolytic therapy in myocardial infarction. *Prog. Cardiovasc. Dis.*, **21**, 342–50

165. Stampfer, M. J., Goldhaber, S. Z., Yusuf, S., Peto, R. and Hennekens, C. H. (1982). Effect of intravenous streptokinase on acute myocardial infarction; pooled results from randomized trials. *N. Engl. J. Med.*, **307**, 1180–2

166. Brochier, M., Raynaud, P. and Plamol, T. (1975). Le traitement par l'urokinase des infarctus du myocarde et syndromes de menace. *Arch. Mal. Cœur*, **68**, 563–9

167. A European Collaborative Study: Controlled treatment of urokinase in myocardial infarction. (1975). *Lancet*, **2**, 624–6

168. Amery, A., Roeher, G. and Vermeulen, H. J. (1969). Single blind randomized multi-centre trial comparing heparin and streptokinase treatment in recent myocardial infarction. *Acta Med. Scand.* (Suppl.), **505**, 114–19

169. European Working Party: Streptokinase in recent myocardial infarction: A controlled multi-centre trial. (1971). *Br. Med. J.*, **3**, 325–31

170. Heikinheimo, R., Ahrenberg, P., Honkapohji, H., Iisalo, E., Kallio, V., Konttinen, Y., Leskinein, O., Mustanienii, H., Reinkainen, M. and Sütonen, L. (1971). Fibrinolytic treatment in acute myocardial infarction. *Acta Med. Scand.*, **189**, 7–13

171. Dioguardia, N., Mannucci, P. M., Lotto, A., Rossi, P., Levi, G.F., Lomanto, B., Rota, M., Mattei, G., Proto, C. and Fiorelli, G. (1971). Controlled trial of streptokinase and heparin in acute myocardial infarction *Lancet*, **2**, 891–5

172. Breddin, K., Ehrly, A. M. and Fechler, L. (1973). Die Kurzzeit-fibrinolyse besin a akuten myokardinfarkt. *Dtsch. Med. Wochenschr.*, **98**, 861–73

173. Bett, H. N., Biggs, J. C., Castaldi, P. A., Chesterman, C. N., Hale, G. S., Hirsh, J., Isbister, J. P., McDonald, I. G., McLean, K. H., Morgan, J. J., O'Sullivan, E. F. and Rosenbaum, M. (1973). Australian multi-centre trial of streptokinase in acute myocardial infarction. *Lancet*, **1**, 57–60

174. Ness, P. M., Simon, T. L., Cole, C. and Walston, A. (1974). A pilot study of streptokinase therapy in acute myocardial infarction. Observations on complications and relation to trial design. *Am. Heart J.*, **88**, 705–12

175. Aber, C. P., Bass, N. M. and Berry, C. L. (1976). Streptokinase in acute myocardial infarction; a controlled multi-centre study in the United Kingdom. *Br. Med. J.*, **2**, 1100–1104

176. Poliwoda, H., Schneider, B. and Avenarins, H. J., (1977). Untersuchungen zum klinischen verlant des akutin myokardinfarktes. Gemeinschaftsstudie an 26 krankenhaus en in Norddeutschland. Test 1: Die fibrinolytische theryne des myokardinfarktes mit streptokinase. *Med. Klin.*, **72**, 451–8

177. Benda, L., Haider, M. and Ambrosch, F., (1977). Ergebnisse de oesterreichischen Herz-infarktstudie mit streptokinase. *Wien. Klin. Wochenschr*, **89**, 779–83

178. European Cooperative Study Group (1979). Streptokinase in acute myocardial infarction. *N. Engl. J. Med.*, **301**, 797–802
179. European Cooperative Study Group (1981). Streptokinase in acute myocardial infarction: Extended report of the European Cooperative trial. *Acta Med. Scand.* (Suppl.), **648**, 7–57
180. Furberg, C. (1984). Clinical value of intra-coronary streptokinase. *Am. J. Cardiol*, **53**, 626–7
181. Kennedy, J. W., Ritchie, J. L., Davis, K. B. and Fritz, J. K. (1983). Western Washington randomized trial of intra-coronary streptokinase in acute myocardial infarction. *N. Engl. J. Med.*, **309**, 1477–82
182. Simoons, M. L., Fioretti, P., Van der Brand, M., Gerruys, P. M., Krauss, X. H., Remme, P., Van der Wall, E. E., Verheught, F., Res, J. and de Neef, K. J. (1983). Randomized trial of thrombolysis with streptokinase in acute myocardial infarction. *Circulation*, **68**, Suppl. III, 480A
183. Collaborative Group (1971). Phenytoin after recovery from myocardial infarction: Controlled trial in 568 patients. *Lancet*, **2**, 1055–7
184. Peter, J., Ross, D., Duffield, A., Luxton, M., Harper, R., Hunt, D. and Sloman, G. (1978). Effect on survival after myocardial infarction of long-term treatment with phenytoin. *Br. Heart J.*, **40**, 1356–60
185. Ryden, L., Arnmen, K., Conradson, T. B., Hofrendahl, S., Mortensen, O. and Smedgard, P. (1980). Prophylaxis of ventricular arrhythmias with intravenous and oral tocainide in patients with and recovery from acute myocardial infarction. *Am. Heart J.*, **100**, 1006–12
186. Bastian, B. C., McFarland, P. W., McLauchlan, J., Ballantyne, D., Clark, R., Hillis, W. S., Rae, A. P. and Hutton, I. (1980). A prospective randomised trial of tocainide in patients following myocardial infarction *Am. Heart J.*, **100**, 1017–22
187. Chamberlain, D. A., Jewitt, D. E., Julian, D. S., Campbell, R. W. F., Boyle, D. McC. and Shanks, R. G. (1980). Oral mexiletine in high risk patients after myocardial infarction. *Lancet*, **2**, 1324–7
188. Impact Research Group (1983). Impact: Report on arrhythmia, mortality and other findings. *Circulation*, **68**, III, 1089A
189. Lubsen, J. (1983). Design of clinical trials with anti-arrhythmic drugs. In Van Durme, J. P., Bogaert, M. G., Julian, D. G. and Kulbertus, (eds) *Chronic Anti-arrhythmic Therapy*, p. 40. (Molndahl: AB Hassle)
190. Myerburg, R. J., Conde, C., Sheps, D. S., Appel, R. A., Kiem, I., Sing, R. J. and Castellanos, A. (1979). Anti-arrhythmic therapy in survivors of prehospital cardiac arrest: Comparison of effects on chronic ventricular arrhythimias and recurrent cardiac arrest. *Circulation*, **59**, 855–63
191. Grayboys, T. B., Lown, B., Podril, P. J. and De Silva, R. (1982). Long-term survival of patients with malignant ventricular arrhythmias treated with anti-arrhythmic drugs. *Am. J. Cardiol.*, **50**, 437–43
192. Hoffman, A., Burkhardt, D., White, R. and Follarth, F. (1983). Anti-arrhythmic drug treatment and survival in patients with coronary artery disease. *Circulation*, **68**, III, 111–416(A)
193. Leren, P. (1970). The Oslo Diet–Heart Study: Eleven year report. *Circulation*, **42**, 935–42
194. Leren, P. (1966). The effect of plasma cholesterol lowering diet in male survivors of myocardial infarction. *Acta Med. Scand.*, **466** (Suppl.), 5–92
195. Report of a Research Committee to the Medical Research Council (1968). Controlled trial of soya-bean oil in myocardial infarction. *Lancet*, **2**, 693–9
196. Oliver, M. F. and Boyd, G. S. (1961). Influence of reduction of serum lipids on prognosis of coronary heart disease. Five year study using oestrogen. *Lancet*, **2**, 499–505
197. Stamler, J., Pick, R., Katz, L. N., Pick, A., Kaplan, B. M., Berkson, D. M. and Century, D (1963). Effectiveness of oestrogens for therapy of myocardial infarction in middle-age men. *J. Am. Med. Assoc.*, **183**, 632–8

198. The Coronary Drug Project Research Group (1970). Initial findings leading to modifications of its research protocol. *J. Am. Med. Assoc.*, **214**, 1303–13

199. The Coronary Drug Project Research Group (1972). Findings leading to further modifications of its protocol with respect to dextrothyroxine. *J. Am. Med. Assoc.*, **220**, 996–1008

200. The Coronary Drug Project Research Group (1973). Findings leading to discontinuation of the 2.5 mg/day oestrogen group. *J. Am. Med. Assoc.*, **226**, 652–7

201. The Coronary Drug Project Research Group (1975). Clofibrate and niacin in coronary heart disease. *J. Am. Med. Assoc.*, **231**, 360–81

202. Detre, K. M. and Show, L. (1974). Long-term changes of serum cholesterol with cholesterol-altering drugs in patients with coronary heart disease: Veterans Administration Drug–Lipid Cooperative Study. *Circulation*, **50**, 998–208

203. Five year study by a group of physicians of the Newcastle-upon-Tyne region (1971). Trial of clofibrate in the treatment of ischaemic heart disease. (1971). *Br. Med. J.*, **4**, 767–75

204. Report by a Research Committee of the Scottish Society of Physicians (1971). Ischaemic heart disease: A secondary prevention trial using clofibrate. *Br. Med. J.*, **4**, 775–84

205. Dewar, H. A. and Oliver, M. F. (1971). Secondary prevention trials using clofibrate: A joint commentary on the Newcastle and Scottish Trials. *Br. Med. J.*, **4**, 784–6

206. Rahlfs, V. W. and Bedall, F. K. (1973). The effect of clofibrate: A comment on two published studies. *J. Chron. Dis.*, **26**, 817–20

207. Carlson, L. A., Danielson, M., Ekberg, I., Klintemar, B. and Rosenheimer, G. (1977). Reduction of myocardial infarction by the combined treatment with clofibrate and nicotinic acid. *Atherosclerosis*, **28**, 81–6

208. Rosenheimer, G. and Carlson, L. A. (1980). Effect of combined clofibrate-nicotinic acid treatment in ischaemic heart disease. *Atherosclerosis*, **37**, 129–38

209. Shaper, A. G. (1976). Primary and secondary prevention trials in coronary heart disease. *Postgrad. Med. J.*, **52**, 464–9

210. Elwood, P. C. and Sweetman, P. M. (1974). Aspirin and secondary mortality after myocardial infarction. *Lancet*, **2**, 1313–15

211. The Coronary Drug Project Research Group (1976). Aspirin in coronary heart disease. *J. Chron. Dis.*, **29**, 625–42

212. Breddin, K. (1977). Multicentre two year prospective study on the prevention of secondary infarction by ASA in comparison with phenprocoumon and placebo. *In* Boissel, J.P. and Klimt, C. R. (eds.) *Multi-centre Controlled Trials: Principles and Problems*, pp. 79–85. (Paris: INSERM)

213. Breddin, K., Loew, D., Lechner, K., Uberla, K. and Walter, E. (1979). Secondary prevention of myocardial infarction. Comparison of acetylsalicylic acid; phenprocoumon and placebo. A multi-centre two year prospective study. *Thromb. Haemost*, **41**, 225–36

214. Elwood, P. C. and Williams, W. O. (1979). A randomized controlled trial of aspirin in the prevention of early mortality in myocardial infarction. *J. R. Coll. Gen. Pract.*, **29**, 413–16

215. Aspirin Myocardial Infarction Study Research Group (1980). A randomized controlled trial of persons recovered from myocardial infarction. *J. Am. Med. Assoc.*, **243**, 661–9

216. The Anturane Reinfarction Trial Research Group (1978). Sulphinpyrazone in the prevention of cardiac deaths after myocardial infarction. *N. Engl. J. Med.*, **298**, 289–95

217. The Anturane Reinfarction Trial Research Group (1980). Sulphinpyrazone in the prevention of sudden death after myocardial infarction. *N. Engl. J. Med.*, **302**, 250–6

218. The Anturane Reinfarction Trial Policy Committee (1982). The Anturane Reinfarction Trial: Re-evaluation of outcome. *N. Engl. J. Med.*, **306**, 1005–1008

219. Temple, R. and Pledger, G. W. (1980). The FDA's critique of the Anturane Reinfarction Trial. *N. Engl. J. Med.*, 303, 1488-92
220. Anturane Reinfarction Italian Study Group (1982). Sulphinpyrazone in post-myocardial infarction. *Lancet*, 1, 237-42
221. Editorial. (1980). Aspirin after myocardial infarction. *Lancet*, 2, 1172-3
222. Marcus, A. J. (1977). Aspirin and thromboembolism - a possible dilemma. *N. Engl. J. Med.*, 297, 1284-5
223. Lewis, H. D., Davis, J. W. and Archibald, D. G. (1984). Aspirin and the risk of myocardial infarction. *N. Engl. J. Med.*, 310, 122-3
224. Fields, W. S., Lemak, N. A., Frankowski, R. F. and Hardy, R. J. (1977). Controlled trial of aspirin in cerebral ischaemia. *Stroke*, 8, 301-16
225. Bousser, M. G., Eschivege, E., Haguenau, M., Lefaucconnier, J. M., Thibault, N., Tonboue, D. and Touboul, P. J. (1983). 'AICLA' controlled trial of aspirin and dipyridamole in the secondary prevention of athero-thrombolic cerebral ischaemia. *Stroke*, 14, 5-14
226. Canadian Cooperative Study Group (1978). A randomized trial of aspirin and sulphinpyrazone in threatened stroke. *N. Engl. J. Med.*, 299, 53-9
227. The Danish Study Group (1984). Verapamil in acute myocardial infarction. *Eur. Heart J.*, 5, 516-28
228. Andersen, M. P., Bechsgaard, P., Fredercksen, J., Hansen, D. A., Jürgensen, H. J., Nielson, B., Pedersen, F., Pedersen-Bjergaad, O. and Rasmussen, S. (1979). Effect of alprenolol on mortality among patients with definite or suspected acute myocardial infarction: Preliminary results. *Lancet*, 2, 865-8
229. McIlmoyle, L., Evans, A., Boyle, D. McC., Cran, G., Barber, J. M., Elwood, H., Salathia, K. and Shanks, R. (1981). Early intervention in myocardial ischaemia with metoprolol. *Proc. Br. Cardiac Soc.* Dec. 1981, 3-4 (Abstr.)
230. Hjalmarson, A., Elmfeldt, D., Herlitz, J., Holmberg, S., Malek, I., Nyberg, G., Ryden, L., Swedberg, K., Vedin, A., Waagstein, F., Waldenström, A., Waldenström, J., Wedel, H. and Wilhelmsen, L. (1981). Effect on mortality of metoprolol in acute myocardial infarction. A double-blind randomized trial. *Lancet*, 2, 823-7
231. Balcon, R., Jewitt, D. E., Davies, J. P. H. and Oram, S. (1966). A controlled trial of propranolol in acute myocardial infarction. *Lancet*, 2, 917-20
232. Clausen, J., Felsby, M., Jorgensen, F. S., Nielsen, B., Rom, J. and Strange, B. (1966). Absence of prophylactic effect of propranolol in myocardial infarction. *Lancet*, 2, 920-4
233. Multi-Centre Trial. Propranolol in acute myocardial infarction (1966). *Lancet*, 2, 1435-8
234. Barber, J. M., Murphy, F. M. and Merrett, J. D. (1977). Clinical trial of propranolol in acute myocardial infarction. *Ulster Med. J.*, 36, 127-30
235. Norris, R. M., Laughey, D. E. and Scott, P. J. (1968). A trial of propranolol in acute myocardial infarction. *Br. Med. J.*, 2, 398-400
236. Briant, R. B. and Norris, R. M. (1970). Alprenolol in acute myocardial infarction: double-blind trial. *NZ Med. J.*, 71, 135-8
237. Lombardo, M., Selvini, A., Motolese, M., Belli, C. and Pedroni, P. (1979). Beta-blocking treatment in 440 cases of acute myocardial infarction: a study with oxprenolol. *Proceedings of Florence International Meeting on Myocardial Infarction*, 8-12 May 1979, 2, 803-807
238. Fuccella, L. M. (1968). Report on the double-blind trial with compound CIBA 3 9089 (Trasicor) in myocardial infarction. Quoted by Sowton, E., in *Prog. Cardiovasc. Dis.*, 10, 561-74
239. Evemy, K. L. and Pentecost, B. L. (1978). Intravenous and oral practolol in the acute stages of myocardial infarction. *Eur. J. Cardiol.*, 7, 391-8
240. Johansson, B. W. (1980). A comparative study of cardioselective beta-blockade and diazepam in patients with acute myocardial infarction and tachycardia. *Acta Med. Scand.*, 207, 47-53
241. Yusuf, S., Sleight, P., Rossi, P. R. F., Ramsdale, D., Peto, R., Furse, L., Motivani, R., Parish, S., Gray, R., Bennett, D. and Bray, C. (1983). Reduction in infarct

size, arrhythmias, chest pain and morbidity by early intravenous beta-blockade in suspected acute myocardial infarction. *Circulation*, **67** (Suppl. I), I-32, I-41

242. International Collaborative Study Group (1984). Reduction of infarct size with the early use of timolol in acute myocardial infarction. *N. Engl. J. Med.*, **310**, 9-15

243. Brown, M.A., Barnaby, P.F., Geary, G.G. and Norris, R.M. (1984). Intravenous propranolol prevents ventricular fibrillation during acute myocardial infarction. *Aust. NZ J. Med.*, (In press)

244. Jurgensen, H.J., Frederiksen, J., Hansen, D.A. and Pedersen-Bjergaard, O. (1981). Limitation of myocardial infarct size in patients less than 66 years, treated with alprenolol. *Br. Heart J.*, **45**, 583-8

245. Boyle, D.McI., Barber, J.M., McIlmoyle, E.Z., Salathia, K.S., Evans, A.E., Cran, G., Elwood, J.H. and Shanks, R.G. (1983). Effect of very early intervention with metoprolol on myocardial infarct size. *Br. Heart J.*, **49**, 229-33

246. Wilcox, R.G., Roland, J.M., Banks, D.C., Hampton, J.R. and Mitchell, J.R.A. (1980). Randomized trial comparing propranolol with atenolol in immediate treatment of suspected myocardial infarction. *Br. Med. J.*, **280**, 885-8

247. Barber, J.M., Boyle, D.McC., Chaturvedi, N.C., Singh, N. and Walsh, M.J. (1976). Practolol in acute myocardial infarction. *Acta. Med. Scand.*, (Suppl.) **587**, 213-19

248. Coronary Prevention Research Group (1981). An early intervention secondary prevention study with oxprenolol following myocardial infarction. *Eur. Heart J.*, **2**, 389-93

249. Rutherford, J.D., Singh, B.N., Ambler, P.K. and Norris, R.M. (1976). Plasma propranolol concentrations in patients with angina and acute myocardial infarction. *Clin. Exp. Pharmacol. Physiol.*, **3**, 297-304

250. Sleight, P., Yusuf, S., Ramsdale, D., Rossi, P. and Peto R. (1982). Early intravenous beta blockade in myocardial infarction. *Br. J. Clin. Pharmacol.*, **14**, 37s-40s

251. Ramsdale, D.R., Faragher, E.B., Bennett, D.H., Bray, C.L., Ward, C., Cruickshank, J.M., Yusuf, S. and Sleight, P. (1982). Ischaemic pain relief in patients with acute myocardial infarction by intravenous atenolol. *Am. Heart J.*, **103**, 459-67

252. Peter, J., Norris, R.M., Clarke, E.D., Heng, M.K., Singh, B.N., Williams, B., Howell, D.R. and Ambler, P.K. (1978). Reduction of enzyme levels by propranolol after acute myocardial infarction. *Circulation*, **57**, 1091-5

253. Muller, J., Roberts, J., Stone, P., Rude, R., Raabe, D., Gold, H., Jaffe, A., Strauss, W., Juri, Z., Hartwell, T., Poole, K., Passamani, E., Willerson, J., Sobel, B., Braunwald, E., MILIS Group. Failure of propranolol administration to limit infarct size in patients with acute myocardial infarction. *Circulation*, **68**, III 1177A

254. Herlitz, J., Hjalmarson, A., Holmberg, S., Swedberg, K., Vedin, A., Waagstein, F., Waldenstrüm, A., Waldenstrüm, J., Wedel, H., Wilhelmsen, L. and Wilhelmsson, C. (1982). Limitation of infarct size in acute myocardial infarction with metoprolol (Abstr.) *Am. J. Cardiol.* **49**, 1004

255. Hertiltz, J., Elmfeldt, D., Hjalmarson, A., Holmberg, S., Malek, I., Nyberg, G., Ryden, L., Swedberg, K., Vedin, A., Waagstein, F., Waldenström, A., Waldenström, J., Wedel, H., Wilhelmsen, L. and Wilhelmsson, C., (1983). Effect of metoprolol on indirect signs of the size and severity of acute myocardial infarction. *Am. J. Cardiol.*, **51**, 1282-8

256. Lloyd, E.A., Gordon, G.P., Mabin, J.A., Charles, R.G., Connerford, P.J. and Opie, L.H. (1982). Intravenous sotalol in acute myocardial infarction. *Circulation*, (Suppl. II) **66**, I-3 Abstr. 10

257. Norris, R.M., Clark, E.D., Samuel, N.L., Smith, W.M. and Williams, B. (1978). Protective effect of propranolol in threatened myocardial infarction. *Lancet*, **2**, 907-909

258. Yusuf, S. (1980). Improvement of electrocardiogram by chronic beta-adrenoceptor blockade during healing phase of clinical and experimental myocardial infarction. *Br. Heart J.*, **43**, 99–103
259. Rossi, P.R., Yusuf, S., Ramsdale, N., Furze, L. and Sleight, P. (1983). Reduction of ventricular arrhythmias by early intravenous atenolol in suspected acute myocardial infarction. *Br. Med. J.*, **286**, 506–510
260. Ryden, L., Amiego, R., Arnmar, K., Herlitz, J., Hjalmarson, A., Holmberg, S., Reyes, C., Smedgard, P., Svedberg, K., Vedin, A., Waagstein, F., Waldenström, A., Wilhelmsson, C., Wedel, H. and Yamamoto, M. (1983). A double blind trial of metoprolol in acute myocardial infarction: effects on ventricular tachycardia. *N. Engl. J. Med.*, **308**, 614–18
261. Gold, H., Lemboch, R. and Maroko, P. (1976). Reduction of myocardial injury in patients with acute infarction by propranolol. *Am. J. Cardiol.*, **38**, 689–95
262. Waagstein, F. and Hjalmarson, A.C. (1976). Double blind study of the effect of cardioselective beta-blockade on chest pain in acute myocardial infarction. *Acta Med. Scand.*, (Suppl.) **587**, 201–11
263. Mueller, H.S. and Herron, R. (1977). How, when and why to use propranolol in acute myocardial infarction. *Cardiovasc. Med.*, **2**, 321–8
264. Bay, G., Lund-Larsen, P., Lorenstein, E. and Sivertssen, E. (1967). Haemodynamic effects of propranolol ('Inderal') in acute myocardial infarction. *Br. Med. J.*, **1**, 141–3
265. Lehmann, H.J., Oeff, M., Witt, E. and Hochrein, H. (1981). The treatment of acute myocardial infarction with beta receptor blockers. ii. Haemodynamic effects of propranolol with and without combination with nitroglycerine. *Z. Kardiol.*, **70**, 748–53
266. Wilhelmsson, C., Vedin, J.A., Wilhelmsen, I., Tibblin, G. and Werko, L. (1974). Reduction in sudden deaths after myocardial infarction by treatment with alprenolol. *Lancet*, **2**, 1157–60
267. Multi-centre International Study Group (1975). Improvement in prognosis of myocardial infarction by long-term beta-adrenoceptor blockade using practolol. *Br. Med. J.*, **3**, 735–40
268. Multi-centre International Study Group (1977). Reduction in mortality after myocardial infarction with long-term beta-adrenoceptor blockade: supplementary report. *Br. Med. J.*, **2**, 419–21
269. Baber, N.S., Evans, D.W., Howett, G., Thomas, M., Wilson, C., Lewis, J.A., Dawes, P.M., Handler, K. and Tuson, R., (1980). Multi-centre post-infarction trial of propranolol in 49 hospitals in United Kingdom, Italy and Yugoslavia. *Br. Heart J.*, **44**, 96–100
270. Rehnquist, N., Ahnve, S. and Erhardt, L. (1980). Effect of metoprolol after acute myocardial infarction. *Proc. Eur. Congr. Cardiol.*, **16** (Abstr.)
271. The Norwegian Multi-Centre Study Group (1981). Timolol-induced reduction in mortality and reinfarction in patients treated with timolol after myocardial infarction. *N. Engl. J. Med.*, **304**, 801–807
272. Taylor, S.H., Silke, B., Ebult, A., Sutton, G.C., Prout, B.J. and Burley, D.M. (1982). A long term prevention study with oxprenolol in coronary heart disease. *N. Engl. J. Med.*, **307**, 1293–1301
273. Hansteen, V., Moinichen, E., Lorensten, E., Andersen, A., Shrøn, O., Søiland, K., Dyrberk, D., Refsum, A.M., Thomsdal, A., Knudsen, K., Eika, C., Bakian, J. Jr., Smith, P. and Hoff, P.I. (1982). One year's treatment with propranolol after myocardial infarction. Preliminary report of Norwegian Multi-centre trial. *Br. Med. J.*, **284**, 155–60
274. Beta-blocker Heart Attack Trial Research Group (1982). A randomized trial of propranolol in patients with acute myocardial infarction: I. Mortality results. *J. Am. Med. Assoc.*, **247**, 1707–14
275. Julian, D.G., Prescott, R.J., Jackson, F.S. and Szekely, P. (1982). Controlled trial of sotalol for one year after myocardial infarction. *Lancet*, **1**, 1142–7
276. Australian and Swedish Pindolol Study Group (1983). The effect of pindolol on

the two years mortality after complicated myocardial infarction. *Eur. Heart J.*, **4**, 367–75

277. Manger Cats V., von Capelle, F.J.L., Lie, K.I. and Durrer, D. (1983). Effects of treatment with 2 × 100 mg metoprolol on mortality in a single-centre study with low placebo-mortality rate after infarction. *Circulation*, **68**, Suppl. III, III–181 (Abstr.)

278. European Infarction Study Group (1984). European Infarction Study (EIS). A secondary prevention study with slow release oxprenolol after myocardial infarction: morbidity and mortality. *Eur. Heart J.*, **5**, 189–202

279. Taylor, S.H., Silke, B., Sutton, G.C., Prout, B.J., Richard, A. (1984). Is there a dose-response effect with beta-blocking drugs in secondary prevention after acute myocardial infarction? *Br. Heart J.*, **51**, 106 (Abstr.)

280. Peto, R., Pike, M.C., Armitage, P., Breslaw, N.E., Cox, D.R., Howard, S.V., Mantel, N., McPherson, K., Peto, J. and Smith, P.G., (1977). Design and analysis of randomized clinical trials requiring prolonged observation of each patient. 11: Analysis and examples. *Br. J. Cancer*, **34**, 1–39

281. Furberg, L.D. and Byington, R.P. (1983). What do subgroup analyses reveal about differential response to beta-blocker therapy. The Beta-Blocker Heart Attack Trial Experience. *Circulation*, **67**, I-98–I-101

282. Griggs, T.R., Wagner, G.S. and Gettes, L.S. (1983). Beta adrenergic blocking agents after myocardial infarction: An undocumented need in patients at lowest risk. *J. Am. Coll. Cardiol.*, **1**, 1530–3

283. Furberg, C.D., Hawkins, C.M. and Lichstein, E. (1984). Effect of propranolol in post infarction patients with mechanical and electrical complications. *Circulation*, **69**, 761–5

284. Opie, L.H. (1984). Drugs and the heart four years on. *Lancet*, **1**, 496–501

285. Herlitz, J., Hjalmarson, A., Holmberg, S., Swedberg, K., Vedin, A., Waagstein, F., Waldenström, A., Wedel, H., Wilhelmsen, L. and Wilhelmsson, C. (1984). Development of congestive heart failure after treatment with metoprolol in acute myocardial infarction. *Br. Heart J.*, **51**, 539–44

286. Goldstein, S., Lichstein, E. and Morgonroth, J. (1983). From: *International Symposium on 'Long term Ambulatory Monitoring'*, *European Society of Cardiology*, Rotterdam, October 13–15, pp. 27–33

4
Drug treatment of cardiac failure

C.J.C. ROBERTS

GENERAL INTRODUCTION

Most patients interpret the term 'heart failure' as carrying a grave prognosis. In fact people may survive for many years following the initial diagnosis of cardiac failure even when a procedure remedial to the cause is not possible. If cardiac failure occurs when the heart's pumping capacity is inadequate for the needs of the body, how can it be that it may carry a remarkably good prognosis? In the first place it is important to realize that an episode of cardiac failure may be precipitated in a patient with diseased myocardium by some acute event such as pneumonia, an intravenous infusion or the taking of a myocardial depressant or fluid retaining drug. These factors may trigger a vicious cycle of events leading to the heart failure syndrome. Spontaneous recovery may not be possible but appropriate therapy will reverse the spiralling deterioration, and allow the heart to regain its previous dimensions and function. Then the patient may be able to continue quite well, perhaps with no drugs at all until the next insult to the myocardium.

The treatment of cardiac failure is changing and yet the cornerstones of therapy are drugs which have been available to doctors for many years – even centuries. Improved understanding of the pathophysiology of the condition together with better knowledge of the drugs' actions and limitations is permitting doctors to tailor therapy more closely to the many different clinical situations so that the beneficial effects are maximized and risks reduced.

The aim of this chapter is to collect together the relevant facts as presently available and to examine how they can lead the physician to a rational choice of therapy.

PATHOPHYSIOLOGY OF CARDIAC FAILURE

There are a host of causes of cardiac failure and some of these are illustrated in Figure 4.1. The most common cause of pump failure is

159

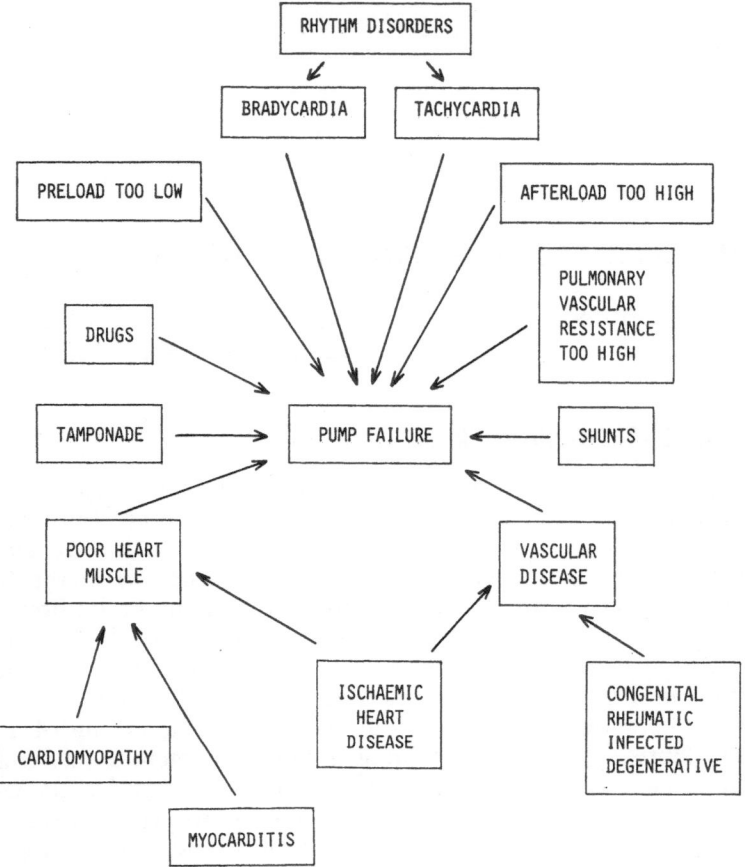

Figure 4.1   Causes of pump failure (after Webb–Peploe, 1979)

a weak myocardium, but it is important to realize that in the absence
of myocardial disease the heart may fail because of an excessive load
being applied. This may occur as a result of valvular stenosis or incompetence, increased resistance as in hypertension, large arterio-
venous shunts or excessive blood volume. Also failure may occur if
there is a disturbance to the mechanism by which the heart responds
to increased load by a rise in rate of contraction. In practice usually a
combination of factors is responsible in the individual for the cardiac
failure event. This explains why considerable improvement can be
achieved in the patient with mitral valve disease by reducing blood
volume, correcting arrhythmias and improving myocardial contractility without any attempt being made to correct the fundamental defect.
In order to understand this we must consider the five major determinants of cardiac function which operate whether or not there is myocardial disease or valvular obstruction. Change in these determinants

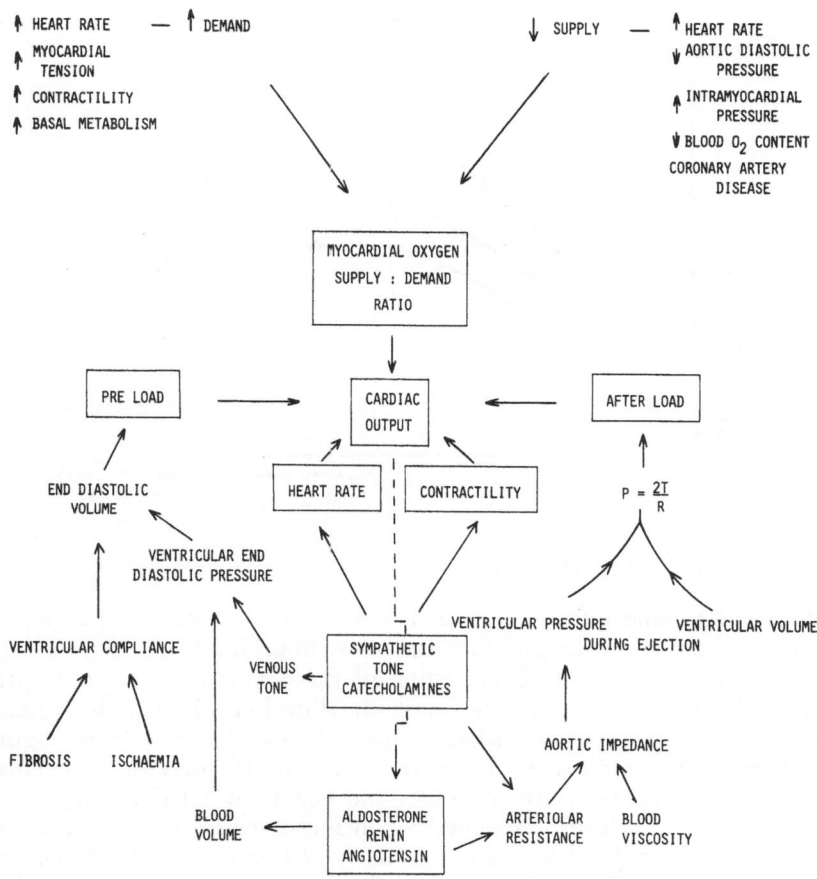

Figure 4.2 Factors determining cardiac output (after Webb–Peploe, 1979)

– preload, afterload, heart rate, myocardial oxygen supply to demand ratio and contractility – may be responsible for the occurrence of heart failure and may occur as part of the compensatory response of the body to circulatory embarrassment (Figure 4.2).

Preload

This term implies myocardial fibre length at the end of diastole, and consequently it reflects end-diastolic ventricular dimensions. It is determined by both ventricular compliance and end-diastolic pressure. Where myocardial compliance is decreased as in the presence of ischaemic damage much higher end-diastolic pressure is required to achieve a similar volume. End-diastolic pressure is determined by the interaction of blood volume and the tone in the capacitance blood vessels (mainly peripheral venous beds). A rise in venous tone will

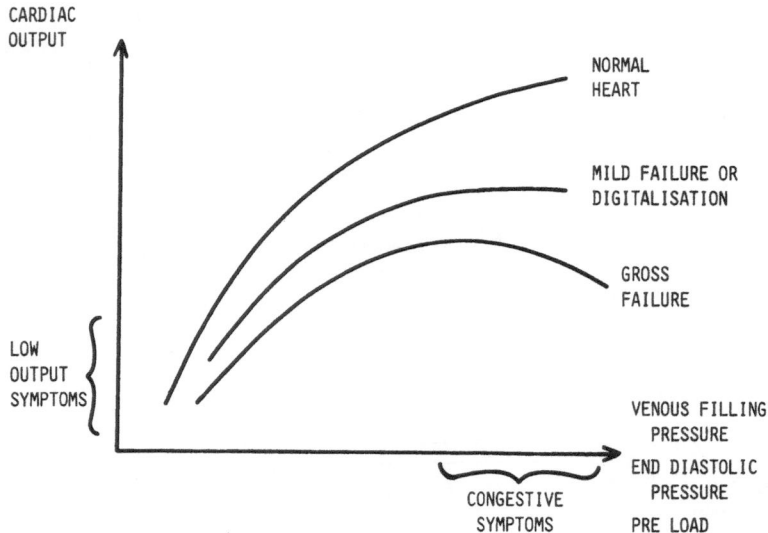

Figure 4.3   The Frank–Starling hypothesis

produce the same effect as an increase in blood volume: that is, an increase in end-diastolic pressure and a rise in preload.

Fundamental to the understanding of the effects of changes in pre-load on haemodynamics is the Frank–Starling hypothesis. This relates end-diastolic pressure to cardiac output. As can be seen from Figure 4.3 increasing end-diastolic pressure results in an increase in cardiac output. As filling pressure increases the effect on cardiac output becomes less until a level is reached when increases in pressure have no further effect on cardiac output and indeed it may fall. When the myocardium is damaged the curve is displaced so that at a given end-diastolic pressure the cardiac output is reduced. Under these circumstances the body compensates by attempting to increase preload. This is achieved by a reduction in the capacitance of the venous system mediated through increased secretion of catecholamines and increased sympathetic tone. There is also an attempt at volume expansion through increased salt and water reabsorption in the kidney. The latter is mediated by both an increase in aldosterone secretion, with the consequent increase in sodium reabsorption in the distal tubule of the nephron, and by a change in proximal tubular sodium handling.

These compensatory effects to increase preload are not always beneficial. Although cardiac output may be maintained it is at the expense of an increasing left ventricular end-diastolic pressure, and this will eventually exceed plasma colloidal oncotic pressure.

It is helpful to consider the relationship between cardiac output and filling pressure in four different situations (Figure 4.4). These are the normal heart, right ventricular failure, left ventricular failure and bi-ventricular failure.

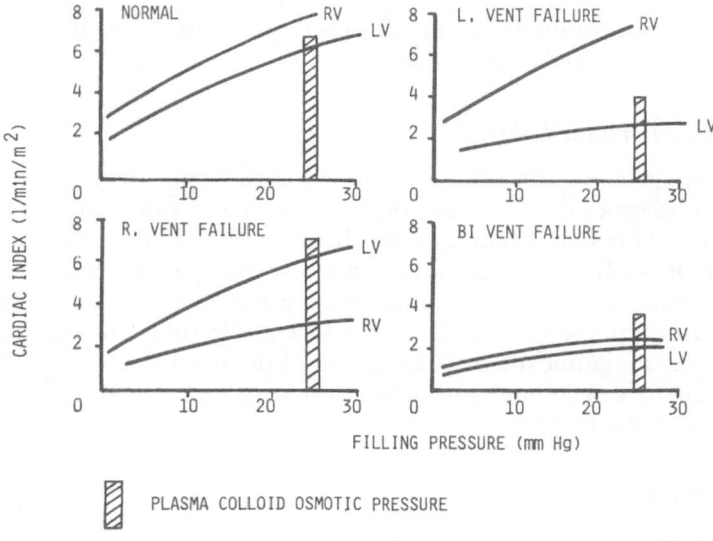

Figure 4.4 Frank–Starling curves in four situations (after Webb-Peploe, 1979)

The normal heart

At a normal cardiac output of about 3 l/min/m² the normal right atrial pressure is about 1 mmHg. Obviously to maintain constant pulmonary and systemic blood volumes and pressures, left and right ventricular outputs must be equal. The right and left ventricular function curves are virtually parallel. It follows therefore that a rise in right atrial pressure will result in a comparable change in left atrial pressure. It is important to realize, however, that even in the normal heart massive over-transfusion with its accompanying rise in filling pressure can result in pulmonary oedema once the filling pressure has exceeded plasma colloidal oncotic pressure. This occurs when cardiac output has been elevated to about 7 l/min. Left ventricular pressure is 30 mmHg, which is well above plasma colloidal oncotic pressure, whereas right atrial filling pressure is approximately 20 mmHg.

Left ventricular failure

In this situation the performance curve for the right ventricle remains normal whereas that for the left ventricle becomes flattened. Thus in order to maintain a normal cardiac output of, say, 3 l/min/m², right atrial pressure may remain normal at around 1 mmHg, whereas that of the left ventricle may rise to approximately 30 mmHg. Again this exceeds the plasma colloidal oncotic pressure and the result is pulmonary oedema. It can easily be seen that a small reduction in right

163

atrial pressure will cause a small reduction in cardiac output but may produce a substantial fall in left ventricular end-diastolic pressure and thereby reduce pulmonary oedema.

Right ventricular failure

In this situation the function curve for the right ventricle is the one which becomes flattened and the left ventricular function curve remains normal. This may occur as a result of increased afterload on the right ventricle such as occurs during massive pulmonary embolism. Right ventricular output is maintained by the rise in right atrial filling pressure. Attempts to reduce filling pressure under these circumstances may produce a significant and disastrous fall in cardiac output. Clearly venodilators or attempts to reduce blood volume could have an adverse effect in these patients.

Biventricular failure

Under these circumstances the function curves for both ventricles remain parallel, and both are flattened. Although filling pressures on both sides of the heart may become substantially elevated in an attempt to maintain cardiac output the patient is relatively protected against pulmonary oedema.

Afterload

Afterload refers to the tension or force per cross-sectional area in the wall of the ventricle during ejection of blood – in other words the tension which must be generated to maintain stroke volume. According to La Place's law, wall tension is proportional to the pressure during systole, multiplied by the diameter of the chamber and divided by the thickness of the wall. If cardiac output is to be maintained in the presence of an increased systemic vascular resistance, then pressure must rise. The rise in pressure must be offset by a rise in wall tension during ejection – that is, a rise in afterload. It is also evident from La Place's law that where the ventricle has become dilated a greater tension must be generated in order to maintain stroke volume and pressure. A normal ventricle ejects more than 50% of its end-diastolic volume. Therefore ventricular dimensions become rapidly reduced during systole, and the wall tension required to maintain the pressure is also rapidly reduced. Thus peak wall tensions are only maintained for a short period of systole. When the ventricle is dilated stroke volume represents a smaller proportion of end-diastolic volume. Thus during systole the change in ventricular dimensions is relatively small. Consequently peak wall tension must be maintained for a longer period of systole. This increased wall tension that the dilated ventricle must develop to maintain normal pressure results in an increased myocardial oxygen demand. The other determinant of wall tension, left ventricular systolic pressure, is determined by aortic impedance which in turn reflects the arteriolar cross-sectional area regulated by sympathetic tone, and to some extent the compliance of arteries, blood viscosity and intra-arterial blood volume.

Let us consider the effects of an increase in afterload on the heart. The normal heart has reserve capacity so that an increase in afterload can be overcome by an increase in left ventricular work. It is important to realize that afterload and preload are interrelated variables, so that a sudden increase in afterload causes an initial increase in left ventricular end-diastolic pressure and volume. There may be a transient fall in cardiac index but this is soon compensated for by an increase in left ventricular work and the normal cardiac dimensions are reassumed. There has been no change in the curve relating filling pressure to cardiac output. Conceptually there has been a downward shift in that curve as a result of the increase in afterload, followed by an upward shift due to an increase in contractility. The end result is no change. The failing left ventricle has no reserve capacity for an increase in contractility; consequently, faced with a sudden increase in afterload it dilates and end-diastolic pressure rises. Cardiac output can only be maintained by the Frank–Starling mechanism – that is, by allowing left ventricular end-diastolic pressure and volume to remain elevated. Thus a new situation arises in which afterload is elevated, preload is elevated and cardiac output is maintained – that is to say that the curve relating filling pressure to cardiac output has been depressed and the left ventricle is functioning at a point to the right on the curve. In severe left ventricular failure when the curve relating cardiac output to filling pressure is almost completely flattened, a further increase in afterload will almost certainly result in a reduction in cardiac output as well as a further rise in left ventricular end-diastolic volume. In cardiac failure increased arterial tone may be necessary to maintain blood pressure in the face of a falling cardiac output and arterial constriction may occur as a result of increased circulating catecholamines. These physiological responses inevitably increase afterload and may cause a depression of myocardial function and a further reduction in cardiac output.

Myocardial contractility

This is the force with which the ventricle can contract independent of heart rate, preload and afterload. It is a difficult commodity to consider or to measure, as myocardial contraction is in fact never independent of these other factors. Nevertheless, it is accepted that an increase in contractility occurs physiologically in the presence of increased sympathetic tone and circulating catecholamines, and can be achieved pharmacologically by the administration of the cardiac glycosides. Stimulation of the vagus decreases contractility as does the administration of drugs which block the sympathetic nervous system. In general a rise in contractility is at the expense of a disproportionately high increase in myocardial oxygen consumption.

Heart rate

Heart rate is under the control of sympathetic and vagal tone and is affected by circulating catecholamines. In the normal person a rise in heart rate *per se* does not necessarily cause an increase in cardiac output. The more likely outcome is a decrease in left ventricular end-diastolic volume, and a reduction in stroke volume. However, in the failing heart stroke volume is less sensitive to changes in filling pressure and cardiac output becomes much more dependent on heart rate.

Myocardial oxygen supply to demand ratio

Clearly myocardial function will be adversely affected by an inadequate supply of oxygen saturated blood to meet the changing oxygen requirements. It is known that the flow of blood per gram of muscle is approximately equally distributed throughout the myocardium. However, there is gradient of pressure in the tissue through the wall of the myocardium. Subendocardial myocardium is subject to the greatest pressure and perfusion of this part of the muscle can only take place during diastole. It follows that coronary arterial resistance in the subendocardial muscle must be lower than that towards the outside of the heart. It also follows that in situations of reduced blood supply the potential for compensating by vasodilatation is much greater towards the outside of the myocardium. Consequently the subendocardial muscle is much more suspectible to ischaemic damage. The demand for oxygen will be increased by a rise in heart rate and contractility. Supply will be reduced in the presence of coronary artery disease or decreased arterial oxygen tension and by an increase in heart rate. A rise in preload and afterload is associated both with an increased demand for oxygen because of the need to increase myocardial tension and a reduction in blood supply to the myocardial cells because of the increased intracardiac pressure.

Conclusions

The relationships between the various factors which determine cardiac output are complex but they carry important implications for choice of therapy for patients with cardiac failure. The following is a list of the most important factors.

(1) The Frank–Starling mechanism relating filling pressure to ventricular output is fundamental to the understanding of therapeutic approaches.

(2) Depression of the curve for the left ventricle in the absence of a change in the curve for the right ventricle can explain the mechanism of pulmonary oedema.

(3) Depression of the curve for the right ventricle in the absence of a change in the curve for the left ventricle accounts for the need to maintain a high filling pressure in acute right ventricular failure.

(4) Parallel depression of both curves explains the relative absence of severe pulmonary oedema in patients with congestive cardiac failure.

(5) Excessive reduction in preload can result in symptoms due to low cardiac output.

(6) Excessive elevation of preload can result in pulmonary oedema in a relatively normal heart.

(7) The curve relating filling pressure to cardiac output can be depressed by excessive peripheral arterial resistance and that can result in a rise in preload and/or a fall in cardiac output.

(8) The curve can be elevated by an increase in myocardial contractility but only at the expense of increased oxygen consumption by the myocardium.

(9) Heart rate *per se* is a determinant of cardiac output only in the presence of depressed contractility.

(10) The physiological responses to myocardial disease which occur in the body and which result in an elevation in preload and an elevation in afterload may in themselves be detrimental to the clinical state of the patient.

THERAPEUTIC APPROACHES

Apart from the definitive therapy of the cause, there are only three ways in which we can improve the clinical state of patients with heart failure. We can reduce preload; we can reduce afterload; and we can increase myocardial contractility.

INOTROPIC AGENTS

Theoretically, drugs which improve myocardial contractility would be of benefit in all forms of cardiac failure. However, this approach to therapy is limited by the small number of drugs available. Some can only be given by intravenous infusion and are therefore only suitable for acute and urgent therapy. Others such as the cardiac glycosides may take too long to act in urgent situations and chronic administration is hampered by the difficulty in tailoring the dose to the exact requirements of the patient. Thus, unless they are managed carefully, toxicity may occur and outweigh benefit. In terms of the Frank-Starling mechanism the administration of a drug with a positive inotropic action will cause the curve to rise so that either cardiac output can increase for a given filling pressure or filling pressure can decrease for a given cardiac output. Over recent years there has been a number of studies showing that digoxin may be unnecessary in patients previously diagnosed as having cardiac failure and in whom sinus rhythm is present. This has led many physicians to believe that digitalis is useless in any patient with sinus rhythm. Such a conclusion is probably a misinterpretation of the available information.

Digitalis – what use is it in heart failure?

There is no controversy over the use of digoxin in patients with cardiac failure and atrial fibrillation with a fast ventricular response. In fact, properly managed digoxin therapy is mandatory in this situation. Stroke volume is limited by inadequate ventricular filling and so the negative chronotropic effect is invaluable in prolonging ventricular diastole and improving cardiac output. This effect is brought about by a slowing of atrioventricular conduction through the bundle of His by a direct effect. Digoxin also slows conduction indirectly by increasing vagal tone and thus, without abolishing atrial fibrillation, the ventricular response is controlled. Occasional patients with atrial fibrillation do convert to sinus rhythm, but this is particularly unusual in the presence of cardiac failure. When patients have in the past had episodes of atrial fibrillation for which there is no acute or remediable cause, it is probably wise to continue the drug indefinitely. The usual recommendation is that patients with a ventricular rate in excess of about 90 beats per minute should receive the drug. Where the ventricular rate is below this, digoxin therapy is not mandatory and it may not offer particular advantage. It is important that atrial fibrillation be accurately diagnosed by electrocardiogram and it is as well to remember that atrial fibrillation may be a manifestation of digoxin toxicity. Where there is doubt the plasma concentration of digoxin should be measured before there is any increase in the dose of drug administered. Digoxin should be administered in a dose sufficient to reduce the ventricular rate to approximately 70–90 beats/min. The ventricular rate provides a good guide to correct dosage and there are very few patients in whom the heart rate cannot be controlled by digoxin alone. In the absence of specific contraindications to the use of digoxin the drug should be continued *ad infinitum*.

In patients with cardiac failure in the presence of sinus rhythm, the decision to use digoxin is much less clear cut and frankly controversial. In this circumstance it is the positive inotropic action of digoxin only which can contribute to the therapeutic effect. A number of years ago this effect was highly valued but during the last 20 years powerful diuretics have become available and our knowledge and skill at using them has greatly improved. Diuretic therapy is therefore likely to be the first line approach in such patients. At present, digoxin occupies the second line of approach. As our experience and understanding of the use of vasodilator drugs to reduce afterload and preload increases, however, it is conceivable that digoxin therapy may be relegated to the third position. Indeed many physicians would prefer to use diuretics and vasodilators before considering digoxin. The confusion about the place of digoxin therapy has been compounded by a number of studies in which the discontinuation of digoxin therapy in patients previously suffering from cardiac failure in sinus rhythm has resulted in no deterioration in their condition. It has been suggested that the inotropic effect of digoxin is only transient, and some have questioned whether it occurs at all. However, before condemning digoxin as useless in the presence of sinus rhythm, it is important to realize the limitations of the studies that have been performed. In the first place, once the patient with acute cardiac failure has settled, and is receiving chronic maintenance therapy, it may well be that diuretics alone will prevent the patient sinking into cardiac failure. Under such circumstances removal of digoxin will cause no deterioration, but that provides no evidence that its inotropic action is lost. In order to demonstrate an inotropic action, with prolonged administration, invasive techniques are really required, as measurement of systolic time interval may be inaccurate and not reproducible. The assessment of digoxin's contribution under these circumstances can therefore only be made clinically. The evidence against digoxin in maintenance therapy in sinus rhythm rests on a number of studies in which digoxin has been withdrawn. Although it has been shown that about 75–94% of patients do not deteriorate with removal of digoxin therapy, there may be a number of reasons for this which are unrelated to the drug's pharmacology. For example, in some of the patients digoxin therapy was instituted for inadequate reasons, such as sinus tachycardia in the absence of infarction or for dependent oedema, without other evidence of cardiac failure. Some of the patients may never have been taking their digoxin in the prescribed doses, as it is known that compliance with instructions for most drugs is around 50%. Some patients may not have been given adequate doses in the first place. As one might expect one study showed that where the plasma digoxin level was very low, there was no deterioration when the drug was withdrawn. It was only in those patients in whom the digoxin concentration was in the therapeutic range that any deterioration was shown. Whilst one can accept that a large number of patients may be receiving maintenance digoxin therapy unnecessarily, it is important to realize that there are a number of patients who appear to need such therapy. At present there is no satisfactory way of identifying those patients. Equally it is important not to be misled into thinking that digoxin has no place in the treatment of heart failure in patients with sinus rhythm.

Digoxin has very little place in the urgent treatment of patients with acute pulmonary oedema, secondary to left ventricular failure. There is no place in modern therapy for the intravenous use of cardiac glycosides, and other approaches to therapy are far more likely to produce rapid results than the use of digoxin.

Conclusions

There is no question that digoxin should be given to patients with atrial fibrillation with a fast ventricular response, who are suffering from cardiac failure. Treatment should be lifelong in the absence of a remediable cause. In these patients digoxin therapy is a first line approach in conjunction with diuretics. In the presence of sinus rhythm in patients with cardiac failure, digoxin should be reserved as a second line therapy, or possibly third line therapy. However, in patients with acute pulmonary oedema, due to left ventricular failure, digoxin is a third line therapy after diuretics and vasodilators. When the episode of cardiac failure has resolved and assuming that the patient has had no episode of atrial fibrillation, digoxin should be cautiously withdrawn after about 3 months. Whether or not the patient's episode of cardiac failure has resolved, it is rational to measure the serum digoxin level and to titrate the dose to achieve a plasma level in the normally accepted therapeutic range. Unless this is performed, the therapeutic trial of digoxin cannot be regarded as adequate. Attempts to withdraw digoxin therapy are particularly important in patients who are elderly, in hepatic and renal dysfunction and in whom the presence of hypokalaemia may make toxicity more likely. Successful withdrawal of digoxin therapy is more likely where there has been no substantial evidence of cardiac failure, or of atrial tachyarrhythmia, and where the clinical state of the patient has been stable for a prolonged period, and where the plasma concentration of digoxin is below the commonly accepted therapeutic range.

Mechanism of action of digoxin

Our understanding of the mechanism of action of the cardiac glycosides is hampered firstly by the fact that there are both direct actions and indirect actions mediated through the vagus nerve. Either of these may predominate in an individual patient. A further complication is the fact that digoxin has a different effect on refractory period in atrial and ventricular muscle (where it is shortened) compared to the conducting system of the heart (where refractory period is lengthened). At a cellular level it is not certain whether a single mode of action can explain both the inotropic and chronotropic effects of the drug or the effects on excitability and automaticity in both atria and ventricles. Nevertheless it is clear that digoxin along with all the cardiac glycosides causes an inhibition of Na,K-ATPase – the enzyme which is

Table 4.1 Actions of digoxin

Direct
(1) A positive inotropic effect
(2) Increased excitability and automaticity in atrial and ventricular myocardial cells
(3) Reduced refractory period in atrial and ventricular myocardial cells
(4) Negative chronotropic effect in the conducting system of the heart
(5) Lengthened refractory period in the conducting system of the heart
Indirect
    Vagal stimulation resulting in sinus bradycardia

---

responsible for the breakdown of Na,K-ATP and therefore mainten-ance of the sodium pump and intracellular and extracellular concen-trations of sodium and potassium. The inotropic effect of digoxin is probably explained by the resulting intracellular accumulation of sodium displacing bound calcium ions which in turn exert the positive inotropic effect. The toxic effect of the cardiac glycosides on excitabil-ity and automaticity can be readily explained by the loss of membrane potential as intracellular potassium is replaced by sodium. Thus, in terms of the action potential, maximum repolarization is reduced and the speed of slow depolarization is increased. Although it would be very satisfying to explain all the direct actions of the cardiac glycosides on the basis of inhibition of Na,K-ATPase there are some objections to this concept. The time course of the actions appears to differ in that the effect on contractility reverses rapidly but inhibition of the enzyme is lost only slowly and improvement in contractility may be demon-strated at concentrations below the threshold for inhibition of the enzyme. A summary of the actions of digoxin is given in Table 4.1.

Managing digoxin therapy

In most of the surveys of drug adverse reactions in recent years, di-goxin has ranked highly as a cause of morbidity. This is because the drug has a very low therapeutic ratio. Clinical monitoring of the drug may be difficult so that the dose required to achieve the therapeutic end point is difficult to achieve. It also reflects the fact that there is wide variability between individuals in the pharmacokinetic handling of the drug and in the sensitivity with which the myocardium responds to the drug's actions. Apart from interindividual variability there are many disease processes, drug interactions and the ageing process itself which compound this variability and predisposes to the development of toxicity. Clearly, if the drug's benefit is to be maximized and risk to be minimized account must be taken of these many variables when prescribing digoxin.

Situations in which there is increased sensitivity to the toxic effects of digoxin

There are a number of myocardial conditions in which digoxin's toxicity is particularly liable to be manifest (Table 4.2). In the immediate postmyocardial infarction period there is an increased risk of producing tachyarrythmias and ventricular fibrillation because of the increased excitability of myocardial tissues. Also in this situation there

Table 4.2   Sources of variability in the pharmacodynamics of digoxin

Increased sensitivity
Hypokalaemia
The aged
Anoxia
Cor pulmonale
Myocardial infarction
Hypertrophic obstructive cardiomyopathy
Hypercalcaemia
Interaction with sympathomimetic amines
Hypothyroidism
Decreased sensitivity
Hyperkalaemia
Hypocalcaemia
Hyperthyroidism

is an increased risk of producing heart block when there is already a conduction defect present. Although acute myocardial infarction cannot be regarded as an absolute contraindication to the use of digoxin, particular care must be taken to avoid the use of the drug in the presence of conduction defects or electrolyte abnormalities, and the patient should be breathing oxygen. In patients with cor pulmonale there is an increased risk of toxicity and the response to digoxin is usually disappointing. This is therefore regarded as another relative contraindication. In patients with hypertrophic obstructive cardiomyopathy, the increase in contractility does nothing to relieve the outflow obstruction and digoxin may increase the hypertrophic defect. The toxicity of digoxin is greatly enhanced in the presence of hypokalaemia. For this reason the plasma potassium level should always be measured in the acutely ill patient before digoxin is administered. If the plasma level of potassium is below 3.0 mmol/l, digoxin therapy should be withheld in the majority of patients until the hypokalaemia has been corrected. Theoretically hypercalcaemia may predispose to the unwanted effects of digoxin. In practice, though, levels of calcium high enough to materially interfere with the effects of digoxin are rarely encountered in patients. Hypoxia itself should be remembered as an important predisposing factor and attempts should be made to oxygenate fully any patient in whom digoxin therapy is to be started or continued. Similarly, concurrent medication with drugs which increase myocardial excitability may predispose to digoxin toxicity.

These include sympathomimetic amines and possibly L-Dopa and tricyclic antidepressants. Other drugs which may interact with digoxin in a pharmacodynamic manner include the β-blockers which may exacerbate the adverse effect of digoxin on the conducting system. Suxamethonium has been reported to induce ventricular irritability in patients receiving digitalis glycosides. The mechanism for the interaction is possibly the sudden release of catecholaminesor sudden shifts of potassium from inside muscle cells into the extracellular space. Naturally diuretics will interact with digoxin through their hypokalaemic and hypomagnesaemic effects and other drugs which induce hypokalaemia such as amphotericin B, and carbenoxolone will similarly interact.

The foregoing have been examples of sources of variability in the sensitivity of the myocardium to cardiac glycosides. However, another major source of variability is due to changes in the pharmacokinetic handling of the drug (Table 4.3).

Table 4.3   Sources of variability in the pharmacokinetics of digoxin

Bioavailability
Differences in pharmaceutical preparations
Drug interactions within the gastrointestinal tract
Acute gastrointestinal upset
Malabsorption syndromes

Reduced clearance
Renal impairment
The elderly
Interaction with spironolactone
Hypothyroidism

Increased clearance
Hyperthyroidism

Reduced apparent volume of distribution
Renal Impairment – acute and chronic
Drug interactions with quinidine, verapamil, and amiodarone
The elderly

Variability in the pharmacokinetics of digoxin

Digoxin is a poorly water soluble drug whose absorption is therefore susceptible to variation. It is widely distributed throughout the body, being taken up by cardiac muscle, voluntary muscle and the liver, so that its apparent volume of distribution is many times total body volume (usually between 500 and 600 litres). The drug is bound to plasma proteins only to the extent of about 50% and it is mostly excreted unchanged by the kidney.

BIOAVAILABILITY
Because of the drug's poor water solubility, digoxin absorption is highly susceptible to pharmaceutical considerations. In the early 1970s

it was shown that there was wide variation between the various preparations of digoxin, as regards the amount which was absorbed from a tablet. This problem has now largely been eradicated by the use of small particle size and standard methods in tablet manufacture. Thus the standard preparation of digoxin (Lanoxin) has a bioavailability in excess of 90%. Nevertheless it should be remembered that the systemic availability of digoxin is highly susceptible to changes in gastrointestinal function. It appears that digoxin's absorption occurs mainly in the duodenum with little further absorption taking place in the ileum. Consequently the drug's bioavailability is highly susceptible to changes in gastrointestinal motility and changes in the mechanism for lipid absorption in the duodenum. Thus malabsorption syndromes, acute gastrointestinal upsets and drugs which speed gastrointestinal motility, such as metoclopramide, may reduce the absorption of digoxin especially when preparations of relatively low bioavailability are used. Under normal circumstances, however, the absorption of digoxin after oral administration is rapid and there is no advantage in giving the drug intravenously. Intramuscular injection confers no advantage and may cause painful local muscle necrosis. The bioavailability of digoxin may also be affected by drugs within the gastrointestinal tract which may bind digoxin. The most obvious example of this is cholestyramine, but also the antidiarrhoeal preparation kaolin pectin has been implicated. A number of antacids have been shown to bind digoxin within the gastrointestinal tract and interference with its absorption has been demonstrated with sulphasalazine, para-aminosalicylic acid and neomycin. The exact mechanisms of these interactions are unknown. From the practical point of view it remains important for patients to continue on the same pharmaceutical preparation of digoxin. In the presence of therapeutic failure a concurrent medication which might be interfering with the drug's absorption should be sought. Where there is gastrointestinal malfunction, particular care must be taken in monitoring digoxin's effect. It should be noted, however, that gastric surgery and duodeno-ileal bypass have been shown to have no effect on digoxin's bioavailability.

BODY DISTRIBUTION
There is considerable interindividual variation in the apparent volume of distribution of digoxin, so that plasma concentrations after a single dose may vary by two and a half fold. In addition disease processes may alter tissue binding of digoxin and therefore reduce the distribution volume. Best studied is acute and chronic renal failure which may reduce the volume of distribution to as low as 200 litres. The consequence of this is that in renal insufficiency the loading dose of digoxin should be drastically reduced, if toxicity is to be avoided. Recently it has become clear that a number of drugs may interact with digoxin by displacing it from tissue binding sites. Thus quinidine may elevate the

plasma level of digoxin, and so may amiodarone. Thyroid disease and the serum potassium concentration may also cause variability.

CLEARANCE

Digoxin is excreted mostly unchanged by the kidney; the main route of administration is glomerular filtration but there is a small amount of tubular secretion and reabsorption. The normal plasma half-life of digoxin is about 1.6 days. Clearance is linearly related to creatinine clearance, and the half-life may be as high as 4.4 days in patients with renal failure. Most of the increase in digoxin half-life associated with the ageing process can be accounted for by a fall-off in renal function. Minor changes in renal clearance of digoxin may be associated with dehydration and transient changes occur in association with adminis-tration of loop diuretics. Spironolactone has been reported to cause a substantial increase in serum digoxin concentrations as a result of inhibition of renal tubular secretion. In hyperthyroidism renal clear-ance of digoxin is increased, and it is reduced in hypothyroidism.

The use of plasma digoxin concentration measurement

Digoxin fulfils many of the criteria which make the plasma level measurement of a drug a worthwhile exercise. It is a drug with a low therapeutic ratio, there is wide pharmacokinetic variability and often the criteria for monitoring the drug clinically are vague. Also it may be difficult or impossible to distinguish the toxic manifestations of digoxin from therapeutic failure and inadequate dosage. In the vast majority of patients there are no active metabolites of digoxin although in about 10–15% the drug may be sufficiently metabolized to produce significant amounts of active compounds. However, as discussed above, there are many sources of pharmacodynamic variability to di-goxin. This variability ruins to some extent the predictability of toxic and therapeutic effects from the plasma digoxin concentration effect relationship. Furthermore it appears there may be variability between the plasma digoxin concentration and the concentration of the drug in myocardial cells. Within individuals there may be a good relationship between plasma digoxin concentration and changes in systolic time interval or in the configuration of the electrocardiogram but the rela-tionship of these changes to the therapeutic and toxic effects of the drug is not clear. The interindividual relationships show much greater variability. Nevertheless, the measurement of the plasma digoxin con-centration can be an extremely useful adjunct to therapy. A radio-immunoassay for performing the measurement is now widely available and provides a reliable and accurate measurement. There is little, if any, point in measuring the plasma concentration of digoxin in patients being treated for atrial fibrillation with a fast ventricular re-sponse, in whom adjusting the dose of digoxin to provide a ventricular rate between 70 and 90 beats/min provides a perfectly acceptable approach. As with all drugs, measurement of the plasma level is useful as a check of compliance with therapy and it may also be very useful in patients in sinus rhythm in whom an episode of cardiac failure has been successfully treated and when the need for continuation of the digoxin therapy is being assessed. Under these circumstances a plasma digoxin level of less than 0.8 ng/ml predicts that it is unlikely that there will be deterioration if the drug is discontinued. Where there is renal impairment and particularly where renal function is changing it is advisable to monitor carefully the plasma digoxin concentration. Renal impairment not only reduces the elimination of digoxin but also reduces considerably the apparent volume of distribution. The concentration achieved by a given dose is therefore quite unpredictable on starting therapy and although at steady state there are some formulae to predict dosage requirement these provide only a very rough guide and do not remove the need for establishing the dose according to plasma level. The aim is to achieve a plasma digoxin concentration 4–6 hours after dose administration of between 1 and 2 ng/ml. Measuring the plasma digoxin concentration can also be useful when patients previously well-controlled deteriorate or develop symptoms which could be manifestations of digoxin toxicity. Some consider it important to measure the level when other therapies have been changed in order to assess possible drug interactions. Plasma digoxin concentrations can be very useful in the diagnosis of digoxin toxicity but they must be interpreted with wisdom. In the first place it is probably advisable always to measure the serum potassium level, because digoxin can manifest toxicity at relatively low levels in the presence of hypokalaemia. There is no doubt that if the clinical diagnosis of digoxin toxicity is suspected a plasma concentration in excess of 3 ng/ml clinches the diagnosis. In the absence of hypokalaemia, a plasma concentration of less than 1.5 ng/ml is unlikely to support the diagnosis of digoxin intoxication. Between these two levels the plasma concentration does not contribute greatly and one must rely on clinical assessment.

Table 4.4 Situations in which the measurement of plasma digoxin concentration can be useful

----

(1) The diagnosis of digoxin overdose
(2) The diagnosis of digoxin toxicity
(3) To assess compliance
(4) To avoid toxicity in patients with renal impairment
(5) In the presence of therapeutic failure or deterioration in the patient's condition or where concurrent therapy has been changed
(6) In the assessment of the need for long term therapy

Therapeutic guidelines

Because digoxin is rapidly absorbed the oral route should be used when possible. Although rapid digitalization can be achieved by slow intravenous infusion of the undiluted drug, this is rarely required. In urgent situations some other positive inotropic drug is usually more appropriate. There may or may not be the need for a loading dose. Because the drug has a relatively long plasma half-life, plasma concentrations may take 1 week or more to achieve steady state. Where the need for digitalization is relatively immediate, a loading dose should be prescribed. Under most circumstances a dose between 0.75 mg and 1.5 mg is sufficient. The loading dose should be given in divided doses approximately 6 h apart and the patient should be observed for early signs of digitalis intoxication. The loading dose should be halved in patients with hypothyroidism or renal disease and in the elderly. Where patients are started off on a maintenance dose of digoxin it appears that knowledge of the serum creatinine or creatinine clearance does not improve the prediction of the plasma level achieved. In most, a maintenance dose of 0.25 mg is an appropriate starting dose and this should be reduced by 50% in the elderly or uraemic patient and in those with severe myocardial ischaemia or where there is concurrent interfering drug therapy. Where there is therapeutic failure or there is difficulty in assessing progress, measurement of the plasma digoxin concentration may be helpful. It should be remembered, however, that this has no predictive value if taken less than 4-5 half-lives after a previous dose change. The following formula can then be used:

$$\text{New dose} = \frac{\text{Previous dose} \times 1.5}{\text{Plasma concentration (ng per ml)P}}$$

Other inotropic agents

The search for a suitable agent which increases the force of contraction of the heart has continued for many years. Ideally such an agent could be administered orally as well as parenterally. It would not predispose to cardiac arrhythmias or increase myocardial oxygen consumption. It would not cause peripheral vasoconstriction and in other ways would be free of serious toxic effects. A number of drugs have been discovered and are available but they all fall short of this ideal in one or more respect. Although a temporary haemodynamic improvement may occur in patients treated with these drugs it is worrying that there is a suggestion that this occurs at the expense of progressive deterioration in the long term. The basis of this suggestion is that increased myocardial oxygen consumption might have an adverse effect on the diseased myocardium. It is possible that increased energy expenditure

Table 4.5 Some guidelines for digoxin administration

(1) Oral administration in the vast majority of instances
(2) Use a preparation of high bioavailability
(3) Use a loading dose in most instances but adjust in the presence of reduced volume of distribution
(4) Adjust dose according to clinical observation and critical use of steady state plasma digoxin concentrations

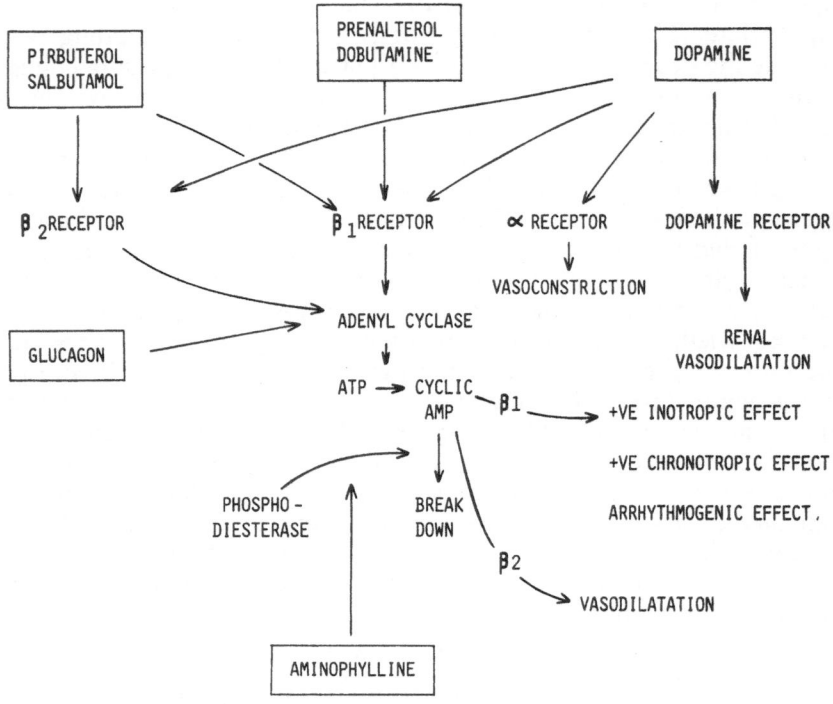

Figure 4.5 Some inotropes used in heart failure

following a forced increase in contraction may accentuate the focal necrosis which leads to diffuse fibrosis in the failing myocardium. Some drugs are available for oral administration so that long term administration is feasible, but presently we lack evidence of lasting benefit derived from their use. For these reasons this group of drugs should be reserved for use in urgent situations such as cardiogenic shock and in patients desperately ill with cardiac failure and hypotension. The classification of some of these agents is illustrated in Figure 4.5.

Drugs acting through the sympathetic nervous system

Sympathomimetic agents could produce a beneficial effect on cardiac function through a number of mechanisms. Firstly β_1-stimulation causes a positive inotropic effect, secondly β_2-stimulation causes a dilatation in peripheral arterioles and therefore a reduction in afterload and, thirdly, stimulation of α-receptors might restore blood pressure in patients who are hypotensive. However the latter effect might equally be adverse by increasing the afterload, as the blood pressure rises. β_1-Stimulation tends to precipitate arrhythmias and also increases myocardial oxygen requirements with the risk of increasing ischaemic damage. Noradrenaline and isoprenaline have been abandoned but a number of other drugs acting through the sympathetic nervous system continue to have a place in therapy.

Dopamine

Dopamine is the precursor of noradrenaline. It acts in part by releasing noradrenaline from the adrenergic neuron terminal in the heart and partly by acting on specific dopamine receptors which dilate the renal, mesenteric, coronary and cerebral beds and increase the blood flow to them. Dopamine is said to have a 'flexible' molecule which accounts for its capacity to stimulate a number of different receptors. At high doses dopamine causes peripheral vasoconstriction through stimulation of α-adrenergic receptors. Under these circumstances peripheral resistance increases, afterload increases and renal blood flow falls. For this reason, the dose of dopamine which is used has to be kept within strict bounds and when used for the therapy of severe heart failure and cardiogenic shock vasodilator therapy should in the majority of cases be administered concurrently. Dopamine is inactive orally and when given intravenously is metabolized within minutes by dopamine β-hydroxylase and monoamine oxidase. Dopamine is indicated in the short term therapy of refractory cardiac failure. The starting dose should be 0.5–1 mg/kg per minute and the dose raised until an acceptable urinary flow or blood pressure or heart rate is achieved. Above a dose of 15 mg/kg per minute, vasoconstriction is likely to occur and, if so an α-blocking agent or direct acting vasodilator should be administered. In patients with cardiogenic shock 5 mg/kg produces a maximum increase in stroke volume, renal flow reaches a peak at 7.5 mg/kg per minute but arrhythmias appear at 10 mg/kg per minute. There is no evidence of long term benefit in patients with cardiogenic shock. Dopamine should not be used in the presence of ventricular arrhythmias or in patients with suspected pheochromocytoma. Recent treatment with monoamine-oxidase inhibitors is also a contraindication.

Dobutamine

Dobutamine is a synthetic analogue of dopamine but with differing pharmacology. It acts directly on β_1-adrenergic receptors, specifically to increase contractility without an effect on heart rate or on the production of arrhythmias. Dobutamine does not directly release noradrenaline within the heart nor does it affect the dopamine receptors in the renal and other vascular beds. It does not therefore dilate renal arteries but renal function may improve as a result of increased cardiac output. Dobutamine stimulates β_2-receptors, but to a lesser extent than does isoprenaline. It therefore reduces peripheral resistance and reduces afterload. Dobutamine has found a place in the treatment of severe low output congestive heart failure when the need is for an inotropic effect together with unloading of the heart. It can be used in patients with myocardial infarction without great risk of increasing infarct size or inducing arrhythmias. Dobutamine has to be given by intravenous infusion and the usual dose is 2.5–10 mg/kg per minute but occasionally up to 40 mg/kg per minute. The drug is rapidly cleared from the bloodstream with a half-life of 2.4 minutes.

Prenalterol

Prenalterol is a specific β_1-adrenoreceptor agonist with relatively little effect on heart rate and little β_2-vasodilator effect. Infusion increases cardiac output without causing a rise in heart rate and apparently without a tendency to produce arrhythmias. Not surprisingly prenalterol is particularly effective where β-receptor blocking drugs have contributed to the heart failure. Some reduction in peripheral resistance has also been reported in acute studies. Some tachyarrhythmias have been reported but precipitation of myocardial ischaemia is uncommon. Prenalterol has been used with benefit in the treatment of heart failure associated with myocardial infarction. The suggested dose is 0.5 mg/min by slow intravenous infusion to a total of not more than 20 mg. There are few studies of chronic oral prenalterol but one study has shown symptomatic and haemodynamic benefit after 2 weeks of oral therapy.

Pirbuterol, salbutamol and rimiterol

Of the β_2-receptor agonists, salbutamol has been the most widely evaluated. Although originally developed and widely used in the treatment of bronchial asthma, both it and rimiterol have been shown to be beneficial in patients with cardiac failure. Recently attention has been focussed on pirbuterol – an agent seven times more specific for β_2-receptors than salbutamol and with a longer half-life. Acutely this drug causes a substantial rise in cardiac output due principally to a reduction in peripheral vascular resistance but also to a small direct inotropic effect. Heart rate, systolic arterial pressure and myocardial oxygen consumption do not change and arrhythmias are uncommon. Pirbuterol reduces pulmonary vascular resistance in patients with chronic airflow obstruction and cor pulmonale, but hypoxia may be worsened. One study found that pirbuterol improved right and left ventricular ejection fractions in such patients but the effect was not greater than that achieved with salbutamol. Reports of chronic oral pirbuterol are conflicting. Sustained haemodynamic response has been shown to continue for 3 months in some patients while loss of clinical effect after only 1 month has been found in others.

Glucagon

Glucagon, the hyperglycaemic pancreatic hormone which increases myocardial cellular cyclic AMP by a mechanism independent of catecholamines, has been shown to increase myocardial contraction and heart rate usually without any tendency to produce arrhythmias. A number of studies have shown improvement in acute cardiac failure but a variable response in patients with chronic congestive heart failure, and it has been shown that the response to glucagon is lost in the papillary muscles taken from patients with congestive heart failure. In patients with severe aortic stenosis accentuation of left ventricular failure has occurred. Early hopes that glucagon would provide an ideal agent have, therefore, not been borne out in practice.

Phosphodiesterase inhibitors

Aminophylline, which has been used for many years in the treatment of heart failure, acts by inhibiting the enzyme phosphodiesterase and consequently causes an accumulation of cyclic AMP in the myocardial cell. This causes a positive inotropic effect but also accounts for the high incidence of arrhythmias produced by this drug. For this reason and the drug's toxic effects on the central nervous system, aminophylline has been abandoned as a line of therapy in acute cardiac failure.

Amrinone

There have been contradictory reports about the effects of this new inotropic agent but experience is limited to short term use in a relatively small number of patients with severe congestive heart failure. The mechanism of action of amrinone appears to be related to alterations in extracellular and intracellular calcium balance, probably mediated by increased levels of tissue cyclic AMP and possibly involving a sodium dependent pathway. It has been shown to have a powerful effect on myocardial contraction without an effect on heart rate and with little fall in arterial blood pressure. However, a significant vasodilator effect has been shown and it has been suggested that part of the haemodynamic improvement is due to a reduction in afterload. Intravenous amrinone seems to give temporary benefit in some patients with severe congestive heart failure, in whom the outlook is generally poor. Thrombocytopenia is an important side-effect (occurring in about 20% of cases) and must be watched for by repetitive platelet counts. It is reversible and asymptomatic and there is a suggestion that it can be avoided by limiting the dose. Amrinone is administered by intravenous bolus injection followed by continuous infusion. Amrinone's place in therapy is not settled, but at present it is indicated only for intravenous use in severe refractory cases of congestive cardiac failure. Although few small studies suggested that haemodynamic improvement may be maintained in some patients with long term treatment, development of the oral preparation has been abandoned because of gastrointestinal intolerance.

PRELOAD REDUCTION

The greatest benefit from drugs which reduce preload occurs in situations where cardiac output is reasonably well maintained at the expense of high filling pressure and consequent pulmonary oedema. This is the common situation in left ventricular failure. Although preload may fall secondary to a reduction in afterload, drugs which reduce blood volume or dilate the venous capacitance vessels will produce the most profound effect.

Diuretics

Diuretic drugs are used in the treatment of heart failure for two main reasons. Firstly, because of their capacity to cause an acute reduction of plasma volume they are of primary importance in the treatment of left ventricular failure. Secondly, they reverse the salt and water retention which is part of the syndrome of congestive cardiac failure. The exact mechanism by which the latter occurs in cardiac failure remains unclear. It is unlikely to be related directly to glomerular filtration rate, as this must be reduced to below approximately 10 ml per minute before sodium retention results. The sodium retention in cardiac failure occurs before there is such a substantial fall. Sodium retention probably results from a change in renal physiology in response to a reduction in renal blood flow. Proximal tubular sodium reabsorption is undoubtedly increased in patients with congestive cardiac failure. There are a number of possible explanations for this. The fall in renal blood flow causes a rise in the proportion of blood which is filtered at the glomerulus (filtration fraction). It is possible that this results in increased peritubular capillary osmotic pressure and decreases the back leak of sodium into the proximal tubule of the nephron. Thus net sodium reabsorption in the proximal tubule is increased. Another possible mechanism which has been postulated is intrarenal redistribution of blood flow. There are two populations of nephrons in the kidney. A cortical group with a juxtaglomerular apparatus maintains perfusion by autoregulation of arterial pressure. A juxtamedullary group is subjected to passive increase in flow as arterial pressure rises. Sodium reabsorption from the latter tends to be greater than from the cortical group. In oedematous states it has been shown that reduced renal blood flow causes a shunting of blood from cortical to juxtamedullary nephrons. The presence of a natriuretic hormone whose action is in the proximal tubule has also been postulated. The renin–angiotensin system probably plays a part in these changes within the kidney

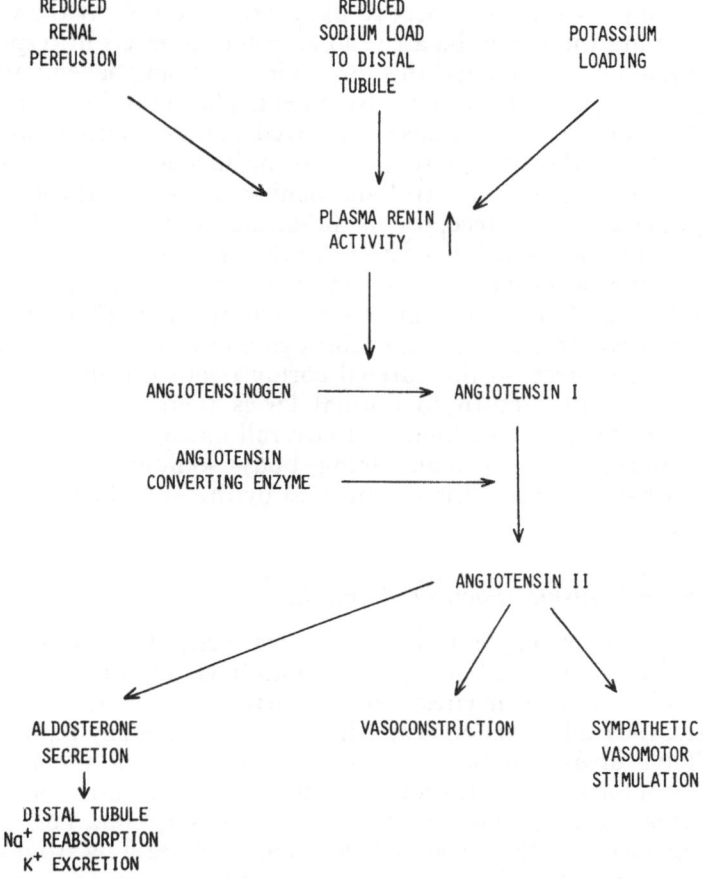

Figure 4.6   The aldosterone feedback control system

although plasma renin activity is not necessarily elevated. Whatever the exact mechanism, it is clear that there is a control of sodium reabsorption in the proximal tubule and that control is sensitive to changes in renal blood flow and changes in plasma and blood volume. Changes in sodium handling also occur in the distal tubule of the nephron in oedematous states. At this site sodium is reabsorbed in exchange for potassium and hydrogen ions both by a mechanism which is dependent on circulating levels of aldosterone and by one which is not. The stimulus for release of aldosterone from the adrenal cortex is angiotensin II. The feedback control mechanism for aldosterone is shown in Figure 4.6. In the past the role of aldosterone in the pathogenesis of oedema has probably been overemphasized. High levels of aldosterone are not found in all patients with oedematous states and in itself high aldosterone secretion does not cause oedema to form. It has been suggested that there are three phases in patients with congestive cardiac failure with respect to aldosterone status. At the onset of cardiac failure there may be a rise in aldosterone levels in response to reduced renal perfusion, and this may help in causing oedema to form. During the response to diuretic treatment, plasma aldosterone levels may fall. This does not reflect improved cardiac output and renal perfusion but rather the presentation of an increased sodium load at the distal tubule. This control mechanism mediated through renin operates via a sodium receptor in the macula densa at the beginning of the distal tubule which is adjacent to the juxtaglomerular apparatus on the afferent arteriole. Reduced plasma potassium concentration in response to the diuresis may also contribute to the inhibition of aldosterone, but whether this operates through a reduction in plasma renin or by a direct effect on the adrenal cortex is not certain. Once body sodium and water return to normal levels there may be a rise in aldosterone. At this stage there is no overall natriuresis. Diuretic therapy is concerned with maintaining body sodium in the face of sodium-retaining mechanisms stimulated by the disturbed cardiac performance.

Site and mechanisms of action of diuretic drugs

The drugs most valuable in the urgent treatment of congestive cardiac failure – frusemide and bumetanide – both have important therapeutic actions other than their effects in the renal tubule. When given intravenously, they dilate venous capacitance vessels, thereby reducing preload. They also increase renal blood flow without a concomitant change in glomerular filtration, thereby decreasing filtration fraction and decreasing proximal tubular sodium reabsorption. There is also some evidence that the intrarenal shunting of blood flow from cortical to juxtamedullary nephrons can be reversed by potent diuretics. It has been postulated that this effect results from the release of a vasoactive substance from the kidney. Prostaglandins, particularly prostacycline (PGI_2), have been implicated since parenterally administered loop diuretics have been shown to cause an increase in the release of PGI_2. Within the tubule of the nephron the loop diuretics inhibit chloride reabsorption in the ascending limb of the loop of Henle and also in the cortical diluting segment – whereas the thiazide diuretics only do so in the latter. It therefore follows that the kidney's capacity to excrete a concentrated urine may be affected by the loop diuretics and its capacity to excrete a dilute urine may be affected by both groups. The thiazide and loop diuretics are all organic acids and highly bound to serum proteins. There is now ample evidence that they act from within the lumen of the tubule. In order to gain access to their site of action they must be transported actively at the organic acid transport pathway of the straight segment of the proximal tubule. Both these groups of drugs cause an increased delivery of sodium to the distal segment of the nephron and this results in a kaliuresis. Although this effect can be demonstrated following the acute administration of a diuretic drug it may not be relevant to long term therapy when aldosterone secretion plays a more important role in the production of hypokalaemia. Although those drugs which act in the distal part of the nephron are of very weak potency, they are assuming increasing importance in the prevention of hypokalaemia due to the other drugs. Amiloride blocks sodium reabsorption in the distal convoluted tubule by a mechanism which is independent of aldosterone. Triamterene has a similar effect in the collecting duct. Spironolactone acts as a competitive blocker of aldosterone.

Choice of diuretic drug

There must be very few instances when frusemide is not the drug of first choice when starting off the treatment of congestive cardiac failure or left ventricular failure. No other loop diuretic has been shown to have any advantage over frusemide and drugs from the other groups are usually too weak for effective management of the acute condition. The greatest danger with frusemide is that it may be continued for too long after the syndrome of congestive cardiac failure has been relieved. In susceptible patients, or when large doses are used sufficiently often, considerable dehydration can result. It is important therefore to assess critically the need for maintenance therapy and to change treatment to a thiazide diuretic at the earliest opportunity.

Dealing with adverse effects

Hypokalaemia. It is important that hypokalaemia should be prevented in patients with congestive cardiac failure whether or not they are receiving digoxin therapy. There is now excellent evidence that the distally acting diuretics are more effective in achieving this than the use of potassium supplements. Of the available distally acting drugs, amiloride and triamterene are of probably equal efficacy and toxicity. Spironolactone is not recommended because of its endocrine side-effects. The risk with these drugs is that they will be given inadvertently to patients with impaired renal function – when dangerous hyperkalaemia may result.

Hyponatraemia. This may be encountered in patients receiving diuretic treatment under two circumstances. The first of these is in the situation of gross cardiac failure with massive oedema refractory to diuretic treatment. Although plasma sodium concentrations are low in these patients, total body sodium is high. It is presumed that reduced renal blood flow results in sodium conservation and with it an inability to excrete a water load. It has been postulated that the central compartment in such patients is relatively depleted and that patients benefit from a period without diuretic treatment, to allow oedema fluid to redistribute. Hyponatraemia is increasingly being encountered in patients receiving maintenance diuretic therapy. They are usually but not invariably elderly and are often receiving a combination of a distally acting and a proximally acting drug. These patients may present with the symptoms of hyponatraemia, such as mental confusion, weakness, nausea and occasionally convulsions. This adverse effect also results from the inability of the kidney to excrete a water load but occurs in the presence of a relative sodium deficiency. Although it has been reported as diuretic-induced syndrome of inappropriate antidiuretic hormone, because elevated levels of antidiuretic hormone have been found, it seems unlikely that this is the primary cause. A more plausible explanation is that, in the presence of a volume deficit, proximal tubular sodium reabsorption is greatly increased and there is failure to deliver a solute load to the cortical diluting segment. This, together with the action of the diuretic in that segment, results in impaired water clearance. Elevation of antidiuretic hormone is in fact appropriate and results from stimulation of volume receptors in the right atrium. Most patients can be managed by fluid restriction although occasionally it is necessary to provide added sodium. Any accompanying potassium deficiency should also be corrected. It is possible that the increased use of distally acting diuretics may increase the incidence of this adverse effect.

Hyperuricaemia and gout. All potent diuretics decrease the renal clearance of uric acid and elevate serum uric acid levels. This effect is almost certainly a consequence of the reduction in extracellular fluid volume. The changes in renal sodium handling which occur in response appear to have a secondary effect on secretion and reabsorption of uric acid in the renal tubule. Renal urate clearance is thus reduced. Chronic hyperuricaemia is less worrying in cardiac failure than when diuretics are used to treat hypertension. Nevertheless an acute attack of gout can be precipitated. In managing this problem it is important to remember that non-steroidal anti-inflammatory drugs may antagonize the effect of the diuretic. One drug – tienilic acid – has been developed which has both diuretic action and a potent uricosuric effect. Unfortunately this drug could not be released generally because of hepatic toxicity, but there would certainly be a place in therapeutics for any such compound which was proved safe.

The impaired carbohydrate tolerance and increase in serum lipids occurring as a result of diuretic treatment is relevant only to the long term management of hypertension.

Diuretic resistance

There are a number of reasons why patients may fail to respond adequately to diuretic treatment. In the first place, it is important to realize that the response to diuretics in any person with reduced cardiac output will be lower than in the normal person or in the patient with left ventricular failure with an adequately maintained cardiac output. The reason for this is the greatly increased proximal tubular sodium reabsorption occurring as a result of reduced renal perfusion, as discussed above. If this effect is sufficiently intense, failure to respond to diuretics is inevitable. Under the circumstances one should aim to maintain therapeutic concentration of the drug at its site of action, continuously. This involves using high doses of loop diuretics administered at frequent intervals. The use of continuous infusions of frusemide has been advocated but it is unlikely that this carries any advantage over repeated intravenous injections. When resistance to the actions of frusemide is encountered parenteral administration of the drug is to be preferred. This is because of the theoretical risk that the absorption of the drug from the gastrointestinal tract may be impaired in patients with oedematous states. However the evidence suggests that the average bioavailability of frusemide is unaffected by congestive cardiac failure, but that there may be wide variability. Where there is diuretic resistance a distally acting drug should certainly also be prescribed. Under these circumstances the drug metolazone should also be considered. Although this drug has been available for many years it has recently gained popularity because many patients appear to respond dramatically to it. This may be because the drug has a significant effect in the proximal tubule of the nephron.

Diuretic resistance may be encountered where there is failure of transport of the drug into the tubule of the nephron. This is probably one of the main reasons for failure to respond to diuretics in patients with moderate renal impairment. In uraemia the accumulated endogenous organic acids apparently block the active transport pathway.

Perhaps one of the most important drug interactions discovered in recent years is that between the non-steroidal anti-inflammatory agents and the diuretics. It is now well documented that the non-steroidal inflammatory agents can cause a degree of salt and water retention in their own right and in a number of studies they have been shown to reduce the response to diuretic drugs. It has been presumed that the mechanism for this interaction is at a tubular level. Prostaglandins appear to inhibit the reabsorption of sodium in the renal tubule. Because many diuretics increase the excretion of prostaglandins it has been presumed that part of their action may be explained through potentiation of prostaglandins. Clearly an antagonistic effect would result from the use of non-steroidal anti-inflammatory drugs which inhibit prostaglandin synthetase. It should also be remembered, however, that the non-steroidal anti-inflammatory drugs are organic acids and may compete with diuretic drugs for secretion in the proximal tubule. Studies have shown that in fact both mechanisms play a part in the interaction.

Vasodilators

Preload may be reduced by vasodilator drugs whose predominant action is on the venous capacitance vessels. The mismatch between circulating volume and blood vessel capacity so produced effectively reduces filling pressure. None of the vasodilator drugs used have a purely venodilator or purely arteriodilator action and a reduction in preload inevitably follows a fall in afterload. It is not possible therefore to classify vasodilators into pure preload reducers or pure afterload reducers, but it is possible to do so on the basis of the predominant effect observed. This distinction is conceptually important because the haemodynamic state of the patient may well dictate the use of one or other type of vasodilator. The drugs most useful for preload reduction in patients with acute left ventricular failure are morphine and the nitrates.

Morphine

Morphine is one of the time-honoured remedies in the treatment of acute left ventricular failure. For many years there was controversy as to its mechanism of action. Some believed that its sedative and mood-elevating properties were responsible for its therapeutic action, whilst others talked of suppression of stretch receptor reflexes in the lungs. Over recent years, however, it has become clear that the single most important pharmacological effect in heart failure is morphine's venous dilating action. Although morphine may still have a minor role in the treatment of acute left ventricular failure its use should be diminishing. There have undoubtedly been many disasters associated with the inappropriate use of this drug. Morphine should not be used in the frail, elderly patient, in whom there is great sensitivity to the sedating effects of the drug, and it has no role where there is considerable reduction in cardiac output. The author has seen a number of patients who have developed opium intoxication as a result of repeated intramuscular injections of morphine to treat heart failure. It should never be given to the exhausted patient. The place of morphine is in the patient who is acutely short of breath and who has good cardiac output but high venous filling pressure and pulmonary oedema. The drug should be given by very slow intravenous injection and injection discontinued at the first signs of relief of the distress. Subsequently other drugs should be used to manage the case.

Nitrates

There is overwhelming evidence that these drugs are effective in the reduction of pulmonary oedema due to left ventricular failure and they should now be regarded as part of the standard therapy of that condition. Marked reductions in pulmonary capillary wedge pressure and right atrial pressure occur but, because of the relatively weak arterial dilating effects, the decrease in systemic vascular resistance and increase in cardiac output are modest. Although their main action is to relax the vascular smooth muscle in the venous capacitance bed, nitrates also dilate large arteries and in particular have a selective vasodilating effect on the pulmonary and coronary circulations. Vasoconstriction may actually occur in the splanchnic beds. If systemic mean arterial pressure is allowed to decrease renal blood flow may also fall. The drugs' effect in the coronary circulation may be important. The large epicardial arteries are dilated but there may be little or no effect on the small intramyocardial arterioles. The latter are responsible for coronary vascular resistance. By dilating diseased coronary arteries and collaterals the abnormal endocardial/epicardial perfusion ratio may be improved with increased blood supply to the subendocardial muscle, even though total blood flow may not increase.

CHOICE OF NITRATE

The pharmacological actions of the nitrates do not differ between the various preparations. Important differences lie in their pharmacokinetics, however. Although glyceryl trinitrate and isosorbide dinitrate are well absorbed from the gastrointestinal tract, they undergo extensive presystemic metabolism in the liver by the enzyme glutathione organic nitrate reductase. Isosorbide dinitrate is metabolized to two active metabolites. These are isosorbide-2-mononitrate and isosorbide-5-mononitrate. Although on average 50% of an oral dose of isosorbide dinitrate circulates as the 5-mononitrate metabolite the proportion varies widely between individuals (22–68%). The elimination half-lives of isosorbide dinitrate and of the 2- and 5-mononitrate metabolites are 0.5, 1.5 and 4.5 hours respectively. It seems therefore that any sustained effect of oral isosorbide dinitrate is due mainly to the 5-mononitrate metabolite. Although slow release isosorbide dinitrate might be expected to provide a continuous effect, there are wide variations in the bioavailability and rate of absorption from the various commercially available preparations. The 5-mononitrate metabolite is now available for therapeutic use. It has the theoretical advantage of 100% bioavailability and more predictable drug concentrations after oral administration. Limited clinical trials have been performed in cardiac failure, comparing the dinitrate and mononitrate preparations, but little advantage has been demonstrated for the latter. Nevertheless common sense would dictate that the mononitrate preparation is to be preferred. Although the topical administration of glyceryl trinitrate in ointment or patch form has been shown to be of benefit in the treatment of congestive cardiac failure, this offers no advantage over the oral administration of either isosorbide dinitrate or isosorbide mononitrate. Nitrates have been found to be useful in treating the cardiac failure complicated by mechanical defects, such as mitral or aortic regurgitation. In these conditions they reduce left ventricular end-diastolic volume and pressure and pulmonary capillary wedge pressure. The volume of blood regurgitated may also be reduced although forward stroke volume may not change. Forward cardiac index may increase in patients with aortic regurgitation as systemic vascular resistance decreases. In patients with mitral stenosis, nitrates can be useful to decrease the symptoms of pulmonary vascular congestion but care must be taken not to lower preload to levels which reduce cardiac output. Nitrates should not be used in patients with predominant right ventricular failure. Under these circumstances right ventricular end-diastolic pressure and volume may be elevated but stroke volume may be decreased and consequently preload to the left ventricle is reduced. A further reduction in venous return can cause a disastrous reduction in preload and fall in stroke volume.

Table 4.6   Vasodilators used in the treatment of heart failure

Drugs affecting predominantly preload	Drugs affecting predominantly afterload	Drugs with a mixed effect
Morphine	Hydralazine	Prazosin
Glyceryl trinitrate	Phentolamine	
Isosorbide dinitrate	Nifedipine	
Isosorbide mononitrate	Captopril	

AFTERLOAD REDUCTION

There is only one method available for the reduction of afterload and that is the administration of drugs with a significant arteriolar dilating activity. The commonly used drugs are shown in Table 4.6. From the Frank–Starling hypothesis it is easy to see that pure afterload reduction must always be beneficial in patients with cardiac failure. The effect is to put the heart onto a higher curve so that either a greater cardiac output can be achieved for a given filling pressure or the same cardiac output can be achieved at a lower filling pressure. Probably the most important danger with arterial vasodilators is the risk of hypotension. When this occurs it can give rise to symptoms due to cerebral under-perfusion or can have an adverse effect on coronary artery perfusion. When using vasodilators it is therefore important to monitor blood pressure and be certain that significant hypotension is not occurring.

Hydralazine

The mechanism of action of hydralazine is related to its direct smooth muscle relaxant effect on the peripheral vascular bed. Some dilatation of venous capacitance vessels occurs but this is insignificant in comparison to the overwhelming effect on the precapillary resistance vessels. Renal and limb blood flow increase but hepatic blood flow remains unchanged. Whilst absorption of hydralazine from the gastrointestinal tract is almost complete, bioavailability is reduced to between 26 and 55% due to variable presystemic acetylation. The effect of hydralazine after oral administration starts within 20-30 min and peak serum concentrations are achieved within 0.5-2 hours. Hydralazine is the prototype of the afterload reducing agents and as expected in patients with chronic congestive cardiac failure, cardiac index, stroke volume index, stroke work index are all significantly increased. When it is administered alone, blood pressure is usually well maintained or falls only slightly. A reflex increase in heart rate usually does not occur, presumably because in the situation of cardiac failure sympathetic drive is maximal anyway. Hydralazine reduces pulmonary vascular resistance, but not to the same extent as would be achieved by preload reducers. Although a positive inotropic effect of hydralazine has been reported in animals, this finding seems unlikely to be relevant to man, as concentrations much greater than those normally achieved are required to produce this effect. Although one would predict wide variation in the dose requirements of hydralazine in patients with cardiac failure, most patients require more than 200 mg/day in divided doses, and the usual range is 300-400 mg/day. Hydralazine is particularly useful where there are mechanical defects contributing to the cause of the congestive cardiac failure. In regurgitant valve lesions (either aortic incompetence or mitral incompetence) afterload reduction reduces the regurgitant volume and increases the forward stroke volume. In patients with congestive cardiac failure hydralazine causes a significant decrease in systemic vascular resistance and a fall in pulmonary vascular resistance, together with a reduction in pulmonary capillary wedge pressure and mean pulmonary arterial pressure, and there is usually an increase in cardiac output without a significant change in heart rate. Particular care must be taken to avoid a reduction in aortic diastolic pressure by too much in those patients with aortic insufficiency, and those with coronary artery disease.

The doses of hydralazine used in patients with heart failure are greater than those normally employed for the treatment of hypertension. This increases the risk of the development of drug induced lupus syndrome. Up to 20% of patients receiving 400 mg of hydralazine per day may develop antinuclear antibodies and the risk of symptomatic lupus syndrome is related to acetylator status. Where long term hydralazine therapy is being considered it is probably advisable to measure acetylator status and to use reduced dosages in patients who are found to be slow acetylators. Patients with severe coronary artery disease may notice an increase in the frequency of their angina, especially if hydralazine causes an increase in heart rate. For this reason blood pressure and heart rate should be monitored in the erect and supine positions. Fluid retention and weight gain occasionally occur, possibly as a result of indirect stimulation of the renin–angiotensin system, but this effect is usually easily counteracted by an increase in diuretic dosage.

Captopril

Captopril is the only presently available angiotensin converting enzyme inhibitor. The drug has been shown to be beneficial in a number of patients with congestive cardiac failure often unresponsive to triple therapy with digoxin diuretics and other vasodilators. Some studies have suggested that those patients who exhibit hyponatraemia are particularly likely to respond to captopril. However it is not clear that suppression of the angiotensin–renin system entirely accounts for the mechanism of the drug's effect. The arteriolar vasodilating action of captopril is not totally explained by the decreased angiotensin II levels which result from inhibition of the conversion of angiotensin I into angiotensin II. In the first place renin and angiotensin levels may not be elevated in severe congestive cardiac failure, and initial systemic vascular resistance is not correlated with plasma renin activity. Although plasma renin activity, aldosterone and angiotensin II have been shown to be elevated in the acute decompensation phase of congestive cardiac failure, they usually return to normal after a steady state situation has been reached. Captopril also inhibits the breakdown of bradykinin, but here again there is no evidence that this mechanism is important in the reduction of systemic vascular resistance brought about by captopril. It is possible that captopril may have its effect through alteration in prostaglandin levels. Captopril has been shown to have a very minor venodilating effect; this probably results from the reduction in angiotensin II levels. The latter has been shown to have a minor venoconstricting effect. Similarly the bradycardia sometimes seen after initiation of captopril therapy may result from loss of the positive chronotropic effect of angiotensin II. Captopril is usually well absorbed from the gastrointestinal tract with a bioavailability of approximately 70%, although this may be reduced if the drug is taken with food. Maximum blood concentrations are achieved within 1.5 h in most patients and the drug is eliminated with a half-life of about 2 h in normal volunteers. Thirty per cent of a dose is excreted unchanged, the remainder being excreted as polar metabolites. The clearance correlates with creatinine clearance and there is a risk of accumulation in patients with renal failure. When captopril is administered to patients with heart failure, cardiac index, stroke work index and stroke volume index all increase in the face of a reduction in systemic vascular resistance. Usually the fall in blood pressure is moderate although occasionally marked hypotension can result after the first dose administration. Because of this it is recommended that initiation of captopril therapy should always be in a situation where careful monitoring is possible. This usually implies a hospital setting. A further reason for this is the marked bradycardia which is sometimes encountered. Captopril appears to produce a relatively selective vasodilatation on the renovascular bed. In one study of the circulatory effects of captopril, cardiac index increased by 16%, hepatic blood flow by 17% and renal blood flow increased by 60%. As glomerular filtration rate did not change this resulted in a decreased filtration fraction and a markedly increased natriuresis. The beneficial haemodynamic effects of captopril last for between 5 and 7 h after oral administration. The drug should therefore be given three times a day and the dose usually ranges between 6.25 and 150 mg three times per day. Captopril therapy is associated with a long list of potentially serious toxic effects but these are extremely rare if the total daily dose is below 150 mg. The profile of adverse reactions is strikingly reminiscent of that which is seen with D-penicillamine and it is possible that it relates to the presence of a sulfhydryl group within the molecule. Proteinuria occurs in about 2% of patients receiving captopril for 8 months or more. In most of these, however, there is already pre-existing renal disease, and the incidence is reduced to 0.4% in patients with normal renal function. Twenty per cent of the patients who develop proteinuria may actually develop the nephrotic syndrome and biopsies may show the presence of membranous glomerulonephritis in some cases. In about 50% of patients who develop nephrotic syndrome on captopril the lesion regresses after the drug is stopped. Clearly, when this drug is used, urinary protein excretion should be monitored and the drug discontinued should proteinuria develop or increase. Neutropenia and agranulocytosis have also been reported and are of some concern. Most of the patients suffered from multiple pathology but a causal relationship is generally accepted. Accumulation of high levels of captopril in patients with renal impairment is implicated. Skin rashes occur. They may be transient but in occasional patients this development necessitates discontinuation of the treatment. Taste disturbance (ageusia) occurs in between 6 and 7% of patients. Hyperkalaemia is a risk especially in the presence of renal impairment.

Nifedipine

The calcium channel blockers, of which nifedipine is one, are assuming increasing importance in the treatments of angina, cardiac arrhythmias and hypertension. Recently investigators have studied the use of nifedipine in patients with congestive cardiac failure. The rationale for this is that nifedipine is a potent arteriodilator and therefore capable of considerable afterload reduction. In comparison to the other calcium channel blockers, nifedipine has minimal negative inotropic effect and it is argued that this is more than offset by the afterload-reducing effect. Nevertheless when doses are large, impairment of myocardial contractility can occur and, although in patients with congestive cardiac failure a moderate increase in cardiac output with some decrease in arterial pressure and systemic vascular resistance has been found, the decrease in left ventricular filling pressure was only modest. When so many arterial vasodilators are available which do not interfere with cardiac function, it seems illogical to choose one with the potential for reducing cardiac contractility. The early use of nifedipine in treatment of heart failure cannot therefore be condoned.

Phentolamine and phenoxybenzamine

These α-adrenoreceptor blockers have been shown in a limited number of patients with congestive cardiac failure to produce beneficial effects. However experience is extremely limited and it is likely that adverse effects such as undue tachycardia and gastrointestinal symptoms will limit their widespread usage.

Minoxidil

This drug is a potent smooth muscle relaxing agent which has predominant effects on the arteriolar resistance vessels. The drug is almost completely absorbed after oral administration achieving a maximum concentration in approximately 1 hour. The elimination half-life of minoxidil is between about 4 and 5 h, but the duration of its haemodynamic effects appears to be longer than that. The haemodynamic effects produced by minoxidil are very similar to those produced by hydralazine. Cardiac index, stroke volume index, stroke work index increase as systemic vascular resistance decreases, often without a significant decrease in blood pressure. Heart rate is usually unchanged or may increase slightly and there is little effect on right or left ventricular filling pressures. The effective dose of minoxidil in patients with cardiac failure has not been accurately determined but single oral doses in the range of 5–20 mg have been effective in achieving haemodynamic benefit. Long term therapy in patients with cardiac failure is associated with salt and water retention and weight gain but this can usually be offset by increased diuretic dosage. Hypertrichosis is the most common side-effect associated with the drug. It comes on usually several weeks after starting therapy and may occur in as many as 30% of cases.

Prazosin

Prazosin is an example of a vasodilator which has both preload and afterload reducing effects. It is a quinazoline derivative which selectively blocks postsynaptic α_1-adrenoreceptors in the walls of the blood vessels. Stimulation of these receptors by noradrenaline causes constriction of both the arterial and venous beds. Conversely blockade of these receptors causes vascular dilatation. The presynaptic α_2-adrenoreceptors located in the adrenergic neurone terminal are unaffected by prazosin. These receptors are responsible for a negative feedback system whereby the neuronal release of noradrenaline is inhibited. This selectivity of prazosin for the α_1-receptor may account for the absence of reflex tachycardia and renin release in response to the administration of prazosin. Prazosin is well absorbed from the gastrointestinal tract with a bioavailability of around 50%. It undergoes extensive metabolism in the liver with only 6% of the drug being excreted unchanged in the urine. The low bioavailability of prazosin is probably explained by hepatic presystemic metabolism and it is likely that the clearance of the drug is sensitive to changes in hepatic blood flow. The mean elimination half-life of prazosin is approximately 2.5 h. However the drug's haemodynamic effect is longer – lasting for about 6 h. Profound hypotension is sometimes encountered in patients following the initial administration of the first dose of prazosin. The effect can be prevented by volume replacement and is unusual on subsequent doses – presumably due to salt and water retention. The pharmacokinetics of prazosin have been shown to be affected by the presence of congestive cardiac failure. Elimination half-life may be considerably prolonged and averages approximately 7 h. The likely explanation for this is that reduced hepatic blood flow decreases clearance from the systemic circulation. There is also prolongation of the elimination of prazosin in patients with renal failure. Because of prazosin's effect on both arterio- and veno-capacitance vessels, it provides an ideal drug where reduction in preload and afterload are both sought. As can be expected, the decrease in systemic vascular resistance is accompanied by an increase in cardiac index, stroke volume index and stroke work index. There is usually a modest reduction in blood pressure in the absence of a significant change in heart rate. Systemic and pulmonary

Table 4.7 Principles in the use of vasodilators in the treatment of cardiac failure

(1) Any patient with significant cardiac failure due to left ventricular dysfunction regardless of the aetiology who has failed to respond to conventional therapy with digoxin and diuretics should be considered for vasodilator therapy
(2) In some patients vasodilator therapy should be considered before the use of positive inotropic agents
(3) Care should be taken in the presence of hypotension and further significant falls in blood pressure should not be allowed to occur
(4) The choice of vasodilator depends on the haemodynamic state of the patient:
  (a) Where there is markedly elevated pulmonary venous pressure and adequate cardiac output a drug with a predominantly venodilator action should be used, e.g. nitrates
  (b) Where cardiac output is markedly reduced and there are signs of an increase in systemic vascular resistance a drug with a predominantly arteriolar dilating action should be used, e.g. hydralazine or minoxidil
  (c) Where cardiac output is low and pulmonary venous pressure is high drugs acting on both the arteriolar and venous systems should be employed cautiously. Thus either prazosin or a combination of hydralazine and nitrates may be employed
(5) Where the currently employed vasodilator fails to produce an adequate response captopril should be tried
(6) The initial dose of vasodilator used should be low and gradually increased according to the haemodynamic response
(7) Late tolerance to the effect of the vasodilator may be explained by fluid retention and weight gain. An increase in diuretic dosage may then be beneficial. An increase in the dose of the vasodilator or a change to another vasodilator should also be considered

venous pressures decrease significantly, and there is a reduction in pulmonary vascular resistance. The usual dose of prazosin for treating congestive cardiac failure is between 3 and 5 mg/day. The haemodynamic effects last for about 6 h and the drug needs to be given in divided doses four times per day. It has been suggested that while short-term use of prazosin produces considerable beneficial effect, many patients become tolerant to the drug and the beneficial effect is lost or increased dosage is required. It is possible that such tolerance relates to increased release of noradrenaline from the neuron terminal, or it may relate to prazosin induced fluid retention. Plasma noradrenaline levels have been shown to be increased and plasma renin activity to be stimulated in patients on long term prazosin therapy. Thus the reduction in vasodilatation could be secondary to increased levels of angiotensin II. It has also been suggested that there is an accumulation of sodium and water in the vascular smooth muscle walls and that that decreases the responsiveness to prazosin. Whatever the mechanism, the delayed tolerance usually responds to diuretic administration with a partial return of the initial beneficial haemodynamic effects. Prazosin is relatively free of serious side-effects. Gastrointestinal symptoms, headache, palpitations, drowsiness, depression and sexual dysfunction occur infrequently. The postural hypotension mentioned above is rarely a problem in patients with congestive cardiac failure. Acute polyarthropathy has also been reported but occurs only rarely.

TOMORROW'S THERAPY

In recent years the most significant advances in the treatment of heart failure have not been due to the development of new drugs. They have been in the increased understanding of the actions, limitations and clinical usefulness of the drugs already available. This is a healthy trend and one which must continue. To many doctors the concept of using vasodilators to treat heart failure is still a foreign one. The logic behind their use is so self-evident that it is amazing that this approach should be a therapeutic innovation. It is not long ago, however, that the use of vasodilators was considered to be safe only in units with special expertise and facilities for invasive investigation. Now we accept that careful clinical monitoring is quite adequate and indeed it is becoming routine practice for patients with severe pulmonary oedema to be given a nitrate along with the intravenous frusemide if not before. Nevertheless our experience is in its infancy. It will not be until general practitioners start to use this line of therapy widely that the true value and perhaps the hidden dangers will be manifest. In the United Kingdom at present there are many, many patients taking digoxin regularly every day for no good reason. Some of these are suffering or will suffer needless morbidity. Yet the principles by which we should prescribe this drug are now well documented. Doctors must learn to use digoxin wisely. Whilst it is exciting to see new drugs on the horizon, let us contain our enthusiasm and concentrate on improving our effectiveness with our present therapeutic armamentarium.

Further Reading

Aronson, J.K. (1983). Indications for the measurement of plasma digoxin concentrations. *Drugs*, 26, 230–42

Awan, N.A., De Maria, A.N. and Mason, D.T. (1982). Therapeutic importance of calcium antagonists in coronary artery disease and congestive heart failure: an overview. *Drugs*, 23, 235–41

Brater, D.C. (1981). Resistance to diuretics: emphasis on a pharmacological perspective. *Drugs*, 22, 477–94

Brown, D.D., Spector, R. and Juhl, R.P. (1980). Drug interactions with digoxin. *Drugs*, 20, 198–206

Davies, D.L. and Wilson, G.M. (1975). Diuretics: mechanism of action and clinical application. *Drugs*, 9, 178–226

El Kayam, U. and Aranow, W.S. (1982). Glyceryl trinitrate (Nitroglycerin) ointment and isosorbide dinitrate: a review of their pharmacological properties and therapeutic use. *Drugs*, 23, 165–94

Hamer, J. (1980). Drugs used in cardiac failure: Digitalis and vasodilators. In Turner, P. and Shand, D.G. (eds.) *Recent Advances in Clinical Pharmocology 2*, pp. 73–100. (Edinburgh, London, Melbourne and New York: Churchill Livingstone)

Hamer J. (1982). *The Modern Management of Congestive Heart Failure*. (London: Lloyd-Luke)

Johnston, G.D. (1980). Digoxin dose precision: prescribing aids or intuition! *Drugs*, 20, 494–9

Lazar, J.D. (1983). Angiotensin-converting enzyme inhibitors. In Turner, P. and Shand, D.G. (eds.) *Recent Advances in Clinical Pharmacology 3*, pp. 81–105. (Edinburgh, London, Melbourne and New York: Churchill Livingstone)

Opie, L.H. (1980). *Drugs and the Heart*. (London: *The Lancet*)

Packer, M. (1982). Selection of vasodilator drugs for patients with severe chronic heart failure: an approach based on a new classification. *Drugs*, 24, 64–74

Reiter, M.J. and Pritchett, E.L.C. (1983). Clinical pharmacology of calcium channel blockers: verapamil, diltiazem, nifedipine. In Turner, P. and Shand, D.G. (eds.) *Recent Advances in Clinical Pharmacology 3*, pp. 107–27. (Edinburgh, London, Melbourne and New York: Churchill Livingstone)

Romankiewicz, J.A., Brogden, R.N., Heel, R.C., Speight, T.M. and Avery, G.S. (1983). Captopril: an update review of its pharmacological properties and therapeutic efficacy in congestive heart failure. *Drugs*, 25, 6–40

Schwartz, A.B. and Chatterjee, K. (1983). Vasodilator therapy in chronic congestive heart failure. *Drugs*, 26, 148–73

Stanaszek, W.F., Kellerman, D., Brogden, R.N. and Romankiewicz, J.A. (1983). Prazosin update: a review of its pharmacological properties and therapeutic use in hypertension and congestive heart failure. *Drugs*, 25, 339–84

Taggart, A.J. and McDevitt, D.G. (1980). Digitalis: its place in modern therapy. *Drugs*, 20, 398–404

Webb-Peploe, M.M. (1979). New approaches to the treatment of heart failure. In Davies, D.M. and Rawlins, M.D. (eds.) *Topics in Therapeutics 5*, pp. 137–61. (Tunbridge Wells: Pitman Medical)

5
Anticoagulants in the treatment of cardiovascular disease

A.K. SCOTT

INTRODUCTION

The history of the discovery of the oral anticoagulants is well known. In the early 1920s Schofield described a severe bleeding disorder in cattle fed on improperly cured sweet clover. Ten years later the defect had been shown to be due to a deficiency of prothrombin and dicoumarol was identified as the toxic agent. Clinical trials of the use of dicoumarol followed in the 1940s. Since then many other chemically related compounds have been studied. Despite 40 years of clinical use there is considerable debate about the value of oral anticoagulants in both medical and surgical disorders. There are also no generally accepted guidelines regarding initiation or duration of therapy.

Warfarin is the most widely used oral anticoagulant and will be considered in detail with only brief reference to other drugs. The clinical pharmacology of warfarin will be discussed initially with particular reference to individual patient factors which may be encountered in the treatment of cardiovascular disorders. Other oral anticoagulants will then be considered. Finally the clinical use of oral anticoagulants will be debated.

WARFARIN – CLINICAL PHARMACOLOGY

Chemistry and analytical methods

Warfarin is a derivative of 4-hydroxycoumarin with structure as illustrated in Figure 5.1. The commercial warfarin used clinically is a racemic mixture of two enantiomers because the molecule has an asymmetric centre (*in Figure 5.1). The R and S enantiomers exhibit different pharmacokinetic properties and potency. This is of considerable clinical importance.

Warfarin concentration was initially measured in biological samples

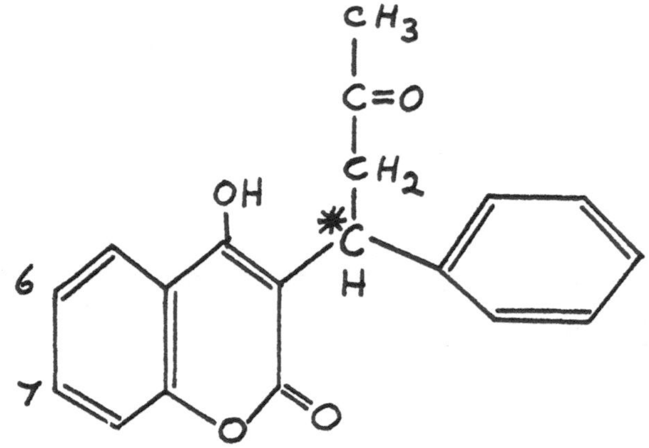

Figure 5.1 Structural formula of warfarin.
*Indicates the asymmetric carbon atom: 6 and 7 indicate the position of hydroxy substitutions of major hydroxylated metabolites

using spectrophotometric techniques[1]. Such methods are non-specific and may suffer from interference from metabolites or other drugs. Later gas liquid chromatographic methods were developed which separated parent drug from the major metabolites[2,3]. These methods involve derivatization and are technically difficult and time consuming.

The analytical method of choice is currently by high performance liquid chromatography (h.p.l.c.) which provides specificity and sensitivity without the need for derivative formation. One suitable method allows measurement of warfarin and its metabolites after a simple extraction at acid pH and elution with a hexane-based solvent[4]. Other methods allow separation and measurement of both the R and S enantiomers of warfarin.

'Pharmacokinetics'

Absorption

Warfarin is almost completely absorbed from the gastrointestinal tract[5,6]. However the methods used in these studies[5,6] were non-specific. It would be of interest to perform a bioavailability study comparing area under the plasma concentration-time curve following oral and intravenous dosing with warfarin using an h.p.l.c. method to evaluate the earlier results. It seems likely however, that bioavailability is high. Rate of absorption is relatively slow, with peak plasma concentration being achieved after 3–9 hours[5]. This is not clinically relevant because it is the extent of absorption which is important in determining steady state concentration[7].

Absorption of warfarin in disease states has not been extensively investigated. It is possible that cardiac failure might reduce warfarin absorption but the effect for such a well absorbed drug is probably small. Other cardiovascular disorders are unlikely to affect warfarin absorption.

Distribution

Warfarin is a highly protein bound drug. Most studies record values of 97–99.5% bound[8–10]. As warfarin is an acidic drug the binding is to plasma albumin[11]. The S-warfarin enantiomer is more highly bound than R warfarin if measurements are made at body temperature[12]. Such a relationship at the receptor could explain the differences in anticoagulant activity of the two enantiomers[13]. Volume of distribution of warfarin is 8–27% of body weight for both enantiomers and roughly equates with that of albumin[14–16].

Serum protein binding shows considerable interindividual variation. Binding of warfarin influences its elimination in both rats[17] and man[18]. Clearance of warfarin is more rapid if there is less protein binding with a higher free fraction. Up to 90% of the interindividual variation in clearance is related to these differences in protein binding[9].

Protein binding may be altered by underlying disease or physiological changes. This has been studied most extensively in renal failure. Warfarin binding is decreased in the presence of uraemia due to the presence of an endogenous protein binding inhibitor[19]. Binding of warfarin is also reduced in the presence of hypoalbuminaemic states, including idiopathic hypoalbuminaemia[20]. Variation in warfarin protein binding with time has been reported in patients with cardiovascular disease but the changes are small in comparison to normal intersubject variation[21]. Despite lower albumin concentrations in the elderly there is no difference in volume of distribution between young and elderly patients[22]. Warfarin is not distributed into breast milk and was not found in the plasma of breast-fed offspring of anticoagulated mothers[23]. The effect of drugs on protein binding is discussed in detail below, in the section on drug interactions.

Elimination

Warfarin has a low hepatic extraction ratio. Elimination for such a drug depends on intrinsic enzyme activity and protein binding[24]. Interindividual variation in protein binding has already been discussed. The metabolic pathways responsible for warfarin excretion also show extensive interindividual variation. A combination of these two factors is responsible for the wide range in warfarin elimination half-life times and clearance values reported from a large number of studies in man[25,26].

Metabolism

The major metabolites of warfarin in man are 6-hydroxywarfarin, 7-hydroxywarfarin and warfarin alcohols, and account for over 90% of a dose[27-29]. The amounts of each metabolite formed differ for the two enantiomers. S-warfarin is mainly metabolized to 7-hydroxywarfarin which is chiefly excreted in the bile. This reaction is cytochrome p-450 dependent and takes place in the liver endoplasmic reticulum. Smaller amounts of an optically active warfarin alcohol are also formed (SS warfarin alcohol). R-warfarin is mainly reduced by soluble enzymes (not cytochrome p-450 dependent) in liver and kidney to form RS warfarin alcohol[30] which is excreted in the urine[29]. Both enantiomers form some 6-hydroxywarfarin. The ring hydroxylated metabolites are probably inactive but the alcohols may have some anticoagulant effect, though considerably less potent than warfarin[31].

Half-life

Plasma elimination half-life of racemic warfarin shows marked inter-individual variation. One study reported values ranging from 10 to 45 h after a single oral dose[6]. The S-enantiomer is more rapidly eliminated than R-warfarin with half-life times of 18–35 h and 20–60 h respectively[13]. Elimination of a drug is more accurately represented by measuring its clearance. Half-life $(T_{\frac{1}{2}})$ may alter because of a change in volume of distribution (Vd) in the absence of change in clearance (Cl). The relationship between these parameters is:

$$T_{\frac{1}{2}} = \frac{0.693 \times \text{Vd}}{\text{Cl}}$$

Clearance values for warfarin are less frequently reported. Accurate measurement requires administration of an intravenous dose to avoid making assumptions about extent of drug absorption. Total plasma warfarin clearance values of 2.5 to 6.4 ml h^{-1} kg^{-1} have been reported[9] following oral administration assuming complete bioavailability[32]. In rats, plasma warfarin clearance is dose dependent due to saturable hepatic uptake[33]. The enzymes responsible for warfarin metabolism do not show saturation within the dose range 0.01–1.0 mg kg^{-1}. It is not known if this occurs in man but it could form the basis of some drug interactions with warfarin[10].

Effects of age and disease

Elderly patients require lower warfarin doses than young adults. However, warfarin pharmacokinetic parameters show no major variation with age[9, 22]. Renal failure results in a reduction in warfarin half-life[19]. This is due to increased clearance as a result of reduced warfarin protein binding rather than an increase in enzymatic activity. Thyroid disease has no effect on warfarin elimination[34]. There is little information regarding the effects of other diseases on warfarin elimination.

Mechanism of action

Warfarin antagonizes the synthesis of vitamin-K-dependent clotting factors (II, VII, IX and X) by γ-carboxylation of glutamyl residues of their precursor proteins[35]. During this reaction vitamin K is converted into vitamin K 2,3-epoxide which is biologically inactive. The epoxide is then reduced back to the active vitamin by microsomal epoxide reductase and this cyclic interconversion is referred to as the vitamin K-epoxide cycle[36,37]. The efficiency of this cycle in conserving vitamin K results in low daily requirements (*ca.* 1 μg/kg) of the vitamin[38,39]. Warfarin inhibits the epoxide reductase to prevent reactivation of vitamin K[40,41]. It is therefore an indirect antagonist of vitamin K.

Interindividual variation in the pharmacodynamic response to warfarin may occur because of variation in receptor affinity or variation in vitamin K availability and the vitamin-K-dependent clotting factors. Differences in receptor affinity for warfarin have been observed in both animals and man. Resistance to the rodenticidal effect of warfarin was first noted in wild rats in Western Scotland[42] but has since been discovered elsewhere in the United Kingdom and in Denmark[25]. The first human kindred with resistance to warfarin was described in 1964[43]. Another family was reported in 1969 and the pattern of inheritance in both cases was compatible with the dominant expression of a single autosomal gene[25]. The dose of warfarin required to achieve a therapeutic effect in the propositus in the first family was 145 mg daily with a plasma warfarin concentration of 55 μg/ml (cf. average dose 8 mg with a plasma concentration around 3 μg/ml).

Variation in vitamin K intake will competitively affect the response to warfarin. Vitamin K is available as vitamin K_1 in the diet and vitamin K_2 from bacterial synthesis in the gut. The diet appears to be the more important source[25]. A very high vitamin K diet will shorten the prothrombin time towards normal in anticoagulated patients[44]. This problem has also been reported in patients on enteral feeds[45] and vegetable-rich, weight reducing diets[46]. Broad spectrum antibiotics reduce gut bacterial synthesis of vitamin K_2 but this appears to affect control of warfarin therapy only if there is also dietary deficiency. Vitamin K deficiency also occurs in malabsorption disorders due to disease of the small intestine or by administration of liquid paraffin but the effect on warfarin control is not well documented[25].

The response to oral anticoagulants is potentiated in liver disease due to defective synthesis of vitamin-K-dependent clotting factors. This may occur in cirrhosis[47], viral hepatitis[48] and hepatic congestion due to congestive heart failure[49]. Hyperthyroidism also results in an increased responsiveness to warfarin. This occurs because of increased degradation of clotting factors[25]. Other proteins also have increased turnover with lower concentrations in serum in hyperthyroidism[50]. Pregnancy may result in relative resistance to anticoagulants[51]. The effect of drugs on clotting factors will be discussed in the following section.

Drug interactions

Documentation of drug interactions with warfarin is extensive and many review articles are available[52–55]. Discussion in this section will be limited to interactions with drugs used in cardiovascular disease and a few other commonly used drugs. Evaluation of interactions with warfarin is difficult because most reported interactions are based on a small number of clinical cases. Relatively few interactions have been studied in detail under controlled conditions.

Drugs used in cardiovascular disease

DIURETICS
Spironolactone reduces the hypoprothrombinaemic effect of warfarin[56]. This is a pharmacodynamic interaction due to increased concentration of clotting factors secondary to a reduction in plasma volume. A second pharmacodynamic mechanism is reduction of hepatic congestion with an improvement in clotting factor synthesis[52]. Chlorthalidone also reduces the effect of warfarin[57]. However the loop diuretics, frusemide and bumetanide, had no effect on warfarin in an acute dosing study[58]. This requires further evaluation in volunteers after chronic dosing and in patients with cardiac failure. No pharmacokinetic interaction between diuretics and warfarin has been reported. Concurrent use of warfarin and diuretics requires great care with regular monitoring of prothrombin time, particularly during initiation of diuretic therapy and improvement of liver congestion.

β-BLOCKERS
Lipid soluble β-blockers have been reported to potentiate the anticoagulant effect of warfarin in a small number of patients. The mechanism was claimed to be inhibition of warfarin metabolism as propranolol reduces antipyrine clearance[59]. Propranolol increased warfarin steady state concentration by 15% in a controlled study in chronically dosed volunteers[10]. This increase is unlikely to be clinically important in most patients but could result in haemorrhage if the patient was controlled at the upper limit of the therapeutic range. Further evaluation of this interaction is necessary in view of current interest in the combined use of β-adrenoceptor blockers and warfarin in the secondary prevention of myocardial infarction.

ANTIARRHYTHMICS

Disopyramide did not interact with warfarin in five patients studied[60]. Amiodarone potentiates the effect of warfarin and the warfarin dose should be reduced with careful monitoring of prothrombin time when the two drugs are prescribed together[61,62]. The mechanism of this interaction may be inhibition of warfarin metabolism[63].

ANTIPLATELET DRUGS

Sulphinpyrazone enhances the anticoagulant effect of warfarin due to a stereoselective inhibition of metabolism of the S-warfarin enantiomer[64,65]. An earlier observation in one patient had suggested that this interaction might be biphasic – initial potentiation followed by antagonism of warfarin effect[66]. The main danger period occurs on starting or stopping sulphinpyrazone medication in a patient on warfarin. Prothrombin time should be measured regularly during that time. Drugs which affect platelet function may potentiate warfarin by an effect on haemostasis[53]. Even small doses of aspirin may do this. High dose aspirin decreases prothrombin synthesis in man[67] and inhibits synthesis of vitamin-K-dependent clotting factors in the rabbit in a manner similar to warfarin[68].

HYPOLIPIDAEMIC DRUGS

Clofibrate potentiates the action of oral anticoagulants, probably by altering receptor sensitivity[69]. Warfarin is displaced from its albumin binding sites by clofibrate but this does not account for the interaction[70]. The transient increase in free warfarin results in an increase in clearance such that the free warfarin concentration returns to its original level. Cholestyramine reduces the anticoagulant effect of warfarin by impairing warfarin absorption and interrupting its enterohepatic recycling[71].

There are no definite reports of interactions of digoxin, vasodilators or calcium channel antagonists with warfarin. However, caution should be observed when giving any drug to a patient taking warfarin, particularly with recently marketed agents.

Non-cardiovascular drugs

INFLUENZA VACCINE

Influenza vaccine may inhibit drug metabolism[72,73]. The effect of influenza vaccination on warfarin is uncertain. An enhanced effect with no change in half-life has been reported[74]. In a controlled study in chronically dosed volunteers, however, the present author and co-workers found neither a kinetic nor a dynamic effect of influenza vaccination on warfarin (unpublished observations). There is some evidence that the type of vaccine used may be important. Further study is necessary as patients with cardiovascular disorders who are taking warfarin are a high risk group who may be advised to undergo vaccination to reduce the risk of influenza and its complications.

SMOKING

Smoking may have a small effect on warfarin kinetics but there is no important effect on warfarin activity[75].

ANALGESICS AND NON-STEROIDAL ANTI-INFLAMMATORY DRUGS

The interaction of phenylbutazone with warfarin is well known. This interaction will rarely be seen in Britain in future, following the limitation of the use of phenylbutazone by the UK Committee on Safety of Medicines. Most non-steroidal anti-inflammatory drugs (NSAIs) have no clinically important effect on warfarin control[76]. Naproxen, fenbufen, flurbiprofen, ibuprofen, diclofenac and diflunisal may be used without the need to alter warfarin dose unless indicated by change in prothrombin time. The response to oral anticoagulants may be enhanced by meclofenamic acid, mefenemic acid, piroxicam and azapropazone. NSAIs may cause peptic ulceration with a risk of haemorrhage in the presence of warfarin. Dextropropoxyphene may inhibit warfarin metabolism and Distalgesic (dextropropoxyphene and paracetamol) has been reported to potentiate the effect of warfarin[77]. Paracetamol administered for 3 weeks has also been reported as potentiating the effect of warfarin but in this study warfarin concentrations were not measured[78]. Further documentation of this interaction would be desirable as paracetamol is often recommended as a safe analgesic for anticoagulated patients.

ORAL CONTRACEPTIVES

Oral contraceptives are thrombogenic and usually contraindicated in patients requiring anticoagulants[53]. If the two drugs are given together the effect on the patient may be a balance between increased clotting factor concentrations and inhibition of oral anticoagulant metabolism[79].

ANTIBACTERIAL AGENTS

Broad spectrum antibiotics may suppress production of vitamin K from the bowel flora but, as discussed above, this is unlikely to be of clinical significance if dietary intake of vitamin K is normal. Cotrimoxazole (trimethoprim-sulphamethoxazole)[80] and metronidazole[81] stereoselectively inhibit the metabolism of S-warfarin. The dose of warfarin should be reduced. Rifampicin induces the metabolism of warfarin and reduces its anticoagulant effect[82].

DRUGS USED FOR PEPTIC ULCERATION

Cimetidine potentiates the action of oral anticoagulants by inhibiting their metabolism[83]. The newer histamine H_2-receptor antagonist, ranitidine, does not have this effect[84]. Antacids do not interfere with warfarin absorption[53]. Anticholinergic drugs will not affect warfarin absorption, though time to reach peak concentration would be delayed. Carbenoxolone also appears not to interact with warfarin[85].

ANTICONVULSANTS

Phenobarbitone, phenytoin and carbamazepine are enzyme inducing drugs. Phenobarbitone administration to a patient on warfarin will result in a reduction of anticoagulant effect within 6 days[86]. Carbamazepine also reduces the effect of warfarin[87]. The interaction with phenytoin is more complex. Phenytoin induces the liver microsomal enzymes which metabolize warfarin but also competes for metabolism. The net result depends on the balance between induction and inhibition in an individual patient. Prothrombin time requires careful monitoring.

PSYCHOTROPIC DRUGS AND ALCOHOL

Tricyclic antidepressants do not inhibit warfarin metabolism in man[88]. Benzodiazepines have no effect on elimination or control of warfarin therapy[89]. Moderate intake of alcohol does not affect anticoagulant control[90].

Summary

Drug interactions with warfarin may be predictable. In many cases, however, the interaction has not been formally studied. When altering concurrent treatment of an anticoagulated patient it is sensible to monitor prothrombin time regularly (alternate days) for the first 2 weeks.

OTHER ANTICOAGULANTS

Dicoumarol

Dicoumarol is slowly and erratically absorbed from the gastrointestinal tract[91]. This may result in drug interaction due to variation in absorption. Elimination half-life is dose dependent[92]. Inhibition of metabolism may result in a large increase in steady state concentration and risk of haemorrhage.

Ethylbiscoumacetate

This is similar to dicoumarol but is well absorbed and less extensively protein bound[93].

Nicoumalone (acenocoumarin)

In contrast to warfarin, the R-enantiomer is the more active[94]. It is highly protein bound and the elimination half-life may be relatively short (8–9 h) if specific methods of measurement are used[95].

Phenprocoumon

Elimination half-life is long (up to 9 days) and it is over 99% bound to plasma proteins[26].

Phenindione

Phenindione and the other indanediones are more liable to cause allergic reactions than the coumarins. They are not recommended as drugs of first choice.

INDICATIONS

Deep venous thrombosis and pulmonary embolism

Findings from two large postmortem studies suggest that 75% of pulmonary emboli (PE) are not suspected clinically and only 7% were formally diagnosed before death[96,97]. In addition, 75% of deaths due to PE occur within 1 hour of embolization before treatment can be started[98]. Nearly all pulmonary emboli begin as deep venous thrombosis (DVT). Treatment should be aimed at prevention of DVT and PE and early treatment of DVT in order to reduce mortality from this condition.

Primary prevention

High risk patients such as those undergoing major surgery or with a medical problem resulting in immobilization should be considered for prophylaxis against DVT. Oral anticoagulants have been shown to reduce thromboembolic disease in patients undergoing major general surgery or elective hip surgery, or with congestive cardiac failure[99]. However widespread use is limited by the risks of haemorrhage. Recent interest has focussed on the use of treatments less likely to cause haemorrhage, such as low-dose subcutaneous heparin, dextran and antiplatelet drugs. Low-dose heparin has been shown to prevent DVT in surgical patients and following myocardial infarction in a large number of trials. It also reduces the incidence of fatal PE[100]. Dextran-70 prevents PE after major surgery[101]. Oral anticoagulants should be used only when alternatives are less effective, such as after orthopaedic surgery, or for long term prophylaxis in medical patients with a low risk of haemorrhage[102].

Established DVT

The aim of treatment is to prevent extension of the thrombus and embolization. However, there is no direct evidence of benefit from the use of anticoagulants in a controlled clinical trial. Accurate diagnosis is a major problem. Bilateral venography will reduce the possibility of using anticoagulants needlessly but many thromboses do not present clinically until embolization has occurred. Indirect evidence of benefit of treatment is available. Untreated DVT (especially proximal to the calf) is associated with PE[103], but PE is rare in anticoagulant-treated DVT if there is an adequate anticoagulant response[99]. In a series of three studies warfarin and heparin have been compared for the treatment of venous thrombosis. The first study reported that fixed dose heparin was not as effective as warfarin in preventing recurrent venous thrombosis[104]. The second study found adjusted doses of heparin were as effective as warfarin and less likely to result in haemorrhage[105]. The final study found that less intensive warfarin treatment was as effective as full dose but less likely to result in haemorrhage[106]. In view of the generally accepted value of anticoagulants in DVT it would be difficult to mount a large controlled trial. On balance it is reasonable to treat DVT with less intensive warfarin (prothrombin time twice normal) for around 3 months after a single episode, as most patients prefer tablets to injections. Heparin is used initially until the warfarin effect occurs. Recurrent DVT may require lifelong warfarin therapy.

Established PE

Anticoagulants are firmly established in the treatment of pulmonary embolism. However, proof of their value in a well-conducted double blind clinical trial is lacking and their value has been critically reviewed[107].

Initial acceptance of oral anticoagulants was widespread, and uncritical by today's standards. A prospective study of anticoagulants versus no treatment reported in 1960 was abandoned after five out of 19 untreated patients died, with no deaths in the treated group[108]. In retrospect, this study could be criticized on the grounds of non-random patient selection, inadequate diagnosis and other disease associated with the recorded deaths. Only one other prospective controlled trial has been published[109]. No deaths and ten recurrent emboli were observed in 308 untreated patients compared with one death and 38 recurrent emboli in 259 anticoagulated patients. This paper shows no benefit from the use of anticoagulants, but is limited in that it deals only with PE following total hip replacement and the diagnosis of PE was made on clinical grounds. Other studies are criticized on their choice of control group – either historical or decision not to treat because of other factors.

The mortality of untreated patients with PE with other disease may be as high as 30%[98]. Many of these patients die of other causes and in others anticoagulants are contraindicated. The overall mortality from PE diagnosed by pulmonary angiography in 144 patients was 8%[110]. The mortality from PE in otherwise fit patients appears to be low[109] and the risk of treatment may outweigh the risk of the disease[111].

Oral anticoagulants are probably of benefit in preventing recurrent emboli in high risk patients with other significant disease and no contraindication to their use. The value of oral anticoagulants for other patients requires re-evaluation and comparison with other methods of treatment. However, it is currently our practice to treat all patients with PE, and no contraindication, with warfarin for 3-6 months.

Myocardial infarction (MI)

Prevention of DVT/PE

Low-dose subcutaneous heparin may prevent venous thromboembolism if started early after myocardial infarction[102]. Oral anticoagulants are not indicated in this situation.

Prevention of systemic embolism

Prophylactic therapy cannot be recommended for all patients but may be useful in a selected high risk group. Patients with extensive infarcts[112] and those with anterior infarction associated with dyskinesis of the ventricular apex[113] should be considered for treatment. There is a high risk of systemic embolism in patients with ventricular aneurysm after myocardial infarction but oral anticoagulants offer only partial protection[102].

Prevention of recurrent MI

Myocardial infarction is the commonest cause of death in Western Europe and North America and is a major cause of morbidity. Even a small reduction in the rate of infarction would be important because of the large numbers of patients involved. Interest has been centred on the use of four drug groups – oral anticoagulants, β-adrenoceptor antagonists, antiplatelet drugs and fibrinolytic agents.

Oral anticoagulants have been evaluated for use following myocardial infarction over the past 30 years. As with most new treatments, early enthusiasm was followed by critical reappraisal. The UK Medical Research Council (MRC) study reported in 1959[114] found an overall death rate after 3 years of 15% in the treated group (195 patients) and 22% in the control group (188 patients). This difference was not statistically significant but unfortunately the study was stopped prematurely on ethical grounds. Continuation of the study might well have avoided current problems regarding prophylactic treatment for myocardial infarction. In the MRC study most benefit was observed in men under 55 years old. Many early clinical trials were inadequately designed. An International Review Group studied several trials which they considered to be of reasonable design[115]. They concluded that there was a 20% reduction in mortality in males aged under 55 with either previous angina or myocardial infarction if oral anticoagulants were used for 1–2 years. This small benefit was set against the hazards and logistic problems of long term oral anticoagulants and their use was generally abandoned.

Interest has recently resurfaced following the report of the Sixty Plus Reinfarction Study Research Group[116]. This was a randomized double-blind multicentre study. Following myocardial infarction, 878 patients over 60 years of age were treated with oral anticoagulants for 6 months. Half then received placebo and half continued on oral anticoagulants (aiming for prothrombin time 2.5–4.0 times normal) for 2 years. Intensive and stable anticoagulant treatment 'substantially reduced the risk of recurrent myocardial infarction and thereby of cardiac death'. Overall death rate was 7.6% in the treated group and 13.4% in the placebo group ($p = 0.017$). Incidence of recurrent MI was 5.7% in the treated group compared to 15.9% in the placebo group ($p = 0.0001$). Major haemorrhage occurred in 27 treated patients but there were no fatal extracranial haemorrhages and intracranial events (haemorrhagic plus non-haemorrhagic) were less common in the treated group.

The Dutch study[116] reopens the question of the use of oral anticoagulants following myocardial infarction. Large, well-conducted trials comparing oral anticoagulants with the other treatments mentioned above are urgently required. We also need information on the level of anticoagulation necessary, as less intensive therapy reduces the risk of haemorrhage. Finally, the question of multiple attack on the pathophysiology of MI has been raised. Pooled data suggest that in selected patients β-blockers reduce mortality following myocardial infarction by 26%[117]. Would an attack on the infarct with β-blocker plus an attack on coagulation with warfarin produce an additive or greater effect on reduction in mortality?

Valvular heart disease and atrial fibrillation

The risk of systemic embolism is increased in patients with mitral valve disease or atrial fibrillation and is most marked in patients with mitral stenosis and atrial fibrillation. Early trials indicated that warfarin was effective in reducing thromboembolism. However, as with the trials for DVT/PE, they are generally of inadequate design by today's standards[118]. Controversy persists regarding the indications for warfarin in this group of patients.

Primary prevention

There is little dispute about treating the high risk patients with mitral stenosis, a large left atrium and atrial fibrillation. Warfarin alone appears to be effective but combination with sulphinpyrazone may give added benefit[118]. Enthusiasm for treating patients in sinus rhythm with mitral valve disease or with atrial fibrillation alone is much less. Short term anticoagulants appear to reduce the risk of embolism during electrical conversion of atrial fibrillation to sinus rhythm[102].

Secondary prevention

Oral anticoagulant treatment is indicated in patients with mitral valve disease or atrial fibrillation after an episode of systemic embolism. Treatment should then be lifelong.

More rational judgement would be possible if results were available from large, well-controlled studies comparing warfarin and antiplatelet drugs alone or in combination in these patients.

Prosthetic heart valves

Anticoagulants are commonly given for life to patients with prosthetic heart valves. Newer types of valve are less likely to cause emboli[99] but even with new valves and use of oral anticoagulants there is a persistant risk of embolism[119]. Combination of warfarin plus an antiplatelet drug may further reduce this risk. After replacement with a mechanical valve, warfarin plus dipyridamole may be superior to warfarin plus aspirin or warfarin alone in reducing thromboembolism[119]. Warfarin plus aspirin resulted in excessive bleeding episodes. In another study aspirin was found to be as effective as warfarin in patients given a porcine bioprosthesis[120]. Further results are awaited to clarify the best combination of drugs and optimum dosage of each for different types of valve replacement.

Systemic embolism

Most arterial emboli originate from the heart. Symptomatic emboli tend to lodge in the cerebral circulation (70%) and have a high risk of recurrence, perhaps up to 75%[121]. The risk of systemic embolism after acute MI is low after the first 6 months but for other causes of systemic emboli treatment with oral anticoagulants should be for life. The decision of when to start treatment after embolic stroke is difficult. There is a risk of recurrence within the first week and treatment may be started within 48 h if intracranial haemorrhage can be excluded by computerized tomographic scan and lumbar puncture if the scan shows no haemorrhage[122,123].

Transient ischaemic attack (TIA)

About 10% of patients presenting with a TIA have a subsequent stroke within 1 year[102]. The consensus of opinion is that oral anticoagulants reduce the incidence of TIA[99,102]. However, there is no good evidence that they reduce the risk of stroke. Most studies suffer from methodological defects and 'the better designed the study the less likely it is to show significant benefit from anticoagulant therapy'[124]. The problems in using warfarin and risk of bleeding at least partly offset the limited benefit and many clinicians would not consider TIA as a primary indication for warfarin. Antiplatelet drugs are also being evaluated for treatment of TIA but present evidence is inconclusive.

Reconstructive artery surgery

Oral anticoagulants appear to offer little benefit in improving long-term patency after coronary artery bypass surgery. Benefit at 8 weeks after operation was reported from a randomized study but there was a relatively low patency rate in the control group[125]. An earlier prospective randomized study in 50 patients found no difference in patency at 6 months after surgery when warfarin was compared with aspirin plus dipyridamole and controls[126]. All three groups had patency rates of around 80%. Most graft occlusions occur within the first 6 months. Further controlled trials in larger numbers of patients are necessary and as discussed previously the possibility of combination therapy needs consideration. There is no evidence that patients with peripheral vascular disease or undergoing reconstructive surgery for peripheral vascular disease benefit from the use of oral anticoagulants.

CONTRAINDICATIONS

The risks of treatment must be balanced against the risks of withholding treatment. Oral anticoagulants are clearly contraindicated where there is active bleeding or if there is a significant risk of bleeding. Some examples are active peptic ulcer, colitis, oesophageal varices, arterial aneurysm, recent undiagnosed stroke, severe hypertension, vascular retinopathy and acute pericarditis. Oral anticoagulants should also be avoided in the presence of clotting factor defects, whether acquired (e.g. liver disease) or congenital. Patient unreliability is important when considering long term treatment. Use of other drugs may be a relative contraindication (e.g. ulcerogenic drugs such as aspirin and indomethacin) but it may be better to stop the other drug rather than withhold warfarin. Extra care should be taken in high risk patients with concurrent disease which alters warfarin response – such as renal failure, hypoalbuminaemia and thyroid disease. Pregnant patients and the elderly also require closer monitoring.

ADVERSE EFFECTS

Bleeding is the only common side-effect from the use of warfarin. Anticoagulants are one of the most often reported causes of drug-related deaths – usually from gastrointestinal or cerebral haemorrhage. The risk of haemorrhage increases as prothrombin time rises. No level is completely safe but the risk of haemorrhage is low if prothrombin time is less than 2.5 times the control value. Careful selection of patients, regular monitoring of prothrombin time and a sound knowledge of the effects of other drugs, disease and physiological change on the response to anticoagulants will considerably reduce the risk of haemorrhage. Other side-effects with warfarin are rare. Skin necrosis within 10 days of starting treatment, alopecia and rash have been recorded. The indanediones are associated with a higher incidence of hypersensitivity reactions and should be avoided.

PREDICTION OF DOSE AND MONITORING TREATMENT

Starting treatment

The response to warfarin is delayed because existing circulating clotting factors must be degraded before the inhibitory effect on hepatic synthesis becomes apparent. If an urgent anticoagulant effect is necessary, heparin is started initially. Warfarin may be started at the same time or delayed until the diagnosis has been confirmed. There is no point in further delaying the use of oral anticoagulants to allow several days treatment with heparin alone[127]. If heparin is given by intravenous infusion rather than bolus it does not interfere with the measurement of prothrombin time either by Thrombotest or British comparative reagent if the kaolin cephalin clotting time is normal[128].

Until recent years warfarin was generally recommended to be given in a loading dose of 20–30 mg with prothrombin time measured 3 days post-dosing. This results in a precipitous drop in Factor VII and a high percentage of patients have prothrombin times outwith the therapeutic range. There is frequently difficulty in stabilizing the maintenance dose of warfarin. The current recommendation is to give 10 mg daily for 3 days and measure prothrombin time from the fourth day. However, by the fourth day 70% of patients are outwith the therapeutic range – roughly half are overtreated and half undertreated[129]. This is hardly surprising, as warfarin is not a suitable drug for such rigid prescribing. Warfarin has a low therapeutic index and the interindividual dose requirements commonly vary by 10- or 20-fold[25]. A more flexible approach is necessary.

Attempts have been made to predict the dose of warfarin necessary for an individual patient but these have met with only partial success. The maintenance dose of warfarin is related to the logarithm of the Thrombotest 64 h after starting treatment with 10 mg warfarin daily[129].

This gave a predictive value of about 80% but has limitations to its use. Plotting prothrombin time against cumulative warfarin dose was found to result in 96% of patients having an average prothrombin time over a 7-day period of between 20 and 24 seconds[130]. A computer-assisted method performed better than a control group[131]. However, it did not appear to be an improvement on the simpler methods discussed above.

The ideal method for starting warfarin treatment and predicting maintenance dose has not been found. There are major economic, medical and social advantages in determining a method which would allow early stabilization of treatment with minimum risk to the patient. Many patients remain in hospital for several days after they would otherwise be fit for discharge, waiting for their warfarin control to reach the therapeutic range. The recommended initial treatment of 10 mg daily still results in a precipitous fall in Factor VII in sensitive patients. This has led some clinicians to initiate treatment with lower doses (Breckenridge, personal communication). Most studies find a mean warfarin dose of between 6 and 9 mg daily. It would be of interest to evaluate initial treatment with a daily dose of 7 or 8 mg in combination with a modification of one of the predictive methods outlined above.

On present evidence, warfarin should be started in a dose of between 5 and 10 mg daily. Prothrombin times should be monitored daily. Dose adjustments should be made by an experienced physician on the basis of the pattern of prothrombin times, perhaps with the aid of a predictive equation. The selected initial dose should be altered in the light of important patient factors – age, disease and drugs.

Monitoring treatment

The maintenance dose of warfarin should be adjusted to achieve a prothrombin time of between two and three times the control value. A standard reference thromboplastin and external quality control are essential. Checks should be frequent until stabilization is assured and repeated at 6–12 week intervals thereafter.

The effects of pharmacokinetic and pharmacodynamic factors on warfarin control have been discussed previously. Other factors – patient compliance, hospital record systems, organization of anticoagulant clinics – are equally important. Patient non-compliance with therapy is an important problem. Suspicion of this is one of the few indications for measurement of plasma warfarin concentration, to differentiate non-compliance from receptor resistance. If unreliability in taking warfarin persists it is generally safer to stop treatment. Hospital record systems are frequently inadequate in providing ready access to information on a patient's previous medical problems and other drug therapy. A structured record system coupled with at least a limited form of problem orientation (master problem list and drug list) offers savings in time and improvement of awareness in dealing with patients seen frequently for review[132]. Allied to this problem, many anticoagulant clinics are staffed by a rota of junior physicians who may not have previously seen the patient. Clinic records frequently do not contain information on the expected duration of therapy. Patients may be attending several clinics concurrently with changes in therapy altering anticoagulant control.

Finally, patient education is vital. A well-informed patient is more likely to take medication regularly. Several booklets are available to aid in this process. Particular attention needs to be paid to the use of other drugs, dietary alterations, regular drug administration and attendance for monitoring of control.

CONCLUSIONS

Oral anticoagulants have been in use for over 40 years. Their role in cardiovascular disorders is based more on anecdotal evidence than reliable clinical trials. We need to learn from past mistakes in trial design and continually re-evaluate the therapeutic role of anticoagulants in comparison to other drugs.

Warfarin is the most widely used drug and is remarkably free from non-haemorrhagic side-effects. Safe usage of warfarin depends on careful individual control of its effect on clotting. Warfarin is administered as a racemic mixture of two pharmacologically distinct drugs – the R and S enantiomers. The S-enantiomer is more often affected by other drugs and disease. It would be of interest to evaluate the use of R-warfarin to determine whether the reduction of pharmacokinetic inter-individual variation would benefit anticoagulant control.

Warfarin use in clinical practice would be further simplified if the ideal therapeutic effect was known and the maintenance dose could be established early in a course of treatment. The work of Hull and colleagues suggests that, at least in some circumstances, benefit is obtained at lower prothrombin times than are frequently used. If a therapeutic effect can be obtained when the prothrombin time is less than 2.5 times normal the risk of haemorrhage is low. A recent study[133] has evaluated more flexible dosing of warfarin during initiation of treatment and demonstrated that all the patients (50) were controlled within 6 days. Further studies are necessary with regard to these points. If the results are confirmed and applied in practice, then the toxicity of warfarin should be reduced and time spent in hospital for stabilization of dosage shortened. The potential cost benefit to the health service and patient is considerable.

References

1. O'Reilly, R.A., Aggeler, P.M., Hoag, M.S. and Leong, L.S. (1962). Studies on the coumarin anticoagulant drugs: assay of warfarin and its biological application. *Thromb. Diath. Haem.*, 8, 82–95

2. Midha, K.K., McGilveray, I.S. and Cooper, J.K. (1974). GLC determination of plasma levels of warfarin. *J. Pharm. Sci.*, **63**, 1725-9
3. Kaiser, D.G. and Martin, R.S. (1974). Determination of warfarin in human plasma. *J. Pharm. Sci.*, **63**, 1579-81
4. Shearer, M.J. (1983). High-performance liquid chromatography of K vitamins and their antagonists. *Adv. Chromatogr.*, **21**, 243-301
5. O'Reilly, R.A., Aggeler, P.M. and Leong, L.S. (1963). Studies on the coumarin anticoagulant drugs: the pharmacodynamics of warfarin in man. *J. Clin. Invest.*, **42**, 1542-51
6. Breckenridge, A. and Orme, M. (1973). Measurement of plasma warfarin concentrations in clinical practice. In Davies, D.S. and Prichard, B.N.C. (eds.) *Biological Effects of Drugs in Relation to their Plasma Concentrations*, pp. 145-51. (London: Macmillan)
7. Scott, A.K. and Hawksworth, G.M. (1981). Drug absorption. *Br. Med. J.*, **282**, 462-3
8. O'Reilly, R.A. (1973). The binding of sodium warfarin to plasma albumin and its displacement by phenylbutazone. *Ann. N.Y. Acad. Sci.*, **226**, 293-308
9. Routledge, P.A., Chapman, P.H., Davies, D.M. and Rawlins, M.D. (1979). Pharmacokinetics and pharmacodynamics of warfarin at steady State. *Br. J. Clin. Pharmacol.*, **8**, 243-7
10. Scott, A.K., Park, B.K. and Breckenridge, A.M. (1984). Interaction between warfarin and propranolol. *Br. J. Clin. Pharmacol.*, **17**, 559-64
11. O'Reilly, R.A. (1969). Interaction of the oral anticoagulant drug warfarin and its metabolites with human plasma albumin. *J. Clin. Invest.*, **48**, 193-202
12. Sellers, E.M. and Koch-Weser, J. (1975). Interaction of warfarin stereoisomers with human albumin. *Pharmacol. Res. Commun.*, **7**, 331-6
13. Hignite, C., Uetrecht, J., Tschanz, C. and Azarnoff, P. (1980). Kinetics of R and S warfarin enantiomers. *Clin. Pharmacol. Ther.*, **28**, 99-105
14. O'Reilly, R.A. (1974). Studies on the optical enantiomers of warfarin in man. *Clin. Pharmacol. Ther.*, **16**, 348-54
15. Hewick, D.S. and McEwan, J. (1973). Plasma half-lives, plasma metabolites and anticoagulant efficacies of the enantiomers of warfarin in man. *J. Pharm. Pharmacol.*, **25**, 458-65.
16. Breckenridge, A., Orme, M., Wesseling, H., Lewis, R. J. and Gibbons, R. (1974). Pharmacokinetics and pharmacodynamics of the enantiomers of warfarin in man. *Clin. Pharmacol. Ther.*, **15**, 424-30
17. Levy, G. and Yacobi, A. (1974). Effect of plasma protein binding on elimination of warfarin. *J. Pharm. Sci.*, **63**, 805-6
18. Yacobi, A., Udall, J.A. and Levy, G. (1976). Serum protein binding as a determinant of warfarin body clearance and anticoagulant effect. *Clin. Pharmacol. Ther.*, **19**, 552-8
19. Bachmann, K., Shapiro, R. and Mackiewicz, J. (1977). Warfarin elimination and responsiveness in patients with renal dysfunction. *J. Clin. Pharmacol.*, **17**, 292-9
20. Piroli, R.J., Passananti, T., Shively, C.A. and Vesell, E.S. (1981). Antipyrine and warfarin disposition in a patient with idiopathic hypoalbuminaemia. *Clin. Pharmacol. Ther.*, **30**, 810-16
21. Yacobi, A., Udall, J.A. and Levy, G. (1976). Intrasubject variation of warfarin binding to protein in serum of patients with cardiovascular diseases. *Clin. Pharmacol. Ther.*, **20**, 300-303
22. Shepherd, A.M.M., Hewick, D.S., Moreland, T.A. and Stevenson, I.H. (1977). Age as a determinant of sensitivity to warfarin. *Br. J. Clin. Pharmacol.*, **4**, 315-20
23. Orme, M.L'E., Lewis, P.J., De Swiet, M., Serlin, M.J., Sibeon, R., Baty, J.D. and Breckenridge, A.M. (1977). May mothers given warfarin breast-feed their infants. *Br. Med. J.*, **1**, 1564-5
24. Wilkinson, G.R. and Shand, D.G. (1975). A physiological approach to hepatic drug clearance. *Clin. Pharmacol. Ther.*, **18**, 377-90

25. Breckenridge, A.M. (1977). Interindividual differences in the response to oral anticoagulants. *Drugs*, **14**, 367-75
26. Kelly, J.G. and O.Malley, K. (1979). Clinical pharmacokinetics of oral anticoagulants. *Clin. Pharmacokin.*, **4**, 1-15
27. Lewis, R.J. and Trager, W.F. (1970). Warfarin metabolism in man: Identification of metabolites in urine. *J. Clin. Invest.*, **49**, 907-13
28. Lewis, R.J. and Trager, W.F. (1971). The metabolic fate of warfarin: Studies on the metabolites in plasma. *Ann. N.Y. Acad. Sci.*, **179**, 205-12
29. Lewis, R.J., Trager, W.F., Chan, K.K., Breckenridge, A., Orme, M., Roland, M. and Schary, W. (1974). Warfarin: Stereochemical aspects of its metabolism and the interaction with phenylbutazone. *J. Clin. Invest.*, **53**, 1607-17
30. Hewick, D.S. and Moreland, T.A. (1975). An NADPH dependent warfarin reductase in human and rat liver and kidney soluble fraction. *Br. J. Pharmacol.*, **53**, 441p
31. Lewis, R.J., Trager, W.F., Robinson, A.S. and Chan, K.K. (1973). Warfarin metabolites: the anticoagulant activity and pharmacology of warfarin alcohols. *J. Lab. Clin. Med.*, **81**, 925-31
32. Breckenridge, A. and Orme, M. (1973). Kinetics of warfarin absorption in man. *Clin. Pharmacol. Ther.*, **13**, 955-61
33. Covel, D.G., Abbrecht, P.H. and Berman, M. (1983). The effect of hepatic uptake on the disappearance of warfarin from the plasma of rats: a kinetic analysis. *J. Pharmacokin. Biopharm.*, **11**, 127-45
34. Eichelbaum, M. (1976). Drug metabolism in thyroid disease. *Clin. Pharmacokin*, **1**, 339-50
35. Stenflo, J. and Suttie, J.W. (1977). Vitamin K-dependent formation of γ-carboxyglutamic acid. *Ann. Rev. Biochem.*, **46**, 154-72
36. Willingham, A.K. and Matschiner, J.T. (1974). Changes in phylloquinone epoxide activity related to prothrombin synthesis and microsomal clotting activity in the rat. *Biochem. J.*, **140**, 435-41
37. Bell, R.G. (1978). Metabolism of vitamin K and prothrombin synthesis-anticoagulants and the vitamin K-epoxide cycle. *Fed. Proc.*, **37**, 2599-2604
38. Frick, P.G., Riedler, G. and Brogli, H. (1967). Dose response and minimal daily requirement of vitamin K in man. *J. Appl. Physiol.*, **23**, 387-9
39. Barkhan, P. and Shearer, M.J. (1977). Metabolism of vitamin K_1 (phylloquinone) in man. *Proc. R. Soc. Med.*, **70**, 93-6
40. Bell, R.G. and Matschiner, J.T. (1972). Warfarin and the inhibition of vitamin K activity by an oxide metabolite. *Nature (Lond.)*, **237**, 32-3
41. Park, B.K., Leck, J.B., Wilson, A.C., Serlin, M.J. and Breckenridge, A.M. (1979). A study of the effect of anticoagulants on [³H] - vitamin K_1 metabolism and prothrombin complex activity in the rabbit. *Biochem. Pharmacol.*, **28**, 1323-9
42. Boyle, C.M. (1960). Case of apparent resistance of Rattus norvegicus Berkenhout to anticoagulant poisons. *Nature (Lond.)*, **188**, 517
43. O'Reilly, R.A., Aggeler, P.M., Hoag, M.S., Leong, L. and Kropatkin, M. (1964). Hereditary transmission of exceptional resistance to coumarin anticoagulant drugs: first reported kindred. *N. Engl. J. Med.*, **271**, 809-15
44. Udall, J.A. (1965). Human sources and absorption of vitamin K in relation to anticoagulant stability. *J. Am. Med. Assoc.*, **194**, 127-9
45. Watson, A.J.M., Pegg, M. and Green, J.R.B. (1984). Enteral feeds may antagonise warfarin. *Br. Med. J.*, **288**, 557
46. Qureshi, G.D., Reinders, T.P., Swint, J.J. and Slate, M.B. (1981). Acquired warfarin resistance and weight-reducing diet. *Arch. Intern. Med.*, **141**, 507-9
47. Brodie, B.B., Burns, J.J. and Weiner, M. (1959). Metabolism of drugs in subjects with Laennec's cirrhosis. *Med. Experimentalis*, **1**, 290-2.
48. Kliesch, W.F., Young, P.C. and Davis, W.D. (1960). Dangers of prolonged anticoagulant therapy in hepatic disease. *J. Am. Med. Assoc.*, **172**, 223-6
49. Killip, T. and Payne, M.A. (1960). High serum transaminase activity in heart disease. *Circulation*, **21**, 646-60

50. Scott, A.K., Khir, A.S.M., Bewsher, P.D. and Hawksworth, G.M. (1984). Oxazepam pharmacokinetics in thyroid disease. *Br. J. Clin. Pharmacol*, **17**, 49-53
51. Field, J.B., Overman, R.S. and Baumann, C.A. (1942). Prothrombin activity during pregnancy and lactation. *Am. J. Physiol.*, **137**, 509-14
52. Koch-Weser, J. and Sellers, E.M. (1971). Drug interactions with coumarin anticoagulants. *N. Engl. J. Med.*, **285**, 487-98 and 547-58
53. Serlin, M.J. and Breckenridge, A.M. (1983). Drug interactions with warfarin. *Drugs*, **25**, 610-20
54. Standing advisory committee for haematology of the Royal College of Pathologists (1982). Drug interaction with coumarin derivative anticoagulants. *Br. Med. J.*, **285**, 274-5
55. Scott, A.K. and Orme, M.C.L'E. (1983). Drug interactions with warfarin - current views. *Adverse Drug Reaction Bull.*, **103**, 380-3
56. O'Reilly, R.A. (1980). Spironolactone and warfarin interaction. *Clin. Pharmacol. Ther.*, **27**, 198-201
57. O'Reilly, R.A., Sahud, M.A. and Aggeler, P.M. (1971). Impact of aspirin and chlorthalidone on the pharmacodynamics of oral anticoagulant drugs in man. *Ann. N.Y. Acad. Sci.*, **179**, 173-86
58. Nilsson, C.M., Horton, E.S. and Robinson, D.S. (1978). The effect of furosemide and bumetanide on warfarin metabolism and anticoagulant response. *J. Clin. Pharmacol*, **18**, 91-4
59. Greenblatt, D.J., Franke, K. and Huffman, D.H. (1978). Impairment of antipyrine clearance in humans by propranolol. *Circulation*, **57**, 1161-4.
60. Sylven, C. and Anderson, P. (1983). Evidence that disopyramide does not interact with warfarin. *Br. Med. J.*, **286**, 1181
61. Martinowitz, U., Rabinovici, J., Goldfarb, D., Many, A. and Bank, H. (1981). Interaction between warfarin sodium and amiodarone. *N. Engl. J. Med.*, **304**, 671-2
62. Hamer, A., Peter, T., Mandel, W.J., Scheinman, M.M. and Weiss, D. (1982). The potentiation of warfarin anticoagulation by amiodarone. *Circulation*, **65**, 1025-9
63. Serlin, M.J., Sibeon, R.G. and Green, G.J. (1981). Dangers of amiodarone and anticoagulant treatment. *Br. Med. J.*, **283**, 58
64. O'Reilly, R.A. (1982). Stereoselective interaction of sulfinpyrazone with racemic warfarin and its separated enantiomorphs in man. *Circulation*, **65**, 202-7
65. Miners, J.O., Foenander, T., Wanwimolruk, S., Gallus, A.S. and Birkett, D.J. (1982). Interaction of sulphinpyrazone with warfarin. *Eur. J. Clin. Pharmacol.*, **22**, 327-31
66. Nenci, G.G., Agnelli, G. and Berrettini, M. (1981). Biphasic sulphinpyrazone - warfarin interaction. *Br. Med. J.*, **282**, 1361-2
67. Quick, A.J. and Clesceri, L. (1960). Influence of acetylsalicylic acid salicylamide on the coagulation of blood. *J. Pharmacol. Exp. Ther.*, **128**, 95-8
68. Park, B.K. and Leck, J.B. (1980). On the mechanism of salicylate-induced hypoprothrombinaemia. *J. Pharm. Pharmacol.*, **33**, 25-8
69. O'Reilly, R.A., Sahud, M.A. and Robinson, A.J. (1972). Studies on the interaction of warfarin and clofibrate in man. *Thromb. Diath. Haem.*, **27**, 309-18
70. Bjornsson, T.D., Meffin, P.J., Swezey, S. and Blaschke, T.F. (1979). Clofibrate displaces warfarin from plasma proteins in man: an example of a pure displacement interaction. *J. Pharmacol. Exp. Ther.*, **210**, 316-21
71. Jahnchen, E., Meinertz, T., Gilfrich, H.-J., Kersting, F. and Groth, U. (1978). Enhanced elimination of warfarin during treatment with cholestyramine. *Br. J. Clin. Pharmacol.*, **5**, 437-40
72. Kramer, P. and McClain, C.J. (1981). Depression of aminopyrine metabolism by influenza vaccination. *N. Engl. J. Med.*, **305**, 1262-4
73. Renton, K.W., Gray, J.D. and Hall, R.I. (1980). Decreased elimination of theophylline after influenza vaccination. *Can. Med. Assoc. J.*, **123**, 288-90
74. Kramer, P., Holtzman, J., Potter, T., and McClain, C. (1982). Influenza vaccin-

ation enhances the anticoagulant effect of warfarin. *Circulation*, **66** (Suppl. II), 302

75. Bachmann, K., Shapiro, R., Fulton, R., Carroll, F.T. and Sullivan, T.J. (1979). Smoking and warfarin disposition. *Clin. Pharmacol. Ther.*, **25**, 309–15

76. Verbeeck, R.K., Blackburn, J.L. and Loewen, G.R. (1983). Clinical pharmacokinetics of non-steroidal anti-inflammatory drugs. *Clin. Pharmacokin.*, **8**, 297–331

77. Orme, M., Breckenridge, A. and Cook, P. (1976). Warfarin and Distalgesic interaction. *Br. Med. J.*, **1**, 200

78. Boeijinga, J.J., Boerstra, E.E., Ris, P., Breimer, D.D. and Jeletich-Bastiaanse, A. (1982). Interaction between paracetamol and coumarin anticoagulants. *Lancet*, **1**, 506

79. de Teresa, E., Vera, A., Ortigosa, J., Pulpon, L.A., Arus, A.P. and de Artaza, M. (1979). Interaction between anticoagulants and contraceptives: an unsuspected finding. *Br. Med. J.*, **2**, 1260–1

80. O'Reilly, R.A. (1980). Stereoselective interaction of trimethoprim-sulfamethoxazole with the separated enantiomorphs of racemic warfarin in man. *N. Engl. J. Med.*, **302**, 33–5

81. O'Reilly, R.A. (1976). The stereoselective interaction of warfarin and metronidazole in man. *N. Engl. J. Med.*, **295**, 354–7

82. O'Reilly, R.A. (1974). Interaction of sodium warfarin and rifampicin. *Ann. Intern. Med.* 81, 337–40

83. Serlin, M.J., Sibeon, R.G., Mossman, S., Breckenridge, A.M., Williams, J.R.B., Atwood, J.L. and Willoughby, J.M.T. (1979). Cimetidine: interaction with oral anticoagulants in man. *Lancet*, **2**, 317–19

84. Serlin, M.J., Sibeon, R.G. and Breckenridge, A.M. (1981). Lack of effect of ranitidine on warfarin action. *Br. J. Clin. Pharmacol.*, **12**, 791–4

85. Thornton, P.C., Papouchado, M. and Reed, P.I. (1980). Carbenoxolone interactions in man – preliminary report. *Scand. J. Gastroenterol.*, **15**, (Suppl. 65), 35–9

86. Breckenridge, A.M. and Orme, M.L'E. (1971). Clinical implications of enzyme induction. *Ann. N.Y. Acad. Sci.*, **179**, 421–31

87. Hansem, J.M., Siersbaek-Neilson, K. and Skovsted, L. (1971). Carbamazepine-induced acceleration of diphenylhydantoin and warfarin metabolism in man. *Clin. Pharmacol. Ther.*, **12**, 539–43

88. Pond, S.M., Graham, G.G., Birkett, D.J. and Wade, D.N. (1975). Effects of tricyclic antidepressants on drug metabolism. *Clin. Pharmacol. Ther.*, **18**, 191–9

89. Orme, M., Breckenridge, A. and Brooks, R.V. (1972). Interactions of benzodiazepines with warfarin. *Br. Med. J.*, **3**, 611–14

90. O'Reilly, R.A. (1979). Lack of effect of mealtime wine on the hypoprothrombinaemia of oral anticoagulants. *Am. J. Med. Sci.*, **277**, 189–94

91. Weiner, M., Shapiro, S., Axelrod, J., Cooper, J.R. and Brodie, B.B. (1950). The physiological disposition of dicoumarol in man. *J. Pharmacol. Exp. Ther.*, **99**, 409–20

92. Vesell, E.S. and Page, J.G. (1968). Genetic control of dicoumarol levels in man. *J. Clin. Invest.*, **47**, 2657–63

93. Brodie, B.B., Weiner, M., Burns, J.J., Simson, G. and Yale, E.K. (1952). The physiological disposition of ethylbiscoumacetate (Tromexan) in man and a method for its estimation in biological material. *J. Pharmacol. Exp. Ther.*, **106**, 453–62.

94. Meinertz, T., Kasper, W., Kahl, C. and Jahnchen, E. (1978). Anticoagulant activity of the enantiomers of acenocoumarol. *Br. J. Clin. Pharmacol.*, **5**, 187–8

95. Dieterle, W., Faigle, J.W., Montigel, C., Sule, M. and Theobald, W. (1977). Biotransformation and pharmacokinetics of acenocoumarol (Sinstrom) in man. *Eur. J. Clin. Pharmacol.*, **11**, 367–75

96. Coon, W.W. and Coller, F.A. (1959). Some epidemiologic considerations of thromboembolism. *Surg. Gynaecol. Obstet.*, **109**, 487–501

97. Coon, W.W. (1976). The spectrum of pulmonary embolism. *Arch. Surg.*, 111, 398–402
98. Dalen, J.E. and Alpert, J.S. (1975). Natural history of pulmonary embolism. *Prog. Cardiovasc. Dis.*, 17, 259–70
99. Lawson, D.H. and Lowe, G.D.O. (1977). Drug therapy reviews: Clinical use of anticoagulant drugs. *Am. J. Hosp. Pharm.*, 34, 1225–34
100. Kakkar, V.V., Corrigan, T.P., Fossard, D.P., Sutherland, I. and Thirwell, J. (1977). Prevention of fatal postoperative pulmonary embolism by low doses of heparin. *Lancet*, 1, 567–9
101. Kline, A., Hughes, L.E., Campbell, H., Williams, A., Zlosnick, J. and Leach, K.G. (1975). Dextran 70 in prophylaxis of thromboembolic disease after surgery: a clinically orientated randomized double-blind trial. *Br. Med. J.*, 2, 109–12
102. Gallus, A.S. (1983). Indications for oral anticoagulant treatment. *Drugs*, 26, 543–9
103. Kakkar, V.V., Howe, C.T., Flanc, C. and Clarke, M.B. (1969). Natural history of postoperative deep-vein thrombosis. *Lancet*, 2, 230–2
104. Hull, R., Delmore, T., Genton, E., Hirsh, J., Gent, M., Sackett, D., McLaughlin, D. and Armstrong, P. (1979). Warfarin sodium versus low-dose heparin in the long-term treatment of venous thrombosis. *N. Engl. J. Med.*, 301, 855–8
105. Hull, R., Delmore, T., Carter, C., Hirsh, J., Genton, E., Gent, M., Turpie, G. and McLaughlin, D. (1982). Adjusted subcutaneous heparin versus warfarin sodium in the long-term treatment of venous thrombosis. *N. Engl. J. Med.*, 306, 189–94
106. Hull, R., Hirsh, J., Jay, R., Carter, C., England, C., Gent, M., Turpie, A.G.G., McLaughlin, D., Dodd, P., Thomas, M., Raskob, G. and Ockelford, P. (1982). Different intensities of oral anticoagulant therapy in the treatment of proximal-vein thrombosis. *N. Engl. J. Med.*, 307, 1676–81
107. Egermayer, P. (1981). Value of anticoagulants in the treatment of pulmonary embolism: a discussion paper. *J. R. Soc. Med.*, 74, 675–81
108. Barritt, D.W. and Jordan, S.C. (1960). Anticoagulant drugs in the treatment of pulmonary embolism. A controlled trial. *Lancet*, 1, 1309–12
109. Johnson, R. and Charnley, J. (1977). Treatment of pulmonary embolism in total hip replacement. *Clin. Orthop. Relat. Res.*, 124, 149–54
110. Alpert, J.S., Smith, R., Carlson, J., Ockene, I.S., Dexter, L. and Dalen, J.E. (1976). Mortality in patients treated for pulmonary embolism. *J. Am. Med. Assoc.*, 236, 1477–80
111. Mant, M.J., O'Brien, B.D., Thong, K.L., Hammond, G.W., Birtwhistle, R.V. and Grace, M.G. (1977). Haemorrhagic complications of heparin therapy. *Lancet*, 1, 1133–5
112. Thompson, P.L. and Robinson, J.S. (1978). Stroke after myocardial infarction: Relation to infarct size. *Br. Med. J.*, 2, 457–9
113. Asinger, R.W., Mikell, F.L., Elsperger, J. and Hodges, M. (1981). Incidence of left ventricular thrombosis after acute transmural myocardial infarction. *N. Engl. J. Med.*, 305, 297–302
114. Medical Research Council (1959). An assessment of long-term anticoagulant administration after cardiac infarction. *Br. Med. J.*, 1, 803–10
115. International Anticoagulant Review Group (1970). Collaborative analysis of long-term anticoagulant administration after acute myocardial infarction. *Lancet*, 1, 203–9
116. Sixty Plus Reinfarction Study Research Group (1980). A double-blind trial to assess long-term oral anticoagulant therapy in elderly patients after myocardial infarction. *Lancet*, 2, 989–93
117. Mitchell, J.R.A. (1982). 'But will it help my patients with myocardial infarction?' The implications of recent trials for everyday country folk. *Br. Med. J.*, 285, 1140–8
118. Goodnight, S.H. (1980). Antiplatelet therapy for mitral stenosis? *Circulation*, 62, 466–8

119. Chesebro, J.H., Fuster, V., Elveback, L.R., McGoon, D.C., Pluth, J.R., Puga, F.J., Wallace, R.B., Danielson, G.K., Orszulak, T.A., Piehler, J.M. and Schaff, H.V. (1983). Trial of combined warfarin plus dipyridamole or aspirin therapy in prosthetic heart valve replacement: danger of aspirin compared with dipyridamole. *Am. J. Cardiol.*, 51, 1537–41

120. Nunez, L., Aguado, M.G., Celemin, D., Iglesias, A. and Larrea, J.L. (1982). Aspirin or coumadin as the drug of choice for valve replacement with porcine bioprosthesis. *Ann. Ther. Surg.*, 33, 354–8

121. Easton, J.D. and Sherman, D.G. (1980). Management of cerebral embolism of cardiac origin. *Stroke*, 2, 433–42

122. Furlan, A.J., Cavalier, S.J., Hobbs, R.E., Weinstein, M.A. and Modic, M.T. (1982). Haemorrhage and anticoagulation after nonseptic embolic brain infarction. *Neurology*, 32, 280–2

123. Koller, R.L. (1982). Recurrent embolic cerebral infarction and anticoagulation. *Neurology*, 32, 283–5

124. Cervantes, F.D. and Schneiderman, L.J. (1975). Anticoagulants in cerebrovascular disease. *Arch. Intern. Med.*, 135, 875–7

125. Gohlke, H., Gohlke-Barwolf, C., Sturzenhofecker, P., Gornandt, L., Ritter, B., Reichelt, M., Buchwalsky, R., Schmuziger, M. and Roskamm, H. (1981). Improved graft patency after aorto-coronary bypass surgery: A prospective, randomised study. *Circulation*, 64 (Suppl. 11), 22–7

126. Pantely, G.A., Goodnight, S.H., Rahimtoola, S.H., Harlan, B.J., De Mots, H., Calvin, L. and Rosch, J. (1979). Failure of antiplatelet and anticoagulant therapy to improve patency of grafts after coronary-artery bypass. *N. Engl. J. Med.*, 301, 962–6

127. Self, T.H., Bauman, J.H., Brown, J.R., Bickers, W.J. and Wood, C.A. (1981). Concurrent initiation of heparin and warfarin therapy. *Am. Heart J.*, 102, 470–1

128. Thomas, P., Fennerty, A., Backhouse, G., Bentley, D.P., Campbell, I.A. and Routledge, P.A. (1984). Monitoring effects of oral anticoagulants during treatment with heparin. *Br. Med. J.*, 288, 191

129. Routledge, P.A., Davis, D.M., Bell, S.M., Cavanagh, J.S. and Rawlins, M.D. (1977). Predicting patients' warfarin requirements. *Lancet*, 2, 854–5

130. Williams, D.B. and Karl, R.C. (1979). A simple technic for predicting daily maintenance dose of warfarin. *Am. J. Surg.* 137, 572–6

131. Abbrecht, P.H., O'Leary, T.J. and Behrendt, D.M. (1982). Evaluation of a computer-assisted method for individualized anticoagulation: retrospective and prospective studies with a pharmacodynamic model. *Clin. Pharmacol. Ther.*, 32, 129–36

132. Petrie, J.C. and McIntyre, N. (1979). *The Problem Orientated Medical Record.* (Edinburgh and London: Churchill Livingstone)

133. Fennerty, A., Dolben, J., Thomas, P., Backhouse, G., Bentley, D.P., Campbell, I.A. and Routledge, P.A. (1984). Flexible induction dose regimen for warfarin and prediction of maintenance dose. *Br. Med. J.*, 288, 1268–70

Index

223